Progress in Pain Research and Management
Volume 18

Pain Imaging

Mission Statement of IASP Press®

The International Association for the Study of Pain (IASP) is a nonprofit, interdisciplinary organization devoted to understanding the mechanisms of pain and improving the care of patients with pain through research, education, and communication. The organization includes scientists and health care professionals dedicated to these goals. The IASP sponsors scientific meetings and publishes newsletters, technical bulletins, the journal *Pain*, and books.

The goal of IASP Press is to provide the IASP membership with timely, high-quality, attractive, low-cost publications relevant to the problem of pain. These publications are also intended to appeal to a wider audience of scientists and clinicians interested in the problem of pain.

Previous volumes in the series
Progress in Pain Research and Management

Progress in Pain Research and Management
Volume 18

Pain Imaging

Editors

Kenneth L. Casey, MD

Departments of Neurology and Physiology, University of Michigan,
and Neurology Service, Veterans Affairs Medical Center,
Ann Arbor, Michigan, USA

M. Catherine Bushnell, PhD

Department of Anesthesiology,
McGill University,
Montreal, Quebec, Canada

IASP PRESS® • SEATTLE

Timely topics in pain research and treatment have been selected for publication, but the information provided and opinions expressed have not involved any verification of the findings, conclusions, and opinions by IASP®. Thus, opinions expressed in *Pain Imaging* do not necessarily reflect those of IASP or of the Officers and Councillors.

No responsibility is assumed by IASP for any injury and/or damage to persons or property as a matter of product liability, negligence, or from any use of any methods, products, instruction, or ideas contained in the material herein. Because of the rapid advances in the medical sciences, the publisher recommends that there should be independent verification of diagnoses and drug dosages.

Library of Congress Cataloging-in-Publication Data

Pain imaging / editors, Kenneth L. Casey, M. Catherine Bushnell.
    p. ; cm. -- (Progress in pain research and management ; v. 18)
  Includes bibliographical references and index.
  ISBN 0-931092-34-5 (alk. paper)
    1. Pain--Imaging. I. Casey, Kenneth L. (Kenneth Lyman), 1935- II. Bushnell, M. Catherine, 1949- III. Series.
    [DNLM: 1. Pain--radionuclide imaging. 2. Diagnostic Imaging--methods.
3. Magnetic Resonance Imaging. 4. Tomography, Emission-Computed, Single-Photon.
5. Tomography, Emission-Computed. WL 704 P1456 2000]
  RB 127 .P33226 2000
  616'.0472--dc21

00-047139

Published by:

IASP Press
International Association for the Study of Pain
909 NE 43rd St., Suite 306
Seattle, WA 98105 USA
Fax: 206-547-1703
www.halcyon.com/iasp
www.painbooks.org

Printed in the United States of America

Contents

Contributing Authors

M. Catherine Bushnell, PhD *Departments of Anesthesia, Dentistry, and Physiology, McGill University, Montreal, Quebec, Canada*

Kenneth L. Casey, MD *Departments of Neurology and Physiology, University of Michigan; and Neurology Service, Veterans Affairs Medical Center, Ann Arbor, Michigan, USA*

Robert C. Coghill, PhD *Department of Neurobiology and Anatomy, Wake Forest University School of Medicine, Winston-Salem, North Carolina, USA*

Donna J. Cross, BSE *Department of Internal Medicine and Neuroscience Program, The University of Michigan Medical School, Ann Arbor, Michigan, USA*

Karen Davis, PhD *Division of Neurosurgery, Toronto Western Research Institute; and Department of Surgery, University of Toronto, Toronto, Ontario, Canada*

Ulrich Dirnagl, MD *Department of Experimental Neurology, Charité Hospital, Berlin, Germany*

Gary H. Duncan, DDS, PhD *Faculty of Dental Medicine, University of Montreal, Montreal, Quebec, Canada*

Oleg Favorov, PhD *Department of Biomedical Engineering, University of North Carolina, Chapel Hill, North Carolina, USA; and Division of Computer Science, University of Central Florida, Orlando, Florida, USA*

Richard D. Hoge, PhD *Nuclear Magnetic Resonance Center, Massachusetts General Hospital; and Department of Radiology, Harvard University Medical School, Charlestown, Massachusetts, USA*

Robert A. Koeppe, PhD *Department of Internal Medicine, The University of Michigan Medical School, Ann Arbor, Michigan, USA*

Adam Kohn, PhD *Department of Cell and Molecular Physiology, University of North Carolina, Chapel Hill, North Carolina, USA*

Ute Lindauer, DVM *Department of Experimental Neurology, Charité Hospital, Berlin, Germany*

Satoshi Minoshima, MD, PhD *Department of Internal Medicine and Neuroscience Program, The University of Michigan Medical School, Ann Arbor, Michigan, USA; currently Department of Radiology, University of Washington Medical School, Seattle, Washington, USA*

Thomas J. Morrow, PhD *Department of Neurology, University of Michigan; and Neurology Research Laboratory, Veterans Affairs Medical Center, Ann Arbor, Michigan, USA*

G. Bruce Pike, PhD *McConnell Brain Imaging Center, Montreal Neurological Institute, McGill University, Montreal, Quebec, Canada*

Pierre Rainville, PhD *Department of Neurology, University of Iowa Hospitals and Clinics, Iowa City, Iowa, USA*

Mark Tommerdahl, PhD *Department of Biomedical Engineering, University of North Carolina, Chapel Hill, North Carolina, USA*

Charles J. Vierck, Jr., PhD *Department of Neuroscience, University of Florida, Gainesville, Florida, USA*

Barry L. Whitsel, PhD *Departments of Cell and Molecular Physiology and Biomedical Engineering, University of North Carolina, Chapel Hill, North Carolina, USA*

Foreword

Kenneth Casey and Catherine Bushnell have brought together the latest advances in the field of brain imaging of pain, a topic that has undergone accelerated growth within the last 10 years. Although the chapters focus on different aspects of pain and brain imaging, the book is an integrated account of what is presently understood in this exciting area of psychology and neuroscience of pain. This volume represents a technically and conceptually oriented treatise on how neural imaging helps us to understand neural representations of pain states. It provides satisfying explanations of the technical issues of neural imaging and of the exciting conceptual breakthroughs in understanding brain mechanisms of pain.

The technical underpinnings of each method used to study pain-related neural activities are eloquently elaborated in several chapters. For example, the close spatial and temporal correlation between neuronal and glial activity, metabolic activity, and regional blood flow, known as neurometabolic and neurovascular coupling, is introduced by Lindauer and Dirnagl (Chapter 2). Candidates for possible mediators of this coupling include metabolic activity associated with synaptic transmission, action potentials, and neurogenic control of local blood vessels. All of these are highly associated. Yet the reader is given the exciting prospect that neural imaging is not destined to be confined to global measures of neural activity but may eventually include measures of activation, release, and effects of specific neural transmitters and neuromodulators (e.g., glutamate, opioids).

A generic and sometimes casual criticism of neural imaging techniques, such as 2-deoxyglucose metabolic imaging, is their inability to distinguish excitatory from inhibitory neural activity. Somehow this criticism is often uniquely associated with these techniques despite the fact that other methods, such as extracellular neural recording, cannot distinguish whether a given neuron serves ultimately to inhibit or excite other neurons within a neural circuit. Yet the capacity to study both excitatory and inhibitory phenomena using neural imaging methodology is convincingly illustrated in Chapter 3. Using optical intrinsic signal imaging techniques, Whitsel and his colleagues show how tactile and nociceptive inputs to different components of the somatosensory cortex (3a and 3b) exert reciprocal inhibitory effects.

Pike and Hoge (Chapter 6) review fMRI technical developments over the past decade, an era in which functional brain imaging has been revolutionized by technical advances. They outline the rationale, theory, and technical aspects of fMRI in demonstrating how this technology is uniquely qualified for investigations of steady-state and transient neuronal responses associated with the different aspects of pain. Karen Davis (Chapter 7) provides a methodological review of how fMRI pain studies are conducted and interpreted. This chapter inspires the view that experimental designs of future brain-imaging studies of pain are likely to be very sophisticated, involving mapping the spatiotemporal profiles of distributed areas of neural activation as well as the connectivities of these areas. Moreover, changes in these profiles and connectivities are likely to be related to different subtle aspects of pain experience and pain behavior. Similarly, Minoshima and colleagues (Chapter 4) review the methodology and execution of brain activation studies involving positron emission tomography (PET) and single photon emission computed tomography (SPECT). They provide an overview of how these technologies can be interfaced with experimental designs, image acquisition, data analysis, and interpretation to result in optimal specific and sensitive localizations of pain-related brain activity.

The chapter by Rainville and his colleagues (Chapter 5) discusses new strategies whereby neural imaging techniques can be used to characterize the neural structures that are differentially involved in the different dimensions of pain experience. This approach is not mere "neurophrenology" but recognizes subtle and complex relationships among cerebral cortical regions involved in pain sensation, attention, regulation of consciousness, premotor functions, memory, and emotions. All of these structures and functions serve to induce and maintain pain-related affect, yet some brain regions such as the anterior cingulate cortex appear to have a pivotal role. This chapter discusses how similar strategies can be used to characterize general mechanisms of pain modulation, including analgesia produced by hypnotic suggestions and brain stimulation.

Appropriately, the last chapter by Coghill and Morrow is about functional imaging of animal models of pain. The unique contributions of these types of studies include much higher spatial resolution of images of neural activity and the capacity to combine neural imaging with neurosurgical, pharmacological, and behavioral interventions. Exploring the relationships between animal and human imaging studies represents a potentially powerful means of characterizing the neural mechanisms of pain and analgesia.

Every chapter offers exciting prospects for the future, because the research on brain imaging of pain is still in its beginning stage. Challenges and puzzles remain, but the old questions now seem much more answerable. As Casey points out, we are witnessing at the beginning of the new century a merging of physiology and psychology of pain, with profound consequences for the field of neuroscience and the care of pain patients.

DONALD D. PRICE, PHD
University of Florida

Preface

During this past decade, we have seen remarkable developments in brain imaging methods. The resolution of routine clinical anatomical brain imaging with magnetic resonance has continued to improve so that, for example, it is now regularly possible to see the pituitary stalk—a highly unrealistic expectation even at the beginning of the 1990s. Functional imaging of the human brain has developed in parallel with advances in anatomical imaging and is based on the pioneering work of Sokoloff and colleagues in the 1970s. Fortunately, our understanding of the neural and psychological aspects of pain has continued to improve, so that we can take advantage of these remarkable advances in functional imaging technology. The result has been an accelerating output of pain imaging studies, beginning with the publication of Talbot and colleagues in 1991 (*Science* 251:1355–1358).

What is pain imaging? In this book, we have focused exclusively on positron emission tomography (PET), functional magnetic resonance imaging (fMRI), and, in animals, quantitative autoradiographic imaging of regional cerebral blood flow (rCBF) and glucose utilization (CMRglu). These functional imaging methods are well suited for the study of chronic pathological pain as they permit the application of stimulus durations longer than several minutes, provide three-dimensional spatial resolution in the millimeter (humans) or micrometer (animals) range, and permit the analysis of multifocal responses in cortical and subcortical structures. The book does not cover electrophysiological approaches to the analysis of central nociceptive processing such as magnetoencephalography and evoked potential mapping with dipole analysis, as recently reviewed by Bromm and Lorenz (*EEG Clin. Neurophysiol.* 1998; 107:227–253). These methods are highly useful and complementary to PET and fMRI because they offer spatial resolution that matches or exceeds these other imaging methods, and their temporal resolution is much higher. However, the technical issues involved in their application, analysis, and interpretation in pain studies are sufficiently complex to warrant special consideration in a separate publication.

Science requires the proper application of technology to answer critical and carefully posed questions. In pain research, the questions arise from what we think we know about the neurobiology of pain at the molecular-through-cognitive levels of function. The ultimate test of our understanding will be the ability to predict how pathological biochemical and neuroanatomical changes relate to pain. We are far from that goal today, but we are creating new knowledge at an accelerating pace in the field of pain imaging. This places a heavy burden on clinicians or neuroscientists who are not engaged in pain imaging research because they will ultimately need to consider the results of these studies while making decisions in the clinical setting or while planning and conducting research. This book is intended to meet the present-day needs of clinicians and neuroscientists by providing the physiological and technical background, critically reviewing some of the contributions made thus far, and suggesting possible directions for future research and applications of pain imaging.

Chapter 1 provides an introduction to pain mechanisms and an overview of pain imaging, and is intended for readers who wish to have some background before proceeding to the chapters covering specific aspects of the subject. Readers with a background in functional imaging may benefit from an overview of pain mechanisms but may wish to skip the section on imaging. Conversely, those with experience in basic or clinical pain research may wish to proceed directly to the section on imaging. The sections on the biological and clinical aspects of pain briefly discuss problems and issues that the study of pain presents in each of those areas. I have emphasized a few of the problems that might be effectively addressed by functional imaging.

All functional imaging depends on the local vascular response to synaptic activity in populations of neurons. There is now evidence that the intensity of this focal hemodynamic response is positively and linearly correlated with action potential activity in neuronal populations. In Chapter 2, Lindauer and Dirnagl discuss the dynamics of neurovascular coupling and consider the evidence for its underlying physiological and biochemical mechanisms. Immediately preceding the vascular response, activity-induced changes occur in the chemical composition of the extracellular space immediately surrounding the neuropil. Whitsel and colleagues show in Chapter 3 how optical imaging spectroscopy allows us to detect and image these changes in the cerebral cortex, thus providing unique information about differential focal cortical responses to innocuous and noxious stimuli. These chapters give an excellent background for the following critical review by Minoshima and colleagues of the acquisition and analysis of rCBF responses during PET scans of the human brain (Chapter 4). Rainville and colleagues show how to apply this information by giving an in-depth, selective review of PET studies of pain (Chapter 5). The focus then moves to the increasingly popular and rapidly advancing use of fMRI. Pike and Hoge present a detailed review of the physical and biological basis of fMRI and consider the technical advantages and shortcomings of this method (Chapter 6). Davis then follows (Chapter 7) with examples of fMRI studies of pain, many of which have been conducted under her scientific direction. She considers these findings in relation to PET and other imaging methods. Although PET and fMRI investigations of human subjects form the foundation of pain imaging, they have several technical limitations, including limited spatial resolution and the inability to perform certain invasive manipulations such as selective anatomical or biochemical lesions. In Chapter 8, Coghill and Morrow show that functional imaging of CMRglu and rCBF can be used in animal models of acute and chronic pain, providing spatial resolution at the histological level and the opportunity to apply invasive manipulations of brain function. These animal-based techniques will allow us to investigate the temporal development of the multifocal central responses to noxious stimuli, tissue damage, or peripheral or central nervous system injury.

KENNETH L. CASEY
M. CATHERINE BUSHNELL

Acknowledgments

We are most grateful for the support and patience of our families and friends, who often have had to wait while we devoted our attention to writing and editing this book. We are pleased to have received the enthusiastic and timely participation of our colleagues, who have contributed scholarly chapters of such high quality. The intersection of research in pain and neural imaging has created a field of scientific endeavor that, within less than a decade, has grown so rapidly it requires special expertise to present an accurate, comprehensive, and useful review of the state of the science. The contributors to this book are part of a much larger—and growing—community of investigators in pain imaging and related areas. It has been our intention to have as inclusive a representation of their work as possible, but we realize we may not have achieved this goal. The editorial staff of IASP Press, led by the able judgment of Editor-in-Chief Howard Fields, has provided the highest quality professional assistance throughout the development and production of this volume. Elizabeth Endres and Roberta Scholz merit special recognition in this regard.

Finally, we gratefully acknowledge the support of the Pfizer Corporation (formerly Parke-Davis division of the Warner-Lambert Company), which provided generous funding for the production of the color plates. A colorless book on pain imaging would be completely unacceptable!

Dr. Casey's research is supported by grants from the U.S. Department of Veteran's Affairs and the National Institutes of Health (USA). Dr. Bushnell's research is supported by grants from the Canadian Institutes of Health Research.

KENNETH L. CASEY
M. CATHERINE BUSHNELL

Pain Imaging, Progress in Pain Research and Management, Vol. 18, edited by Kenneth L. Casey and M. Catherine Bushnell, IASP Press, Seattle, © 2000.

1

The Imaging of Pain: Background and Rationale

Kenneth L. Casey

Department of Neurology, University of Michigan; and Neurology Service, Veterans Affairs Medical Center, Ann Arbor, Michigan, USA

Pain and functional imaging each have unique and interesting scientific and technical problems; their combination is especially challenging. Pain is a complex experience that normally follows the stimulation of receptors and afferent fibers that respond specifically to stimuli that are actually or potentially damaging. However, such stimulation is neither necessary nor sufficient to produce pain in all circumstances, including many situations that are clinically important. Pain is an experience, and personal experience is determined by neurophysiological mechanisms within the brain. We now have the ability to analyze, qualitatively and quantitatively, the multifocal activity of the conscious human brain during pain or under conditions intended to evoke pain. We can correlate this brain activity with the report of that person's experience. We can reasonably assume that we are correlating some measure of that experience with the synaptic processes mediating it. However, we do not completely understand the neurophysiological processes we are measuring or how they are generated. Moreover, we do not yet know how best to determine the role played, if any, by each active area of the brain in producing pain. Nonetheless, the solution to these problems is within our grasp—if not now, then in the foreseeable future. Then we will have merged the physiology and psychology of pain, with profound consequences for neuroscience and to the great benefit of patients.

AN OVERVIEW OF PAIN MECHANISMS

THE DEFINITION OF PAIN

According to the definition of pain proposed by the International Association for the Study of Pain (IASP), pain is "an unpleasant sensory and emotional experience associated with actual or potential tissue damage, or described in terms of such damage" (Merskey and Bogduk 1994, p. 210). By this definition, the normal experience of pain recruits neural mechanisms that mediate both sensory and hedonic functions. The *sensory* component of pain includes the ability to localize the stimulus in space and time and to discriminate among different intensities and physical qualities of noxious stimuli. The sensory aspect of pain, by itself, lacks emotional color. In contrast, the *hedonic* or *affective* component of pain lacks sensory characteristics and imparts aversive qualities to noxious stimuli, motivating attempts to escape and avoid them (Melzack and Casey 1968). Pain always has some hedonic aspects. Under unusual and special circumstances, it may assume rewarding and even pleasurable characteristics.

According to the IASP definition, a noxious stimulus is not necessarily painful. Pain is an experience and thus requires the participation of neural mechanisms that are available only within a nervous system that is capable of mediating personal experience. Noxious stimuli are those that are capable of "actual or potential tissue damage" (Merskey and Bogduk 1994) and could, therefore, produce pain; however, in the absence of personal experience, these stimuli do not cause pain. If it is unclear whether a noxious stimulus has produced pain, the terms *nociception* or *nociceptive* are commonly used in reference to the behavioral or neurophysiological responses produced.

The IASP definition includes the possibility that pain may occur in the absence of noxious stimulation or, for that matter, without any stimulation at all. In certain pathological circumstances (discussed below), innocuous stimuli, such as touch or cold, may be painful. Pain also may occur without external stimuli as a consequence of central nervous system (CNS) trauma or disease (central pain syndromes).

The IASP definition of pain appropriately ignores unconscious physiological responses that are evoked by noxious stimuli. These responses, sometimes referred to as nociceptive or nocifensive reflexes, include cardiovascular, respiratory, neuroendocrine, and somatomotor activities that may be observed in unconscious, as well as conscious, animals and humans.

NOCICEPTORS

All extraneural tissues that can evoke pain following noxious stimuli are innervated by *nociceptors,* a class of receptors that normally respond only to such stimuli (Burgess and Perl 1973; Handwerker and Reeh 1994; Cesare and McNaughton 1997). The physiological properties of nociceptors are studied by recording the action potentials of the sensory fibers that innervate them and that transmit impulses to the CNS. Nociceptive afferents have the smallest diameter of all somatic, muscular, or visceral sensory fibers. The nociceptive fibers conduct action potentials at average velocities of about 1 meter/second (unmyelinated C fibers) or 15 m/s (finely myelinated Aδ fibers), which is quite slow compared to the conduction velocity of afferent fibers innervating tactile or muscle stretch receptors (75–100 m/s). The cell bodies of nociceptive afferent fibers are found in the sensory ganglia of the dorsal roots of the spinal cord (bodily and visceral sensation) or the trigeminal ganglion of the brainstem (orofacial sensation).

Some nociceptive afferents are physiologically specialized to respond to mechanical, thermal, or chemical stimuli. Others respond to a variety of physical stimuli and are referred to as *polymodal* nociceptors. The response properties of nociceptors vary with the type of tissue being innervated. For example, pinching or burning activates nociceptors in the skin but is ineffective for nociceptors innervating visceral organs, such as the bowel or bladder, where stretching by increased intravesicular pressure is effective (Cervero 1994). Some properties of all nociceptors, such as the activation threshold or the type of excitatory stimulus, may be altered by tissue damage, inflammation, or damage to the sensory nerve itself (Cesare and McNaughton 1997; Woolf and Salter 2000).

CENTRAL CONNECTIONS OF NOCICEPTIVE AFFERENTS

The central processes of nociceptive afferents terminate in the superficial gray matter of the dorsal spinal cord (dorsal horn) or in the caudal portion of the trigeminal sensory nucleus in the brainstem (medullary dorsal horn). The terminals of nociceptive afferents contain the amino-acid-derived neurotransmitter glutamate and a peptide, substance P, both of which are considered major, but not necessarily exclusive, nociceptive neurotransmitters. Other putative nociceptive neurotransmitters include calcitonin gene-related peptide (CGRP) and vasoactive intestinal peptide (VIP), the latter found primarily in visceral afferent fibers (Levine et al. 1993; Cervero 1994).

Through interneuronal connections with spinal and brainstem motoneurons, nociceptive afferents activate somatic reflexes, including the brainstem corneal and jaw-opening reflexes, and spinally mediated flexion reflexes of the limbs (Matthews 1985; Schouenborg et al. 1994). These reflexes are normally suppressed by inhibitory influences descending from the brainstem and forebrain and are best observed when these supraspinal effects are removed by surgery, cooling, or drugs in animal experiments, or by pathological processes in human patients.

ASCENDING PATHWAYS

Two main types of spinal and trigeminal sensory neurons receive input from nociceptive afferents and transmit information to supraspinal sites (Willis and Coggeshall 1978; Yaksh and Hammond 1982; Fields 1987; Willis and Westlund 1997). Most *nociceptive-specific* (NS) cells are located within the superficial dorsal horn; they respond exclusively to noxious somatic or visceral stimuli. *Wide-dynamic-range* (WDR) neurons respond, as the name implies, to somatic or visceral stimuli with intensities ranging from innocuous to clearly noxious. The action potential discharge frequency of WDR cells increases progressively with stimulus intensity. Like the nociceptive afferent fibers, NS and WDR cells may be physiologically specialized to respond to different forms of stimuli, such as heat, cold, or mechanical pressure. Both NS and WDR cells respond to glutamate and substance P released by nociceptive afferent terminals. Glutamate activates postsynaptic N-methyl-D-aspartate (NMDA) receptors, which produce postsynaptic potentials that are relatively brief (100 ms or less) and rapid in onset. Substance P, however, activates neurokinin-1 (NK-1) receptors, which are associated with prolonged depolarizing synaptic potentials (several hundred milliseconds). The co-release of these neurotransmitters is thought to be responsible for the temporal summation of nociceptive inputs and consequently for the temporal summation of pain intensity following repetitive noxious stimuli (Ruda et al. 1986; Todd and Spike 1993). Craig and colleagues recently presented evidence that spinal and trigeminal nociceptive neurons are morphologically and neurochemically distinct from non-nociceptive cells (Craig et al. 1999; Yu et al. 1999; Blomqvist et al. 2000).

The axons of WDR and NS cells ascend and descend ipsilaterally within the tract of Lissauer for two to three spinal cord segments and form synaptic connections within the substantia gelatinosa of these neighboring segments. This spatial distribution is responsible for the spatial summation of pain, which is sometimes experienced as the spread of painful sensations beyond the region of injury (Handwerker and Kobal 1993).

THE SENSORY-DISCRIMINATIVE COMPONENT OF PAIN

Normal humans can identify the onset, duration, and location of painful stimuli and are able to distinguish accurately among different intensities and physical properties, such as thermal and mechanical stimuli. These behavioral abilities comprise the sensory-discriminative component of pain, which is mediated by a system of physiologically specialized neurons (Melzack and Casey 1968). Clinical experience has shown that lesions within the ventroposterolateral (VPL) thalamus and immediately adjacent thalamic nuclei impair the localization, perceived intensity, and identification of innocuous and noxious somatic and visceral stimuli (Fisher 1982; Melo and Bogousslavsky 1992). The ability to identify noxious stimuli is variously affected by different cortical lesions, including those of the primary somatosensory cortex. In a unique case reported by Ploner and colleagues (1999), focal infarction of the right primary (S1) and secondary (S2) somatosensory cortex markedly impaired all aspects of spatial, temporal, and intensive discrimination of innocuous and noxious cutaneous stimuli. Definite impairment of these functions has also been reported following lesions of the insula, the supramarginal gyrus, and the parietal operculum (Berthier et al. 1988; Greenspan and Winfield 1992; Bassetti et al. 1993). However, such lesions have little or no influence on clinical or experimentally produced intense, deep pain. Furthermore, the hedonic component of pain may also be unaffected (Ploner et al. 1999).

Both WDR and NS spinal and trigeminal sensory neurons contribute axons to ascending pathways in the anterolateral and anteroventral quadrants of the spinal cord and the lateral brainstem. Spinothalamic or trigeminothalamic tract neurons form synaptic connections within the VPL or ventroposterior medial (VPM) thalamus. Within these structures and adjacent smaller thalamic nuclei are cells that respond either exclusively or differentially to noxious stimuli applied to small contralateral regions (receptive fields) of the body (VPL) or face (VPM) (Mountcastle and Henneman 1952; Rose and Mountcastle 1954; Kniffki and Mizumura 1983; Casey and Morrow 1983; Chung et al. 1986; Simone et al. 1993). Some of these cells also respond to presumably noxious visceral stimuli (Chandler et al. 1992; Berkley et al. 1993; Kawakita et al. 1993; Brüggemann et al. 1994; Al-Chaer et al. 1996). VPL and VPM neurons send axons to the S1 cortex, where cells are spatially organized into somatotopically separated regions and have small contralateral receptive fields. The physiological properties of spinothalamic or trigeminothalamic cells and of the thalamic and cortical neurons they excite suggest that these cells mediate the discriminative aspects of pain.

THE HEDONIC COMPONENT OF PAIN

The limbic system was originally defined anatomically as the cortex and associated cortical afferents that form a ring (limbus) around the thalamus and upper brainstem. The cortical structures in this ring include the cingulate and entorhinal cortices, which provide the major afferent and efferent connections to the hippocampal gyrus and amygdaloid nuclei of the temporal lobe. These latter structures, in turn, are major sources of inputs to the hypothalamus (Papez 1937; MacLean 1949). The limbic system includes the medial and anterior thalamic nuclei, which send projections to the limbic cortex, and the periaqueductal gray matter (PAG) in the midbrain, which sends afferents to the medial thalamus and hypothalamus (MacLean 1955; Nauta and Kuypers 1958). Rodents have direct projections from the spinal cord to the hypothalamus, but a similar connection has yet to be identified in humans (Burstein et al. 1987).

The functional significance of identifying this anatomical system was shown by clinical observations and experimental studies that revealed behavioral changes following stimulation or suppression of neuronal activity within one or more limbic system structures (MacLean 1957; Olds and Olds 1963). Although the behavioral changes vary with the nature and location of the functional lesion, they commonly result in an altered expression of rewarding, aversive, appetitive, and social interactive behaviors, which humans associate with affective or hedonic experience (Damasio et al. 1994). Numerous clinical observations have implicated the cingulate and mesial prefrontal cortex in the mediation of hedonic aspects of pain (Foltz and White 1962; Hurt and Ballantine 1973; Degos et al. 1993; Davis et al. 1994; Devinsky et al. 1995). Perception of the hedonic component of pain is correlated with regional cerebral blood flow (rCBF) responses in a portion of the human anterior cingulate cortex, as revealed by recent positron emission tomographic (PET) studies in normal humans (Rainville et al. 1997) (see Chapter 5). In addition to these complex behaviors, limbic system structures mediate or modulate autonomic and neuroendocrine responses to noxious stimulation through their oligosynaptic connections with the hypothalamus. The autonomic reactions, which include increases in blood pressure, heart rate, and respiratory rate and volume, may be combined with neuroendocrine changes, such as increases in circulating adrenocorticotrophic hormone, cortisone, and norepinephrine, producing a physiological condition that closely resembles the stress response (Saper et al. 1976; Saper 1982; Holstege et al. 1996).

Spinoreticular or trigeminoreticular neurons of the dorsal horn form synaptic connections with cells in the brainstem reticular formation of the medulla, pons, and midbrain. Many postsynaptic reticular formation cells emit prolonged responses to a variety of noxious stimuli applied to the viscera or to large and sometimes bilateral areas (receptive fields) of the body or face (Segundo 1967; Burton 1968; Casey 1969; Fields et al. 1975; Blair et al. 1991; Roy et al. 1992; Ness et al. 1998). These cells are thus unlikely to contribute to spatial, temporal, or qualitative discriminative functions. Spinoreticular and spinothalamic neurons, and their trigeminal counterparts, have direct or oligosynaptic connections with several limbic system structures (MacLean 1955; Morrell et al. 1981; Meyer et al. 1986; Holstege 1987; Bernard and Besson 1990; Price 2000). These structures include the midbrain PAG, the amygdala, and the medial and intralaminar thalamus, as well as ventrolateral and ventromedial thalamic cells that project to the perisylvian insular, S2, and inferior parietal cortices (Craig et al. 1994; Blomqvist et al. 2000). These perisylvian cortical regions, in particular the insula, provide a direct link between the S1 somatosensory and parietal association cortex and limbic system structures, such as the hippocampus, of the temporal lobe (Mesulam and Mufson 1982; Friedman et al. 1986; Price 2000). Patients with cortical lesions that include the insula, for example, may have a condition known as "pain asymbolia" in which the spatial, intensive, and qualitative components of pain are recognized, but the emotional responses to both applied and threatened noxious stimuli—anywhere on the body—are attenuated or absent (Berthier et al. 1988). This functional and anatomical relationship between the limbic system and nociceptive afferents underlies the effectiveness of pain as a strong negative potentiating influence for learning and memory. Apparently, integrity of the S1 and S2 cortices is not critical for the hedonic aspect of pain because a patient with an infarction involving S1 and S2 continued to experience the unpleasantness of a noxious laser stimulus (Ploner et al. 1999). As would be expected from the behavioral functions they mediate, neurons within these cortical and subcortical structures can be activated by various sensory inputs, including, but not limited to, noxious stimuli. Based on clinical, neurophysiological, and anatomical evidence, it is reasonable to conclude that the hedonic component of pain may be mediated via the nociceptive activation of limbic system structures (Melzack and Casey 1968; Price 2000).

MODULATION OF NOCICEPTIVE PROCESSES AND PAIN

Numerous psychophysical studies have shown that the lowest intensity at which a stimulus is perceived as painful (the pain threshold) shows little variation among normal subjects examined in a laboratory setting. This observation applies to a variety of stimulus types such as heat, cold, pressure, pinch, and electrical stimulation of the skin or muscle. Furthermore, groups of normal subjects will give very similar subjective ratings of the changes in pain intensity as the applied stimulus intensity increases above pain threshold levels. Similar results are obtained with psychophysical measurements of the hedonic component of pain, during which the subject is usually asked to rate the degree of perceived stimulus unpleasantness, as distinguished from intensity. These laboratory-based experimental studies show that the nervous systems of humans and animals have the capacity to function in a mode that takes full advantage of the peripherally transmitted information about the physical characteristics of the applied stimulus (Gracely et al. 1978; Price et al. 1980; Price 1988).

However, common experience and clinical observation outside the setting of the psychophysical laboratory show that the perception of all components of pain, including intensity, intrinsic unpleasantness, and the emotional and cognitive elaboration of the painful experience, can be greatly modified by the environment in which the noxious stimulus is applied. A common experience is that tissue-damaging injuries may be sustained without awareness of the event until the wound is noticed later under different environmental conditions. Dramatic examples are documented in anecdotal accounts of profound analgesia during life-threatening situations, participation in sporting events, or during religious rituals (Clark and Clark 1980; Price 1988). In the laboratory, the analgesic effect of hypnotic suggestion has been quantified in several studies (Hilgard 1975; Spanos et al. 1989; Danziger et al. 1998). In the clinical setting, the placebo effect, produced by suggestions and the environment, has been so well documented and measured that the efficacy of treatments, especially analgesics, must be measured against a placebo control (Levine et al. 1978, 1979; Turner et al. 1994; Amanzio and Benedetti 1999). Although most attention has focused on the analgesic side of pain modulation, substantial evidence indicates that all aspects of perceived pain can be enhanced by environmental and cognitive influences. This phenomenon has been demonstrated in the laboratory, particularly with the use of hypnotic suggestion (Staats et al. 1998). In the clinical setting, the perceived intensity and unpleasantness of pain and the autonomic and neuroendocrine reactions to the noxious stimulus increase if the pain is perceived to threaten personal integrity or survival (Price et al. 1980, 1987).

Experimental studies have provided information about the neurophysiological basis for pain modulation (Dubner and Ren 1999; Mason 1999). Early neurophysiological experiments showed that certain cortical and bulbospinal pathways could suppress ascending impulses evoked by noxious stimulation (Hagbarth and Fex 1959; Holmquist et al. 1960; Lundberg et al. 1963; Lundberg 1964). Bulbospinal modulation of spinal sensory processing can be evoked by electrical or pharmacological stimulation within the midbrain PAG or the medullary reticular formation in animal experiments. The behaviorally observed analgesia that can be produced by direct stimulation within the PAG is probably mediated through reciprocally interacting medullary bulbospinal neurons that modulate the excitability of nociceptive reflexes (Fields and Basbaum 1978; Fields et al. 1983; Fields 1987; Heinricher et al. 1989). Subsequent neurophysiological and neuroanatomical investigations revealed that both excitatory and inhibitory effects are transmitted through cortical and subcortical pathways to the thalamus, brainstem, or to nociceptive spinal or trigeminal sensory cells. Neurophysiological stimulation studies reveal direct corticothalamic and corticospinal effects on nociceptive transmission at spinal and other subcortical levels (Gerhart et al. 1983; Yezierski et al. 1983; Yuan et al. 1985, 1986; Zhang et al. 1991, 1996). Other investigations in awake monkeys have directly related descending effects to more complex pain-related behavior. The nociceptive responses of cells in the trigeminal nucleus of awake monkeys, for example, can be enhanced or suppressed by altering the experimental conditions for obtaining a food reward. These influences undoubtedly involve the participation of forebrain mechanisms (Dubner et al. 1981; Hayes et al. 1981; Hoffman et al. 1981; Bushnell et al. 1984; Duncan et al. 1987).

The importance of the forebrain as a source of modulatory influence is emphasized by the observation that it comprises 85% of CNS volume in humans compared to 44% in the rodent (Swanson 1995). The human corticospinal tract, which contains $0.8-1 \times 10^6$ fibers, innervates the dorsal horn origin of the spinothalamic tract, which is composed of only $2-5 \times 10^3$ axons (Blinkov and Glezer 1968; Towe 1995). Within the forebrain, only 15% of the estimated 6×10^3 synapses on a VPL thalamocortical neuron originate from ascending inputs; the remaining 85% originate either from (presumed inhibitory) interneurons (35%) or corticothalamic neurons (50%) (Liu et al. 1995). Consequently, normal or pathological changes in forebrain activity may have profound effects on pain and nociceptive processing at all levels (Casey 1999).

Neurochemical and neuropharmacological investigations reveal the neurotransmitter mechanisms through which descending influences modulate central nociceptive processing and pain (Fields et al. 1991). The discovery of several types of opioid receptors and compounds in the mammalian CNS stimulated numerous investigations into the neurotransmitter basis for endogenous (environmentally produced) analgesia. Some of the anatomical locations of the endogenous opioid receptors, such as the spinal afferent terminals, spinal dorsal gray, brainstem PAG, and limbic cortex, are consistent with the mediation of endogenous analgesia. The functional significance of the high concentration of opioid receptors and compounds in such areas as the basal ganglia is less evident (Bourgoin et al. 1994; Jensen 1997; Yaksh 1997). At the human clinical level, the placebo effect is significantly attenuated by systemic injections of naloxone, an opioid receptor antagonist (Levine et al. 1978; Amanzio and Benedetti 1999). Animal experiments show that bulbospinal antinociceptive effects are mediated through both opioid and nonopioid compounds that include norepinephrine, serotonin, and the inhibitory neurotransmitter γ-aminobutyric acid (GABA) (Gebhart 1986; Hammond 1986; Fields et al. 1991). The neurotransmitter mechanisms that mediate nociceptive modulation through corticobulbar or corticospinal pathways are unknown.

PAIN AS A SUBJECT OF BASIC BIOLOGICAL INTEREST

PAIN AS A SENSORY SYSTEM

Similar to any of the other sensory systems, pain presents the problem of how stimulus features are encoded as neuronal activity. Common experience and sophisticated psychophysical studies show that humans and other animals can discriminate among different intensities of noxious stimuli and identify the spatial and temporal features of noxious somatic, muscular, and visceral stimuli. Other physical characteristics of the stimulus, such as thermal, mechanical, or chemical, also can be distinguished (Price 1988). These features of noxious stimuli are encoded through the combined physiological actions of the nociceptors, peripheral afferent fibers, and central neurons. Each level of neural processing contributes to discriminative capacity by transforming the physical event of the stimulus into neuronal discharge patterns that are further transformed and distributed through the CNS. We do not know, however, what the critical transformations are for most discriminative functions—nor do we know how these transformations are centrally distributed. The finding of convergent inputs in the CNS presents an especially difficult conceptual problem. For example, most central neurons that respond to cutaneous somatic stimuli also respond to stimulation of deep subcutaneous and visceral structures (Berkley et al. 1993; Brüggemann et al. 1994; Al-Chaer et al. 1996). Because we can identify and distinguish among noxious stimuli applied to these tissues, there must be a central coding mechanism that represents this discriminative function. At present, we do not know the critical neural code(s) that subserve this function. Another example of this problem is our lack of knowledge about the neural mechanisms mediating the full range of our thermal discriminative capacities. The neural mechanism for encoding different intensities of innocuous warmth, and for distinguishing warmth from noxious heat, seems relatively simple at the peripheral level, but becomes unclear when central mechanisms are investigated (Poulos and Benjamin 1968; Darian-Smith et al. 1979). Recent PET studies by Craig and colleagues (2000), however, have begun to elucidate some of the thermosensory properties of human cortical responses. To answer these and related questions, measures of discriminative function and central neuronal activity must be monitored simultaneously in awake animals and humans.

PAIN AS A GATEWAY TO OTHER BEHAVIORS

The activation of nociceptive afferents induces a wide variety of behaviors, ranging from unconscious reflexive responses to highly cognitive processes. Early investigators quickly recognized the physiological and functional significance of flexor reflexes. The afferent fibers evoking these somatic reflexes, termed flexor reflex afferents, consist largely of what we now recognize as nociceptive afferent fibers (Lundberg 1964). Much remains to be learned about the neurophysiology of nociceptive spinal somatic and autonomic reflexes, especially the supraspinal mechanisms that modulate their excitability.

Of course, pain is not a reflex. By definition, it is an experience that includes hedonic components and the associated behaviors of escape and avoidance. Noxious stimuli have been used for many years to evoke these behaviors in animals and humans and thus gain some insight into the neural mechanisms that mediate them. In special conditions, such as chronic, unavoidable pain, neuroendocrine changes occur that may be accompanied by dramatic changes in behavioral responses to noxious stimuli (Valentino and Curtis 1991; Aloisi et al. 1995). Various forms of stress, also accompanied by neuroendocrine responses, may be associated with profound analgesic states, some of which may be reversed by systemically administered naloxone and thus presumably are mediated by endogenous opioid mechanisms (Beecher 1956; Clark and Clark 1980; Willer 1981; Pitman et al. 1990; Vaccarino et al. 1992; Hawranko et al. 1994; Yamada and Nabeshima 1995). Hedonically weighted stimuli also facilitate learning, so noxious stimuli are used to activate neural mechanisms that mediate long-term changes in synaptic transmission, including mnemonic functions (Lavond et al. 1993; LeDoux 1993; Watkins et al. 1993; Gabriel and Poremba 1995; Poremba and Gabriel 1997; Shi and Davis 1999). These observations emphasize the importance of supraspinal systems in the elaboration and control of the nociceptive processing that leads to pain and pain-modulated behaviors.

PAIN AS A CLINICAL PROBLEM

ACUTE PAIN

Pain caused by the transient activation of nociceptors by stimuli that produce little or no tissue damage does not present a serious clinical problem. Tissue damage, however, evokes an inflammatory response. The physiological and biochemical basis of inflammation is among the most complex subjects in biological pathology. Pain is one of the cardinal clinical features of inflammation. The chemical basis for the inflammatory activation and sensitization of nociceptors is a very active area of study (Levine et al. 1993b; Handwerker and Reeh 1994; Green et al. 1995; Millan 1999; Woolf and Costigan 1999). With few exceptions, the pain of acute tissue injury subsides as the wound heals.

Acute pain presents a clinical problem when it is recurrent. Such pain may be due to recurrent acute inflammatory processes such as various forms of arthritis, or to the recurrent activation of nociceptors, as in the different headache syndromes such as migraine. Although recurrent episodes of acute pain may be frequent and severely disabling, they do not leave clinically significant neuropathology in their wake when the exacerbation spontaneously subsides or is relieved by agents that attenuate the inflammatory activation of nociceptors (Malow and Olson 1981).

CHRONIC PAIN

According to the definition proposed by IASP, pain should be considered chronic when it has persisted nearly continuously for 3 months or longer (Merskey and Bogduk 1994). Depending on its intensity, location, unpleasantness, and other factors, there is little doubt that pain of this duration, or perhaps even less, produces clinically significant functional impairment.

Non-neuropathic pain. Chronic pain may follow tissue damage that does not injure major peripheral nerve branches or the CNS. For example, a persistent inflammatory response or structural abnormality may continually stimulate nociceptors that respond to chemical (inflammatory) or mechanical stimuli. Rarely, apparently minor non-neural tissue damage leads to a chronic condition known as complex regional pain syndrome type I (CRPS-I, also termed reflex sympathetic dystrophy), in which the pain is accompanied by changes in blood flow, temperature, and sweating within the injured region and even beyond. Normally innocuous tactile or thermal stimuli may become painful (allodynia), and the pain of noxious stimuli is exaggerated (hyperalgesia). There may be atrophy of the skin, abnormalities in hair growth, and demineralization of bone within the symptomatic area (van der Laan et al. 1998). In some cases, the pain of CRPS-I depends upon the continuous efferent activity of sympathetic nerves (sympathetically maintained pain [SMP]) (Merskey and Bogduk 1994). If this is the case, pain may be relieved for variable periods of time by surgical or pharmacological blockade of efferent sympathetic activity. The results of some experiments, however, indicate that pain may be independent of sympathetic efferent activity (Baron et al. 1999). The pathophysiology of CRPS-I is unknown, but many clinicians and investigators suspect nociceptively induced changes in the CNS. This speculation is supported by animal experiments showing that inflammation can lead to the expression of substance P, a putative nociceptive neurotransmitter, in large-diameter myelinated tactile afferent fibers innervating the spinal cord dorsal horn (Neumann et al. 1996). In addition, inflammation can sensitize spinal cord dorsal horn neurons, in part through mechanisms that enhance the effect of the neurotransmitter glutamate on postsynaptic NMDA receptors (Dubner and Ruda 1992; Sluka et al. 1992, 1994; Allen et al. 1999; Woolf and Salter 2000).

Neuropathic pain. Damage to peripheral sensory nerves may produce a painful neuropathy, usually characterized by nearly constant pain within the somatic area innervated by the nerve. The extreme form of this condition, originally called causalgia and now designated complex regional pain syndrome type II (CRPS-II) (Merskey and Bogduk 1994), consists of constant, burning pain that is typically severe and debilitating. Allodynia and hyperalgesia are always present and usually extend beyond the area innervated by the damaged nerve. Consequently, patients immobilize and protect a limb affected by CRPS-II. Sudomotor abnormalities and trophic changes are invariably seen in CRPS-II. Medical or surgical sympatholytic treatments frequently relieve the symptoms of CRPS-II, at least temporarily, suggesting that the pain of this condition is sympathetically maintained in many cases (Kim and Chung 1991; Sato and Perl 1991; Hannington-Kiff 1992; Schott 1994; Rowbotham 1998). The overall effectiveness of sympatholysis is difficult to evaluate due to considerable variability in patients' response to treatment and in the long-term, natural course of the untreated condition (Dellemijn et al. 1994; Verdugo and Ochoa 1994; Verdugo et al. 1994; Blumberg et al. 1997). The pathophysiology of CRPS-II, like that of CRPS-I, is unknown. However, animal experiments have shown that nerve damage may trigger an anatomical reorganization of the afferent innervation of spinal sensory neurons, perhaps permitting tactile afferents to excite specifically nociceptive central cells (Woolf et al. 1992). Some cases of CRPS-II provide clinical evidence for CNS involvement because the condition is profoundly affected by emotional state and attention and spreads well beyond the area innervated by the damaged nerve, sometimes even affecting contralateral sites (Rommel et al. 1999; Sieweke et al. 1999). Rarely, CRPS-II may follow injury to the CNS alone (Schott 1986, 1996).

In the more common forms of painful neuropathy caused by trauma or by metabolic, infectious, immunological, or degenerative diseases, trophic and sudomotor changes are absent and there is little or no clinical evidence for SMP. Allodynia and hyperalgesia are often, but not always, present, and the pain is usually confined to the innervation area of the involved nerve (mononeuropathy) or nerves (polyneuropathy). Patients almost always have sensory loss, which may affect tactile, thermal, and nociceptive senses together or selectively. As in CRPS-I and II, the CNS may be secondarily affected, possibly prolonging the condition, limiting the effectiveness of treatment, and exaggerating the perceived intensity and unpleasantness of pain.

Damage or disease that affects the CNS at any level from the spinal cord to the brain may cause central pain (CP) (for review, see Casey 1991; Boivie 1994; Gonzales 1995; Bowsher 1998). A wide variety of CNS lesions can cause CP, which affects an estimated 2–8% of patients with stroke, 20–44% of multiple sclerosis patients, and 31% of patients with spinal cord injury. CP is also increasingly recognized as an occasional complication of Parkinson's disease (Schott 1985). The pain of CP is usually delayed, sometimes for many months, following the CNS injury. The quality of the pain varies among individuals, as does its intensity and unpleasantness. The pain is often described as deep and aching, and always affects the site of neurological disability. Most, but not all, patients have impaired thermal and pain sensation within the affected area. Allodynia and hyperalgesia to thermal or mechanical stimulation are frequently present. The intensity and unpleasantness of the pain are typically increased by anger, anxiety, and depression and are ameliorated, to variable degrees, by relaxation, diversion, and positive emotional states. Although tricyclic antidepressant drugs provide some relief in many cases, CP is widely recognized as one of the most difficult conditions to treat. Various neuroablative procedures have been used in severe cases, but the overall record of success is generally discouraging. Electrical stimulation within the thalamus and motor cortex is reportedly effective in some cases (Tsubokawa et al. 1993).

THE CONTRIBUTION OF IMAGING

In this book, "imaging" refers to the ability to create an image of central neurophysiological processes, usually with a duration of several sec-

onds, that can be localized within several millimeters. This restriction eliminates consideration of electrophysiological events lasting for milliseconds,
such as action or evoked potentials, and of most transient magnetic fields as
recorded in magnetoencephalography, even if these can be located precisely.

PHYSIOLOGICAL BACKGROUND

Imaging devices visualize physiological responses to the activity of
populations of synapses (see Chapters 2 and 3). Several experiments have
demonstrated the close coupling of glucose utilization and synaptic activity
(Schwartz et al. 1979; Mata et al. 1980; Sokoloff 1991). Magistretti and
Pellerin (1997) have reviewed evidence linking the presynaptic release of
glutamate, through the activation of Na^+-K^+ ATPase, to astrocytic glucose
and neuronal pyruvate metabolism with the production of ATP. The close
link between synaptic neurotransmitter release, recycling, and glucose utilization is the physiological rationale for imaging studies of this metabolic
activity. Accordingly, positron emission tomography (PET) and single photon emission computed tomography (SPECT) are used in humans to detect
the product of radiolabeled fluorodeoxyglucose (FDG) metabolism that is
accumulated and trapped within active presynaptic terminals. Similarly, labeled 2-deoxyglucose (2-DG) is used for quantitative radioautography studies in animals to estimate the regional metabolic rate of glucose (CMRglc)
(Kennedy et al. 1975) (see Chapter 8). In both humans and animals, the
synaptic membrane receptors that bind neurotransmitters and drugs can be
labeled with radioactive ligands to identify their distribution and concentration using PET or SPECT (Sadzot and Franck 1990; Frost 1993). In some
cases, it is possible to determine changes in ligand binding associated with
drug or neurotransmitter activity. However, these metabolic and pharmacological investigations are not suitable for studying the effect of brief periods
of stimulation because the duration of the processes under investigation is
many minutes or hours. For example, in a 2-DG study in a rat, the stimulus
must usually be applied for approximately 45 minutes (Mao et al. 1992,
1993). For imaging investigations that require brief periods of stimulation, a
focal process that has a rapid onset and can be repeatedly activated is more
desirable (see Chapters 4 and 7).

The energy demand created by synaptic activity requires the rapid delivery of glucose and oxygen through increases in local blood flow. Approximately a century ago, the experiments of Roy and Sherrington (1890)
provided evidence that global cerebral blood flow (CBF) increases in response to brain activity and the chemical products of brain metabolism. The
physiology of this relationship is now studied at the microscopic level (see

Chapter 3). Special optical sensors and cameras can detect changes in the reflectance of different wavelengths of light as synaptic populations respond to specific stimuli or changing physiological conditions. The signals detected through this *optical imaging* can occur within a few hundred microns of evoked synaptic activity and are thus capable of detecting the anatomical boundaries and organization of the synaptic neuropil. The earliest signal (intrinsic signal) is thought to represent synaptically induced changes in the volume and chemical composition of the extracellular space (see Chapter 3). The intrinsic signal is followed, within several hundred milliseconds, by the first evidence for localized increased blood flow. The earliest increase in blood flow is highly localized, but spreads over several millimeters within 2–3 seconds, so that it is more appropriate to refer to it as *regional cerebral blood flow* (rCBF). Several optical imaging studies have demonstrated the close temporal and anatomical link between synaptic activity and increased local or regional CBF (Malonek and Grinvald 1996; Tommerdahl et al. 1996; Wang et al. 1996; MacVicar 1997). We do not yet know the mechanism that couples synaptic activity and rCBF, but it is likely that several chemical mediators are involved (Chapter 2). The astrocyte, which provides a close anatomical communication between neurons and capillaries, is probably an important component of the mechanism that signals the need for an energy substrate (Magistretti and Pellerin 1997).

    The close spatial and temporal link between synaptic energy demand and increases in rCBF is the basis for cerebral PET and SPECT activation studies. The synaptic activity generated by sensory, motor, and cognitive events generates increases in rCBF, the magnitude of which can be correlated with functional measures of neuronal activity such as motor force, cognitive demand, and the perceived intensity and unpleasantness of noxious stimuli (Fox and Raichle 1984; Pardo et al. 1991; Jonides et al. 1993; Dettmers et al. 1995; Casey et al. 1996; Derbyshire et al. 1997; Rainville et al. 1997; Coghill et al. 1999). An increase in rCBF can be detected within 2–3 seconds of the activating stimulus. Most PET activation studies use radio-labeled water or CO_2, and the accumulated count of radioactive emissions provides an estimate of the regional cerebral perfusion during the scan (about 1 minute). This value is compared across conditions (e.g., pain or no pain) to obtain estimates of task- or stimulus-related changes in rCBF (see Chapter 4). Although decreases in rCBF also can be observed, the physiological interpretation of this event is still uncertain. The contribution of the activity of inhibitory interneurons and synapses to increased (or decreased) rCBF is unknown. Specifically, there is no evidence that decreased rCBF marks the site of inhibitory neuronal activity or even of decreased excitatory activity.

    When a population of active synapses uses oxygen, oxyhemoglobin is changed locally to deoxyhemoglobin. Within approximately 2 seconds, however, a marked microvascular response occurs, which raises oxyhemoglobin levels and rapidly increases the oxyhemoglobin/deoxyhemoglobin ratio. Because these two forms of hemoglobin have different magnetic resonance signals, magnetic imaging devices detect the local shift from one to the other. This magnetic blood-oxygenation-level-dependent (BOLD) signal is the basis for functional magnetic resonance imaging (fMRI) of the brain (Ogawa et al. 1990, 1992; Neil 1993; see Chapters 6 and 7). The amplitude of the signal is proportional to rCBF, which, as in PET studies, can be correlated highly with functional measures of neuronal activity. Indeed, Rees and colleagues (2000) have now demonstrated a strong linear relationship between the magnitude of the fMRI BOLD signal in the human V5 cortex and the discharge of neuronal populations in the same region of monkey cortex.

Among the advantages of fMRI is the lack of radiation, which creates the opportunity to repeat studies of individual subjects frequently. In addition, the spatial resolution of MRI is superior to that of PET or SPECT, allowing investigators to more accurately locate activation within an individual. For many studies, it is not necessary to perform group averaging of the activation responses or to transpose them onto a standard stereotactic atlas for analysis. A disadvantage of fMRI is that ferromagnetic materials, as used in most electronic devices, stimulators, and other recording instruments, cannot be brought into the area of the scanner. Subjects with implanted ferromagnetic metal prostheses or other devices thus cannot be studied with fMRI. Another disadvantage of fMRI is that the imaging and statistical analysis of whole-brain responses are less well established than in PET. In part, this drawback is attributable to various sources of noise that are associated uniquely with fMRI. In addition, metabolic and pharmacological receptor activation and distribution studies cannot be performed with fMRI. Finally, fMRI cannot be used to detect abnormal resting or baseline rCBF, which is likely to be present in pathological conditions such as neuropathic pain (Cesaro et al. 1991; Hsieh et al. 1995; Iadarola et al. 1995). The recent development of quantitative radioautographic studies of rCBF in animals, in addition to CMRglc, offers an opportunity to use animal models for close comparison with the results of similar human studies (Morrow et al. 1998, 2000; Paulson et al. 2000). Currently, animal fMRI is not available, so the same comparison cannot be made with fMRI. Radioautographic techniques provide histological-level spatial resolution to use in conjunction with well-established animal models of neuropathic pain. In addition, invasive techniques, such as the intracerebral injection of drugs or the selective placement of lesions, can be used in animals to investigate the dynamics of inter-regional networks and the development of plastic reorganization in the brain. Rather than regarding PET, SPECT, and fMRI as competing technologies, however, it is better to consider them complementary modes of investigation.

IMAGING NORMAL PAIN

Because imaging presents information about the activity of multiple supraspinal structures ranging from the brainstem to the forebrain, it is especially suited for an analysis of the neurophysiology of pain and pain-related physiological events (see Chapter 5). The supraspinal processing of nociceptive information activates somatic and autonomic reflexes, neuroendocrine responses, attention, arousal, an analysis of the spatio-temporal and physical characteristics of the stimulus, hedonic experience, mnemonic functions, cognitive processes, and the ascending and descending control systems that mediate and modulate each of these activities and their interactions. Information about detailed cellular and molecular mechanisms that participate in one or more aspects of nociceptive activity is critical for a full understanding of these responses to noxious stimulation. However, an understanding of how each of these neuronal populations contributes to one or more nociceptive responses, and how they interact to produce, in unity, the essential components of pain, requires a method that permits a conjoint analysis of conscious behavior and the activity of multiple synaptic populations. This is a serious challenge, but the neurophysiology of pain cannot be understood at the molecular, atomic, or subatomic level alone; the function of the system must be studied also.

Careful behavioral analysis is a critical component of imaging studies of pain. In humans, this method usually requires psychophysical data; in animals, other behavioral measures must be employed. Otherwise, it is impossible to relate behavioral events to changes in rCBF within multiple or single structures. In some cases, the behavioral event of interest may be an autonomic response such as an increase in blood pressure, heart rate, or sudomotor activity. In other experiments, somatic reflexes, voluntary movements, or cognitive processes may be the critical measurements. In either case, it is possible to design the experiment around specific hypotheses about the activity of one or more structures or pathways activated by nociceptive stimulation. Functional brain imaging also permits the simultaneous analysis of the effects of cognitive processes, such as the placebo effect, drugs, hypnosis, counterstimulation, or focal lesions, on nociceptively evoked activity and pain. The development of imaging methods in animals (Chapter 8) and well-validated models of pain behavior allow investigators to use invasive procedures to manipulate these effects.

IMAGING PATHOLOGICAL PAIN

Pain may persist well beyond wound healing in some cases, as discussed above with regard to CRPS-I and -II. The pathophysiology of these painful conditions is not known. Evidence indicates that non-neuronal tissue damage occasionally produces long-lasting increases in the excitability of spinal and supraspinal sensory neurons. In animal models of inflammatory pain, these physiological changes may persist for hours. In human cases of CRPS-I, however, post-injury pain may continue for months and years, sometimes accompanied by changes in sudomotor activity, osteoporosis, and atrophy of skin and muscle. Often, sensory and autonomic function is altered well beyond the site of injury, in rare cases including the homotopic contralateral body site. These observations suggest lasting alterations in the excitability of central neurons, certainly including the spinal cord, and possibly extending to supraspinal sites. These plastic changes might be caused or facilitated by prolonged input from normal nociceptive afferent fibers in cases of CRPS-I where there is no evidence of nerve damage.

In cases of CRPS-II, however, there is, by definition, clinical evidence for direct nerve damage. Animal models of neuropathic pain show that continuing afferent activity can originate spontaneously from damaged nerve fibers, including presumed nociceptive afferents, and from the cell bodies of afferent fibers in the dorsal root ganglion (Devor and Wall 1990). The clinical picture is similar to that of CRPS-I, except that the condition is likely to be more persistent, severe, and widespread, and to be strongly influenced by environmental stress and emotional state. These observations constitute additional evidence that long-term changes have occurred in the physiology of spinal and supraspinal neurons, perhaps exaggerated by abnormal inputs from damaged peripheral nerves. There are several examples of functional reorganization of sensory neurons in the spinal cord, thalamus, and cerebral cortex of animals following peripheral injury with or without nerve damage, but these findings have not been related to a condition of chronic pain (Garraghty and Kaas 1991; Kaas 1991; Pons et al. 1991; Florence et al. 1996, 1998; Jones and Pons 1998; Woolf and Salter 2000). However, Flor and colleagues (1995) were able to demonstrate that the intensity of pain experienced by amputees with a phantom limb correlated well with the extent of functional reorganization of the somatosensory cortex. This study was a direct demonstration that peripheral damage can cause pain-related central changes in the human forebrain. Finally, as previously discussed, central lesions alone may cause pain in the absence of nociceptive input or pathology, as in the case of central pain.

The above examples emphasize the need to obtain information about the immediate and long-term responses of supraspinal systems, including the forebrain, in studying patients with pathological pain of peripheral or central origin (Casey 1999). There is little doubt that neural systems at the highest level of the neuraxis can undergo plastic reorganization that either causes or prolongs the pain of chronic neurological disease. At the first stage, pathological signals emanating from the periphery can reorganize spinal sensory processing. This reorganization, in turn, transmits abnormal signals rostrally, perhaps failing to trigger normal bulbospinal control mechanisms while activating maladaptive reorganization in the thalamus and cortex. The final stage involves a disruption of both ascending and descending systems that normally mediate nociceptive processing and pain. The imaging of pain can provide unique, behaviorally related information about the anatomical and physiological changes that underlie the pathology of chronic non-neuropathic and neuropathic pain.

THERAPEUTIC IMPLICATIONS OF PAIN IMAGING

Ideally, a full understanding of the central pathophysiology of chronic, severely painful conditions such as those discussed above would facilitate the development of measures to prevent them. This desirable outcome first requires researchers to distinguish between adaptive, neutral, and maladaptive reorganization at different levels of the nervous system. Then they must identify the specific conditions that lead to a maladaptive response. Genetic factors could be strong determinants of this process because no clinically obvious reason explains why nearly identical anatomical pathology leads to the development of pain in one patient but not in another. However, the detection of hidden anatomical and physiological differences among such patients may require the development of new technologies or simply more detailed information using current methods. Future physical or pharmacological methods may specifically target conditions that lead to maladaptive central adaptations. These interventions could include the application of aggressive physical and behavioral methods, the delivery of specific stimulators or suppressors of local growth factors (Humpel et al. 1995; Rocamora et al. 1996; Cho et al. 1997), and neurosurgical stimulation or ablative procedures. Once a chronic pain condition has developed, an understanding of the causal pathophysiology in each patient may inspire the development of similar interventions targeting specific sites and pathways, based in part on information obtained by the imaging of pain mechanisms.

REFERENCES

Al-Chaer ED, Lawand NB, Westlund KN, Willis WD. Visceral nociceptive input into the ventral posterolateral nucleus of the thalamus: a new function for the dorsal column pathway. *J Neurophysiol* 1996; 762:661–2674.

Allen BJ, Li J, Menning PM, et al. Primary afferent fibers that contribute to increased substance P receptor internalization in the spinal cord after injury. *J Neurophysiol* 1999; 81:1379–1390.

Aloisi AM, Albonetti ME, Muscettola M, et al. Effects of formalin-induced pain on ACTH, beta-endorphin, corticosterone and interleukin-6 plasma levels in rats. *Neuroendocrinology* 1995; 62:13–18.

Amanzio M, Benedetti F. Neuropharmacological dissection of placebo analgesia: Expectation-activated opioid systems versus conditioning-activated specific subsystems. *J Neurosci* 1999; 19:484–494.

Baron R, Wasner G, Borgstedt R, et al. Effect of sympathetic activity on capsaicin-evoked pain, hyperalgesia, and vasodilatation. *Neurology* 1999; 52:923–932.

Bassetti C, Bogousslavsky J, Regli F. Sensory syndromes in parietal stroke. *Neurology* 1993; 43:1942–1949.

Beecher HK. Relationship of significance of wound to pain experienced. *JAMA* 1956; 161:1609–1613.

Berkley KJ, Guilbaud G, Benoist JM, Gautron M. Responses of neurons in and near the thalamic ventrobasal complex of the rat to stimulation of uterus, cervix, vagina, colon, and skin. *J Neurophysiol* 1993; 69:557–568.

Bernard JF, Besson JM. The spino(trigemino)pontoamygdaloid pathway: electrophysiological evidence for an involvement in pain processes. *J Neurophysiol* 1990; 63:473–490.

Berthier M, Starkstein S, Leiguarda R. Asymbolia for pain: a sensory-limbic disconnection syndrome. *Ann Neurol* 1988; 24:41–49.

Blair RW, Evans AR, Thompson J. Responses of medullary raphespinal neurons to electrical stimulation of thoracic sympathetic afferents, vagal afferents, and to other sensory inputs in cats. *J Neurophysiol* 1991; 66:2084–2094.

Blinkov SM, Glezer II. *The Human Brain in Figures and Tables*. New York: Plenum Press, 1968.

Blomqvist A, Zhang ET, Craig AD. Cytoarchitectonic and immunohistochemical characterization of a specific pain and temperature relay, the posterior portion of the ventral medial nucleus, in the human thalamus. *Brain* 2000; 123:601–619.

Blumberg H, Hoffmann U, Mohadjer M, Scheremet R. Sympathetic nervous system and pain: a clinical reappraisal. *Behav Brain Sci* 1997; 20:426–434.

Boivie J. Central pain. In: Wall PD, Melzack R (Eds). *Textbook of Pain*. Edinburgh: Churchill-Livingstone, 1994.

Bourgoin S, Benoliel JJ, Collin, E, et al. Opioidergic control of the spinal release of neuropeptides. Possible significance for the analgesic effects of opioids. *Fundam Clin Pharmacol* 1994; 8:307–321.

Bowsher D. Pathophysiology of central pain. *Pain Forum* 1998; 7:15–17.

Brüggemann J, Shi T, Apkarian AV. Squirrel monkey lateral thalamus. II. Viscerosomatic convergent representation of urinary bladder, colon, esophagus. *J Neurosci* 1994; 14:6796–6814.

Burgess PR, Perl ER. Cutaneous mechanoreceptors and nociceptors. In: Iggo A (Ed). *Somatosensory System*. Handbook of Sensory Physiology, Vol. II. Berlin: Springer-Verlag, 1973, pp 59–69.

Burstein R, Cliffer KD, Giesler GJ Jr. Direct somatosensory projections from the spinal cord to the hypothalamus and telencephalon. *Neuroscience* 1987; 7:4159–4164.

Burton H. Somatic sensory properties of caudal bulbar reticular neurons in the cat. *Brain Res* 1968; 11:357–372.

Bushnell MC, Duncan GH, Dubner R, He LF. Activity of trigeminothalamic neurons in medullary dorsal horn of awake monkeys trained in a thermal discrimination task. *J Neurophysiol* 1984; 52:170–187.

Casey KL. Somatic stimuli, spinal pathways, and size of cutaneous fibers influencing unit activity in the medial medullary reticular formation. *Exp Neurol* 1969; 25:35–56.

Casey KL. *Pain and Central Nervous System Disease: The Central Pain Syndromes.* New York: Raven Press, 1991.

Casey KL. Forebrain mechanisms of nociception and pain: analysis through imaging. *Proc Natl Acad Sci USA* 1999; 96:7668–7674.

Casey KL, Minoshima S, Morrow TJ, Koeppe RA. Comparison of human cerebral activation patterns during cutaneous warmth, heat pain, and deep cold pain. *J Neurophysiol* 1996; 76:571–581.

Casey KL, Morrow TJ. Ventral posterior thalamic neurons differentially responsive to noxious stimulation of the awake monkey. *Science* 1983; 221:675–677.

Cervero F. Sensory innervation of the viscera: peripheral basis of visceral pain. *Physiol Rev* 1994; 74:95–138.

Cesare P, McNaughton P. Peripheral pain mechanisms. *Curr Opin Neurobiol* 1997; 7:493–499.

Cesaro P, Mann MW, Moretti JL, et al. Central pain and thalamic hyperactivity: a single photon emission computerized tomographic study. *Pain* 1991; 47:329–336.

Chandler MJ, Hobbs SF, Fu Q-G, et al. Responses of neurons in ventroposterolateral nucleus of primate thalamus to urinary bladder distension. *Brain Res* 1992; 571:26–34.

Cho HJ, Kim SY, Park MJ, et al. Expression of mRNA for brain-derived neurotrophic factor in the dorsal root ganglion following peripheral inflammation. *Brain Res* 1997; 749:358–362.

Chung JM, Lee KH, Surmeier DJ, et al. Response characteristics of neurons in the ventral posterior lateral nucleus of the monkey thalamus. *J Neurophysiol* 1986; 56:370–390.

Clark WC, Clark SB. Pain responses in Nepalese Porters. *Science* 1980; 209:410–412.

Coghill RC, Sang CN, Maisog JH, Iadarola MJ. Pain intensity processing within the human brain: a bilateral, distributed mechanism. *J Neurophysiol* 1999; 82:1934–1943.

Craig AD, Bushnell MC, Zhang E-T, Blomqvist A. A thalamic nucleus specific for pain and temperature sensation. *Nature* 1994; 372:770–773.

Craig AD, Zhang ET, Blomqvist A. A distinct thermoreceptive subregion of lamina I in nucleus caudalis of the owl monkey. *J Comp Neurol* 1999; 404:221–234.

Craig AD, Chen K, Bandy D, Reiman EM. Thermosensory activation of insular cortex. *Nat Neurosci* 2000; 3:184–190.

Damasio H, Grabowski T, Frank R, Galaburda AM, Damasio AR. The return of Phineas Gage: clues about the brain from the skull of a famous patient. *Science* 1994; 264:1102–1105.

Danziger N, Fournier E, Bouhassira D, et al. Different strategies of modulation can be operative during hypnotic analgesia: a neurophysiological study. *Pain* 1998; 75:85–92.

Darian-Smith I, Johnson KO, LaMotte C, et al. Coding of incremental changes in skin temperature by single warm fibers in the monkey. *J Neurophysiol* 1979; 42:1316–1331.

Davis KD, Hutchison WD, Lozano AM, Dostrovsky JO. Altered pain and temperature perception following cingulotomy and capsulotomy in a patient with schizoaffective disorder. *Pain* 1994; 59:189–199.

Degos JD, da Fonseca N, Gray F, Cesaro P. Severe frontal syndrome associated with infarcts of the left anterior cingulate gyrus and the head of the right caudate nucleus. A clinicopathological case. *Brain* 1993; 116:1541–1548.

Dellemijn PLI, Fields HL, Allen RR, McKay WR, Rowbotham MC. The interpretation of pain relief and sensory changes following sympathetic blockade. *Brain* 1994; 117:1475–1487.

Derbyshire SW, Jones AK, Gyulai F, et al. Pain processing during three levels of noxious stimulation produces differential patterns of central activity. *Pain* 1997; 73:431–445.

Dettmers C, Fink GR, Lemon RN, et al. Relation between cerebral activity and force in the motor areas of the human brain. *J Neurophysiol* 1995; 74:802–815.

Devinsky O, Morrell MJ, Vogt BA. Contributions of anterior cingulate cortex to behaviour. *Brain* 1995; 118:279–306.

Devor M, Wall PD. Cross-excitation in dorsal root ganglia of nerve-injured and intact rats. *J Neurophysiol* 1990; 64:1733–1746.

Dubner R, Ren K. Endogenous mechanisms of sensory modulation. *Pain* 1999; (Suppl. 6)S45–S53.

Dubner R, Ruda MA. Activity-dependent neuronal plasticity following tissue injury and inflammation. *Trends Neurosci* 1992; 15:96–103.

Dubner R, Hoffman DS, Hayes RL. Neuronal activity in medullary dorsal horn of awake monkeys trained in a thermal discrimination task. III. Task-related responses and their functional role. *J Neurophysiol* 1981; 46:444–464.

Duncan GH, Bushnell MC, Bates R, Dubner R. Task-related responses of monkey medullary dorsal horn neurons, *J Neurophysiol* 1987; 57:289–310.

Fields HL. *Pain.* McGraw-Hill, New York, 1987.

Fields HL, Basbaum AI. Brain stem control of spinal pain-transmission neurons. *Ann Rev Physiol* 1978; 40:217–248.

Fields HL, Wagner GM, Anderson SD. Some properties of spinal neurons projecting to the medial brain-stem reticular formation. *Exp Neurol* 1975; 47:118–134.

Fields HL, Bry J, Hentall I, Zorman G. The activity of neurons in the rostral medulla of the rat during withdrawal from noxious heat. *J Neurosci* 1983; 3:2545–2552.

Fields HL, Heinricher MM, Mason P. Neurotransmitters in nociceptive modulatory circuits. *Annu Rev Neurosci* 1991; 14:219–245.

Fisher CM. Lacunar strokes and infarcts: a review. *Neurology* 1982; 32:871–876.

Flor H, Elbert T, Knecht S, et al. Phantom-limb pain as a perceptual correlate of cortical reorganization following arm amputation. *Nature* 1995; 375:482–484.

Florence SL, Jain N, Pospichal MW, et al. Central reorganization of sensory pathways following peripheral nerve regeneration in fetal monkeys. *Nature* 1996; 381:69–71.

Florence SL, Taub HB, Kaas JH. Large-scale sprouting of cortical connections after peripheral injury in adult macaque monkeys. *Science* 1998; 282:1117–1121.

Foltz EL, White LE. Pain "relief" by frontal cingulumotomy. *J Neurosurg* 1962; 19:89–100.

Fox PT, Raichle ME. Stimulus rate dependence of regional cerebral blood flow in human striate cortex, demonstrated by positron emission tomography. *J Neurophysiol* 1984; 51:1109–1120.

Friedman DP, Murray EA, O'Neill JB, Mishkin M. Cortical connections of the somatosensory fields of the lateral sulcus of macaques: evidence for a corticolimbic pathway for touch. *J Comp Neurol* 1986; 252:323–347.

Frost JJ. Receptor imaging by PET and SPECT: focus on the opiate receptor. *J Recept Res* 1993; 13:39–53.

Gabriel M, Poremba A. The role of pain in cingulate cortical and limbic thalamic mediation of avoidance learning. In: Besson J-M, Guilbaud G, Ollat H (Eds). Forebrain areas involved in pain processing. Montrouge: John Libbey, 1995, pp 197–212.

Garraghty PE, Kaas JH. Large-scale functional reorganization in adult monkey cortex after peripheral nerve injury. *Proc Natl Acad Sci USA* 1991; 88:6976–6980.

Gebhart GF. Modulatory effects of descending systems on spinal dorsal horn neurons. In: Yaksh TL (Ed). *Spinal Afferent Processing.* New York: Plenum Press, 1986, pp 391–416.

Gerhart KD, Yezierski RP, Fang ZR, Willis WD. Inhibition of primate spinothalamic tract neurons by stimulation in ventral posterior lateral (VPL) thalamic nucleus: possible mechanisms. *J Neurophysiol* 1983; 49:406–423.

Gonzales GR. Central pain: diagnosis and treatment strategies. *Neurology* 1995; 45:S11–S16.

Gracely RH, McGrath P, Dubner R. Ratio scales of sensory and affective verbal pain descriptors. *Pain* 1978; 5:5–18.

Green PG, Miao FJP, Jänig W, Levine JD. Negative feedback neuroendocrine control of the inflammatory response in rats. *J Neurosci* 1995; 15:4678–4686.

Greenspan JD, Winfield JA. Reversible pain and tactile deficits associated with a cerebral tumor compressing the posterior insula and parietal operculum. *Pain* 1992; 50:29–39.

Hagbarth KE, Fex J. Centrifugal influences on single unit activity in spinal sensory paths. *J Neurophysiol* 1959; 22:321–338.

Hammond DL. Control systems for nociceptive afferent processing: The descending inhibitory pathways. In: Yaksh TL (Ed). *Spinal Afferent Processing*. New York: Plenum Press, 1986, pp 363–390.

Handwerker HO, Kobal G. Psychophysiology of experimentally induced pain. *Physiol Rev* 1993; 73:639–671.

Handwerker HO, Reeh PW. Nociceptors in animals. In: Besson J-M, Guilbaud G, Ollat H (Eds). *Peripheral Neurons in Nociception: Physio-Pharmacological Aspects*. Paris: John Libbey, 1994, pp 1–12.

Hannington-Kiff JG. Pain: sympathetic maintenance and central nervous sensitization. *Anaesth Rev* 1992; 9:112–126.

Hawranko AA, Monroe PJ, Smith DJ. Repetitive exposure to the hot-plate test produces stress induced analgesia and alters β-endorphin neuronal transmission within the periaqueductal gray of the rat. *Brain Res* 1994; 667:283–286.

Hayes RL, Dubner R, Hoffman DS. Neuronal activity in medullary dorsal horn of awake monkeys trained in a thermal discrimination task. II. Behavioral modulation of responses to thermal and mechanical stimuli. *J Neurophysiol* 1981; 46:428–443.

Heinricher MM, Barbaro NM, Fields HL. Putative nociceptive modulating neurons in the rostral ventromedial medulla of the rat: Firing of on- and off-cells is related to nociceptive responsiveness. *Somatosens Res* 1989; 6:427–439.

Hilgard ER. Hypnosis. *Ann Rev Psychol* 1975; 26:19.

Hoffman DS, Dubner R, Hayes RL, Medlin TP. Neuronal activity in medullary dorsal horn of awake monkeys trained in a thermal discrimination task. I. Responses to innocuous and noxious thermal stimuli. *J Neurophysiol* 1981; 46:409–427.

Holmquist B, Lundberg A, Oscarsson O. Supraspinal inhibitory control of transmission to three ascending pathways influenced by the flexion reflex afferents. *Arch Ital Biol* 1960; 98:60–80.

Holstege G. Some anatomical observations on the projections from the hypothalamus to brainstem and spinal cord: an HRP and autoradiographic tracing study in the cat. *J Comp Neurol* 1987; 260:98–126.

Holstege G, Bandler R, Saper CB. The emotional motor system. *Prog Brain Res* 1996; 107:3–6.

Hsieh J-C, Belfrage M, Stone-Elander S, Hansson P, Ingvar M. Central representation of chronic ongoing neuropathic pain studied by positron emission tomography. *Pain* 1995; 63:225–236.

Humpel C, Lindqvist E, Soderstrom S, et al. Monitoring release of neurotrophic activity in the brains of awake rats. *Science* 1995; 269:552–554.

Hurt RW, Ballantine HT. Stereotactic anterior cingulate lesions for persistent pain: a report on 68 cases. *Clin Neurosurg* 1973; 21:334–351.

Iadarola MJ, Max MB, Berman KF, et al. Unilateral decrease in thalamic activity observed with positron emission tomography in patients with chronic neuropathic pain. *Pain* 1995; 63:55–64.

Jensen TS. Opioids in the brain: supraspinal mechanisms in pain control. *Acta Anaesthesiol Scand* 1997; 41:123–132.

Jones EG, Pons TP. Thalamic and brainstem contributions to large-scale plasticity of primate somatosensory cortex. *Science* 1998; 282:1121–1125.

Jonides J, Smith EE, Koeppe RA, et al. Spatial working memory in humans as revealed by PET. *Nature* 1993; 363:623–625.

Kaas JH. Plasticity of sensory and motor maps in adult mammals. *Annu Rev Neurosci* 1991; 14:137–167.

Kawakita K, Dostrovsky JO, Tang JS, Chiang CY. Responses of neurons in the rat thalamic nucleus submedius to cutaneous, muscle and visceral nociceptive stimuli. *Pain* 1993; 55:327–338.

Kennedy C, Des Rosiers MH, Jehle JW, et al. Mapping of functional neural pathways by autoradiographic survey of local metabolic rate with (14C) deoxyglucose. *Science* 1975; 187:850–853.

Kim SH, Chung JM. Sympathectomy alleviates mechanical allodynia in an experimental animal model for neuropathy in the rat. *Neurosci Lett* 1991; 134:131–134.

Kniffki KD, Mizumura K. Responses of neurons in VPL and VPL-VL region of the cat to algesic stimulation of muscle and tendon. *J Neurophysiol* 1983; 49:649–661.

Lavond DG, Kim JJ, Thompson RF. Mammalian brain substrates of aversive classical conditioning. *Annu Rev Psychol* 1993; 44:317–342.

LeDoux JE. Emotional memory: in search of systems and synapses. *Ann NY Acad Sci* 1993; 702:149–157.

Levine JD, Gordon NC, Fields HL. The mechanism of placebo analgesia. *Lancet* 1978; 2:654–657.

Levine JD, Gordon NC, Bornstein JC, Fields HL. Role of pain in placebo analgesia. *Proc Natl Acad Sci USA* 1979; 76:3528–3531.

Levine JD, Fields HL, Basbaum AI. Peptides and the primary afferent nociceptor. *J Neurosci* 1993; 13:2273–2286.

Liu XB, Honda CN, Jones EG. Distribution of four types of synapse on physiologically identified relay neurons in the ventral posterior thalamic nucleus of the cat. *J Comp Neurol* 1995; 352:69–91.

Lundberg A. Supraspinal control of transmission in reflex paths to motoneurones and primary afferents. *Prog Brain Res* 1964; 12:197–221.

Lundberg A, Norrsell U, Voorhoeve P. Effects from the sensorimotor cortex on ascending spinal pathways. *Acta Physiol Scand* 1963; 59:462–473.

MacLean PD. Psychosomatic disease and the "visceral brain." *Psychosom Med* 1949; 11:338–353.

MacLean PD. The limbic system ("visceral brain") in relation to the central gray and reticulum of the brain stem. *Psychosom Med* 1955; 17:355–366.

MacLean PD. Visceral functions of the nervous system. *Ann Rev Physiol* 1957; 19:397–416.

MacVicar BA. Mapping neuronal activity by imaging intrinsic optical signals. *Neuroscientist* 1997; 3:381–388.

Magistretti PJ, Pellerin L. The cellular bases of functional brain imaging: evidence for astrocyte-neuron metabolic coupling. *Neuroscientist* 1997; 3:361–365.

Malonek D, Grinvald A. Interactions between electrical activity and cortical microcirculation revealed by imaging spectroscopy: implications for functional brain mapping. *Science* 1996; 272:551–554.

Malow RM, Olson RE. Changes in pain perception after treatment for chronic pain. *Pain* 1981; 11:65–72.

Mao J, Mayer DJ, Price DD. Patterns of increased brain activity indicative of pain in a rat model of peripheral mononeuropathy. *J Neurosci* 1993; 13:2689–2702.

Mao J, Price DD, Coghill RC, Mayer DJ, Hayes RL. Spatial patterns of spinal cord [^{14}C]-2-deoxyglucose metabolic activity in a rat model of painful peripheral mononeuropathy. *Pain* 1992; 50:89–100.

Mason P. Central mechanisms of pain modulation. *Curr Opin Neurobiol* 1999; 9:436–441.

Mata M, Fink DJ, Gainer H, et al. Activity-dependent energy metabolism in rat posterior pituitary primarily reflects sodium pump activity. *J Neurochem* 1980; 34:213–215.

Matthews B. Peripheral and central aspects of trigeminal nociceptive systems. *Philos Trans R Soc Lond B Biol Sci* 1985; 308:313–324.

Melo TP, Bogousslavsky J. Hemiataxia-hypesthesia: a thalamic stroke syndrome. *J Neurol Neurosurg Psychiat* 1992; 55:581–584.

Melzack R, Casey KL. Sensory, motivational, and central control determinants of pain. In: Kenshalo DR (Ed). *The Skin Senses*. Springfield: CC Thomas, 1968, pp 423–439.

Merskey H, Bogduk N. *Classification of Chronic Pain: Descriptions of Chronic Pain Syndromes and Definitions of Pain Terms*. Seattle: IASP Press, 1994.

Mesulam MM, Mufson EJ. Insula of the old world monkey: III. Efferent cortical input and comments on function. *J Comp Neurol* 1982; 212:38–52.

Meyer G, Galindo-Mireles D, Gonzalez-Hernandez T, et al. Direct projections from the reticular formation of the medulla oblongata to the anterior cingulate cortex in the mouse and the rat. *Brain Res* 1986; 398:207–211.

Millan MJ. The induction of pain: an integrative review. *Prog Neurobiol* 1999; 57:1–164.

Morrell JH, Greenberger LM, Pfaff DW. Hypothalamic, other diencephalic, and telencephalic neurons that project to the dorsal midbrain. *J Comp Neurol* 1981; 201:589–620.

Morrow TJ, Paulson PE, Danneman PJ, Casey KL. Regional changes in forebrain activation during the early and late phase of formalin nociception: analysis using cerebral blood flow in the rat. *Pain* 1998; 75:355–365.

Morrow TJ, Paulson PE, Brewer KL, Yezierski RP, Casey KL. Chronic, selective forebrain responses to excitotoxic dorsal horn injury. *Exp Neurol* 2000; 161:220–226.

Mountcastle VB, Henneman E. The representation of tactile sensibility in the thalamus of the monkey. *J Comp Neurol* 1952; 97:409–440.

Nauta WJH, Kuypers HGJM. Some ascending pathways in the brain stem reticular formation of the cat. In: Jasper HH, Proctor LD (Eds). *Reticular Formation of the Brain*. Boston: Little, Brown, 1958, pp 3–30.

Neil JJ. Functional imaging of the central nervous system using magnetic resonance imaging and positron emission tomography. *Curr Opin Neurol* 1993; 6:927–933.

Ness TJ, Follett KA, Piper J, Dirks BA. Characterization of neurons in the area of the medullary lateral reticular nucleus responsive to noxious visceral and cutaneous stimuli. *Brain Res* 1998; 802:163–174.

Neumann S, Doubell TP, Leslie T, Woolf CJ. Inflammatory pain hypersensitivity mediated by phenotypic switch in myelinated primary sensory neurons. *Nature* 1996; 384:360–364.

Ogawa S, Lee T-M, Kay AR, Tank D. Brain magnetic resonance imaging with contrast dependent on blood oxygenation. *Proc Natl Acad Sci USA* 1990; 87:9868–9872.

Ogawa S, Tank DW, Menon R, et al. Intrinsic signal changes accompanying sensory stimulation: functional brain mapping with magnetic resonance imaging. *Proc Natl Acad Sci USA* 1992; 89:5951–5955.

Olds ME, Olds J. Approach-avoidance analysis of rat diencephalon. *J Comp Neurol* 1963; 120:259–295.

Papez JW. A proposed mechanism of emotion. *Arch Neurol Psychiat* 1937; 38:725–743.

Pardo JV, Fox PT, Raichle ME. Localization of a human system for sustained attention by positron emission tomography. *Nature* 1991; 349:61–64.

Paulson PE, Morrow TJ, Casey KL. Bilateral behavioral and regional cerebral blood flow changes during painful peripheral mononeuropathy in the rat. *Pain* 2000; 84:233–245.

Pitman RK, van der Kolk BA, Orr SP, Greenberg MS. Naloxone-reversible analgesic response to combat-related stimuli in post-traumatic stress disorder. *Arch Gen Psychiatry* 1990; 47:541–544.

Ploner M, Freund HJ, Schnitzler A. Pain affect without pain sensation in a patient with a postcentral lesion. *Pain* 1999; 81:211–214.

Pons TP, Garraghty PE, Ommaya AK, et al. Massive cortical reorganization after sensory deafferentation in adult macaques. *Science* 1991; 252:1857–1860.

Poremba A, Gabriel M. Amygdalar lesions block discriminative avoidance learning and cingulothalamic training-induced neuronal plasticity in rabbits. *J Neurosci* 1997; 17:5237–5244.

Poulos DA, Benjamin RM. Response of thalamic neurons to thermal stimulation of the tongue. *J Neurophysiol* 1968; 31:28–43.

Price DD. *Psychological and Neural Mechanisms of Pain*. New York: Raven Press, 1988.

Price DD. Psychological and neural mechanisms of the affective dimension of pain. *Science* 2000; 288:1769–1772.

Price DD, Barrell JJ, Gracely RH. A psychophysical analysis of experiential factors that selectively influence the affective dimension of pain. *Pain* 1980; 8:137–150.

Price DD, Harkins SW, Baker C. Sensory-affective relationships among different types of clinical and experimental pain. *Pain* 1987; 28:297–307.

Rainville P, Duncan GH, Price DD, Carrier M, Bushnell MC. Pain affect encoded in human anterior cingulate but not somatosensory cortex. *Science* 1997; 277:968–971.

Rees G, Friston K, Koch C. A direct quantitative relationship between the functional properties of human and macaque V5. *Nat Neurosci* 2000; 3:716–723.

Rocamora N, Welker E, Pascual M, Soriano E. Upregulation of BDNF mRNA expression in the barrel cortex of adult mice after sensory stimulation. *J Neurosci* 1996; 16:4411–4419.

Rommel O, Gehling M, Dertwinkel R, et al. Hemisensory impairment in patients with complex regional pain syndrome. *Pain* 1999; 80:95–101.

Rose JE, Mountcastle VB. Activity of single neurons in the tactile thalamic region of the cat in response to a transient peripheral stimulus. *Bull Johns Hopkins Hosp* 1954; 94:238–282.

Rowbotham MC. Complex regional pain syndrome type I (reflex sympathetic dystrophy): more than a myth. *Neurology* 1998; 51:4–5.

Roy CS, Sherrington CS. On the regulation of the blood-supply of the brain. *J Physiol (Lond)* 1890; 11:85–108.

Roy J-C, Bing Z, Villanueva L, Le Bars D. Convergence of visceral and somatic inputs onto subnucleus reticularis dorsalis neurones in the rat medulla. *J Physiol* 1992; 458:235–246.

Ruda MA, Bennett GJ, Dubner R. Neurochemistry and neural circuitry in the dorsal horn. *Prog Brain Res* 1986; 66:219–268.

Sadzot B, Franck G. Non-invasive methods to study drug disposition: positron emission tomography. Detection and quantification of brain receptors in man. *Eur J Drug Metab Pharmacokinet* 1990; 15:135–142.

Saper CB. Convergence of autonomic and limbic connections in the insular cortex of the rat. *J Comp Neurol* 1982; 210:163–173.

Saper CB, Loewy AD, Swanson LW, Cowan WM. Direct hypothalamic-autonomic connections. *Brain Res* 1976; 117:305.

Sato J, Perl ER. Adrenergic excitation of cutaneous pain receptors induced by peripheral nerve injury. *Science* 1991; 251:1608–1610.

Schott GD. Pain in Parkinson's disease. *Pain* 1985; 22:407–411.

Schott GD. Mechanisms of causalgia and related clinical conditions: the role of the central and of the sympathetic nervous systems. *Brain* 1986; 109:717–738.

Schott GD. Visceral afferents: their contribution to sympathetic dependent pain. *Brain* 1994; 117:397–413.

Schott GD. From thalamic syndrome to central poststroke pain. *J Neurol Neurosurg Psychiatry* 1996; 61:560–564.

Schouenborg J, Weng H-R, Holmberg H. Modular organization of spinal nociceptive reflexes: a new hypothesis. *News Physiol Sci* 1994; 9:261–266.

Schwartz WJ, Smith CB, Davidsen L. Metabolic mapping of functional activity in the hypothalamo-neurohypophysial system of the rat. *Science* 1979; 205:723–725.

Segundo JP. Somatic sensory properties of bulbar reticular neurons. *J Neurophysiol* 1967; 30:1221–1221.

Shi CJ, Davis M. Pain pathways involved in fear conditioning measured with fear-potentiated startle: lesion studies. *J Neurosci* 1999; 19:420–430.

Sieweke N, Birklein F, Riedl B, Neundörfer B, Handwerker HO. Patterns of hyperalgesia in complex regional pain syndrome. *Pain* 1999; 80:171–177.

Simone DA, Hanson ME, Bernau NA, Pubols BH Jr. Nociceptive neurons of the raccoon lateral thalamus. *J Neurophysiol* 1993; 69:318–328.

Sluka KA, Dougherty PM, Sorkin LS, Willis WD, Westlund KN. Neural changes in acute arthritis in monkeys. III. Changes in substance P, calcitonin gene-related peptide and glutamate in the dorsal horn of the spinal cord. *Brain Res Rev* 1992; 17:29–38.

Sluka KA, Jordan HH, Willis WD, Westlund KN. Differential effects of *N*-methyl-D-aspartate (NMDA) and non-NMDA receptor antagonists on spinal release of amino acids after development of acute arthritis in rats. *Brain Res* 1994; 664:77–84.

Sokoloff L. Relationship between functional activity and energy metabolism in the nervous system: whether, where and why? In: Lassen NA, Ingvar DH, Raichle ME, Friberg L (Eds). *Brain Work and Mental Activity*, Vol. 31. Copenhagen: Munksgaard, 1991, pp 52–64.

Spanos NP, Perlini AH, Robertson LA. Hypnosis, suggestion, and placebo in the reduction of experimental pain. *J Abnorm Psychol* 1989; 98:285–293.

Staats P, Hekmat H, Staats A. Suggestion/placebo effects on pain: negative as well as positive. *J Pain Symptom Manage* 1998; 15:235–243.

Swanson LW. Mapping the human brain: past, present, and future. *Trends Neurosci* 1995; 18:471–474.

Todd AJ, Spike RC. The localization of classical transmitters and neuropeptides within neurons in laminae I-III of the mammalian spinal dorsal horn. *Prog Neurobiol* 1993; 41:609–638.

Tommerdahl M, Delemos KA, Vierck CJ Jr, Favorov OV. Whitsel BL. Anterior parietal cortical response to tactile and skin-heating stimuli applied to the same skin site. *J Neurophysiol* 1996; 75:2662–2670.

Towe AL. Pyramidal tract fiber spectrum in rats, with comments on cat and man. *J Brain Res* 1995; 36:393–398.

Tsubokawa T, Katayama Y, Yamamoto T, Hirayama T, Koyama S. Chronic motor cortex stimulation in patients with thalamic pain. *J Neurosurg* 1993; 78:393–401.

Turner JA, Deyo RA, Loeser JD, Von Korff M, Fordyce WE. The importance of placebo effects in pain treatment and research. *JAMA* 1994; 271:1609–1614.

Vaccarino AL, Marek P, Liebeskind JC. Stress-induced analgesia prevents the development of the tonic, late phase of pain produced by subcutaneous formalin. *Brain Res* 1992; 572:250–252.

Valentino RJ, Curtis AL. Pharmacology of locus coeruleus spontaneous and sensory-evoked activity. *Prog Brain Res* 1991; 88:249–256.

van der Laan L, ter Laak HJ, Gabreels-Festen A, Gabreels F, Goris RJA. Complex regional pain syndrome type I (RSD): pathology of skeletal muscle and peripheral nerve. *Neurology* 1998; 51:20–25.

Verdugo RJ, Ochoa JL. 'Sympathetically maintained pain.' I. Phentolamine block questions the concept. *Neurology* 1994; 44:1003–1010.

Verdugo RJ, Campero M, Ochoa JL. Phentolamine sympathetic block in painful polyneuropathies. II. Further questioning of the concept of sympathetically maintained pain. *Neurology* 1994; 44:1010–1014.

Wang G, Tanaka K, Tanifuji M. Optical imaging of functional organization in the monkey inferotemporal cortex. *Science* 1996; 272:1665–1668.

Watkins LR, Wiertelak EP, Maier SF. The amygdala is necessary for the expression of conditioned but not unconditioned analgesia. *Behav Neurosci* 1993; 107:402–405.

Willer JC. Stress-induced analgesia in humans: endogenous opioids and naloxone-reversible depression of pain reflexes. *Science* 1981; 212:689–690.

Willis WD, Coggeshall RE. *Sensory Mechanisms of the Spinal Cord.* New York: Plenum, 1978, p 485.

Willis WD, Westlund KN. Neuroanatomy of the pain system and of the pathways that modulate pain. *J Clin Neurophysiol* 1997; 14:2–31.

Woolf CJ, Costigan M. Transcriptional and posttranslational plasticity and the generation of inflammatory pain. *Proc Natl Acad Sci USA* 1999; 96:7723–7730.

Woolf CJ, Salter MW. Neuronal plasticity: increasing the gain in pain. *Science* 2000; 288:1765–1768.

Woolf CJ, Shortland P, Coggeshall RE. Peripheral nerve injury triggers central sprouting of myelinated afferents. *Nature* 1992; 355:75–78.

Yaksh TL. Pharmacology and mechanisms of opioid analgesic activity. *Acta Anaesthesiol Scand* 1997; 41:94–111.

Yaksh TL, Hammond DL. Peripheral and central substrates involved in the rostrad transmission of nociceptive information. *Pain* 1982; 13:1–86.

Yamada K, Nabeshima T. Stress-induced behavioral responses and multiple opioid systems in the brain. *Behav Brain Res* 1995; 67:133–145.

Yezierski RP, Gerhart KD, Schrock BJ, Willis WD. A further examination of effects of cortical stimulation on primate spinothalamic tract cells. *J Neurophysiol* 1983; 49:424–441.

Yu XH, Zhang ET, Craig AD, et al. NK-1 receptor immunoreactivity in distinct morphological types of lamina I neurons of the primate spinal cord. *J Neurosci* 1999; 19:3545–3555.

Yuan B, Morrow TJ, Casey KL. Responsiveness of ventrobasal thalamic neurons after suppression of S1 cortex in the anesthetized rat. *J Neurosci* 1985; 5:2971–2978.

Yuan B, Morrow TJ, Casey KL. Corticofugal influences of S1 cortex on ventrobasal thalamic neurons in the awake rat. *J Neurosci* 1986; 6:3611–3617.

Zhang D, Owens CM, Willis WD. Short-latency excitatory postsynaptic potentials are evoked in primate spinothalamic tract neurons by corticospinal tract volleys. *Pain* 1991; 45:197–201.

Zhang YQ, Tang JS, Yuan B. Inhibitory effects of electrical stimulation of thalamic nucleus submedius on the nociceptive responses of spinal dorsal horn neurons in the rat. *Brain Res* 1996; 737:16–24.

Correspondence to: Kenneth L. Casey, MD, Neurology Service, Veterans Affairs Medical Center, 2215 Fuller Rd, Ann Arbor, MI 48105, USA. Tel: 734-761-7562; Fax: 734-769-7035; email: kencasey@umich.edu.

Pain Imaging, Progress in Pain Research and Management, Vol. 18, edited by Kenneth L. Casey and M. Catherine Bushnell, IASP Press, Seattle, © 2000.

2

Synaptic Activity and Regional Blood Flow: Physiology and Metabolism

Ute Lindauer and Ulrich Dirnagl

Department of Experimental Neurology, Charité Hospital, Berlin, Germany

Modern functional brain-imaging techniques such as functional magnetic resonance imaging (fMRI), optical imaging spectroscopy, positron emission tomography (PET), and near-infrared spectroscopy (NIRS) allow us to visualize the working of the human or animal brain. However, these techniques do not directly measure neuronal and glial activity, but show associated changes in regional blood flow, blood oxygenation, or energy metabolism. The concept of a close spatial and temporal correlation between neuronal and glial activity, metabolic activity, and blood flow was introduced by Roy and Sherrington (1890). This intricate relationship is known as neurometabolic and neurovascular coupling (Fig. 1). An understanding of the physiology of neurometabolic and neurovascular coupling is essential if we are to take full advantage of the potential of modern functional brain imaging, which uses vascular responses to map brain activity. Any pathological disturbance of neurovascular coupling may contribute to tissue damage in the central nervous system (CNS). A thorough elucidation of the physiology and pathophysiology of neurometabolic and neurovascular coupling may facilitate the development of treatment strategies in acute and chronic CNS disorders.

NEUROMETABOLIC COUPLING

In the brain, approximately 10% of the glucose content of arterial blood is transported into the tissue. During functional activation, the glucose concentration of brain tissue decreases by 10–30% (Ueki et al. 1988; Merboldt et al. 1992; Silver and Erecinska 1994; Chen et al. 1994), and then may increase by about the same magnitude (Silver and Erecinska 1994). The cerebral metabolic rate of glucose (CMRglc) increases in parallel with regional

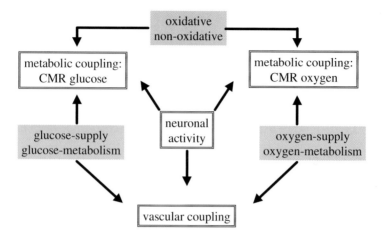

Fig. 1. Neurometabolic and neurovascular coupling: the relationship between neuronal activity, neuronal and glial energy metabolism, and brain vasculature, which is influenced by substrate supply and substrate metabolism and by type of metabolism (oxidative or nonoxidative). CMR = cerebral metabolic rate.

cerebral blood flow (rCBF) during increased neuronal and glial activity (Fox and Raichle 1986). Several energy-consuming neurochemical processes occur during the information transfer from neurons to other neurons and astrocytes: action potentials, neurotransmitter release and re-uptake, and the pre- and postsynaptic activity of excitatory and inhibitory neurons, recorded as somatosensory evoked potentials (Fig. 2). Within these processes, the uptake of the main excitatory and inhibitory neurotransmitters glutamate and γ-aminobutyric acid (GABA) by astrocytes at the synaptic cleft, followed by recycling in neurons, has recently been thoroughly investigated. The release of glutamate by neurons, the re-uptake and glutamate conversion to glutamine by astrocytes, and finally the release, re-uptake, and conversion of glutamine back to glutamate in neurons consume 80–90% of oxidized glucose (Magistretti and Pellerin 1996; Shen et al. 1999). One molecule of glucose is consumed for each glutamate molecule, which is recycled in the glutamate/glutamine cycle (Magistretti et al. 1999). Therefore, nearly all glucose metabolized in brain tissue is used for synaptic activity and for the processing of the two major neurotransmitters. Both excitatory and inhibitory synaptic activity consume energy and are accompanied by increased metabolic activity, which lends complexity to the term "brain activation."

Changes in local blood flow associated with increased neuronal activity closely match fluctuations in local glucose supply, which in turn matches local adenosine triphosphate (ATP) demand. The brain's high rate of aerobic metabolism at rest and its respiratory quotient of 1 indicate that carbo-

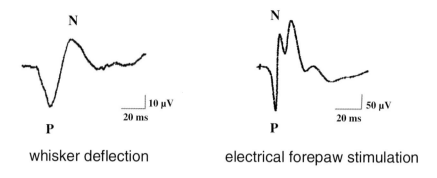

whisker deflection   electrical forepaw stimulation

Fig. 2. Somatosensory evoked potentials: recording of functional activation (action potentials, pre- and postsynaptic activity of excitatory and inhibitory neurons) during whisker deflection (30 s, 3 Hz) or electrical forepaw stimulation (30 s, 3 Hz) in the rat. Reprinted from Lindauer et al. (1996), with permission from Elsevier Science.

hydrates are the substrate of oxidative metabolism. However, some investigators have questioned whether oxidative metabolism is the only form of metabolism in the brain during increased neuronal activity (Fox and Raichle 1986; Hoge et al. 1999). Calculations of the cerebral metabolic rate of oxygen ($CMRO_2$) compared to CMRglc indicate that glycolysis, the nonoxidative metabolism of glucose, may occur during high levels of neuronal activity (Fox and Raichle 1986; Fox et al. 1988; Woolsey et al. 1996; Davis et al. 1998; Mandeville et al. 1999).

NEUROVASCULAR COUPLING

Regional cerebral blood flow is spatially as well as temporally coupled to brain activity. During increased neuronal activity, rCBF increases within the first 2–3 seconds, reaching a peak response after 5–6 seconds, followed by a plateau somewhat lower than the peak response until the end of stimulation, as shown for the somatosensory stimulation of the whisker system in rats (Fig. 3A; Lindauer et al. 1993).

The rCBF response to functional activation of brain tissue induces changes in hemoglobin oxygenation. During neurovascular coupling, oxygen supply to activated brain areas increases and a hyperoxygenation occurs, such that deoxygenated hemoglobin decreases and oxygenated hemoglobin increases (Villringer et al. 1993; Malonek and Grinvald 1996; Malonek et al. 1997). This increased blood oxygenation may be interpreted as a diffusion limitation of oxygen (Buxton and Frank 1997; Buxton et al. 1998), and was postulated by Gjedde et al. (1991) to limit the rate of oxidative phosphorylation in the brain.

A Cerebral blood flow changes

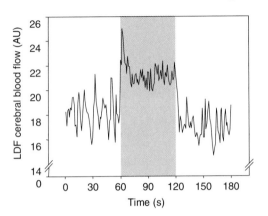

B Hemoglobin oxygenation changes

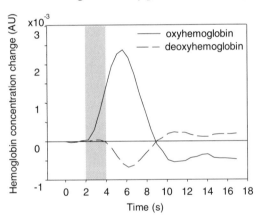

Fig. 3. (A) Vascular coupling: cerebral blood flow (CBF) changes during whisker deflection (60 s, 3 Hz) in the rat, measured with laser Doppler flowmetry (LDF). A significant increase (~17%) in regional CBF occurs during the whole stimulation period. (B) Vascular coupling: hemoglobin oxygenation changes during whisker deflection (2 s, 3 Hz) in the rat using optical imaging spectroscopy. A hyperoxygenation occurs, characterized by an increase in oxygenated hemoglobin and a decrease in deoxygenated hemoglobin. AU = arbitrary units.

Recently, a controversy has developed as to whether the rise in blood oxygenation during activation may be preceded by a very early and transient increase in deoxygenated hemoglobin. Evidence for this oxygenation "dip" was recently derived from reflectance changes at the exposed cortical surface at wavelengths sensitive to hemoglobin oxygenation during activation (Malonek and Grinvald 1996; Malonek et al. 1997; Mayhew et al. 1999).

However, these findings were not confirmed in the whisker system in rats when we used an improved algorithm for the deconvolution of the spectra (Lindauer et al. 1999a; Fig. 3B). Studies using different magnetic resonance approaches also show discrepant results concerning the supposed oxygenation dip (Ernst and Hennig 1994; Menon et al. 1995; Hu et al. 1997; Fransson et al. 1998; Marota et al. 1999; Logothetis et al. 1999; Kim et al. 2000; Silva et al. 2000). The inconsistent findings may be due to the limitations of fMRI technology, as blood-oxygenation-level-dependent (BOLD) measurements on the order of 0.5–1.5 T may be insufficiently sensitive to such small deoxyhemoglobin concentration changes in the cerebral microcirculation. Other explanations must be considered, such as species differences, morphological and functional variations in activated brain areas, and inconsistency of stimulation paradigms (single-condition mapping versus differential mapping; Grinvald et al. 2000). In addition, an early deoxygenation may be masked by the rapid and prominent hyperoxygenation caused by the blood flow response in healthy and well-oxygenated tissue, and perhaps the early dip can only be detected when the rCBF response is delayed or reduced. Further research is needed to resolve this issue.

After more than a century of research (since Roy and Sherrington 1890), we still do not fully understand the physiology of the rCBF response to increased cerebral activity. Vascular coupling provides a constant glucose and oxygen supply to the activated brain tissue, but removal of tissue metabolites such as lactate may be the driving force for vasodilation. In addition, it remains unclear which signal initiates the very early blood flow response, and which factors or mechanisms mediate the sustained increase in rCBF during increased neuronal activity.

WHAT ARE THE MEDIATORS OF NEUROVASCULAR COUPLING?

Since the publication of Roy and Sherrington (1890), it has been generally accepted that vasodilator products accumulate during increased neuronal activity. These metabolites are thought to diffuse to the blood vessels, which then dilate to increase local CBF. The chemical mediators that have received the most intense attention are CO_2 and H^+ (Lassen 1968), K^+ (Kuschinsky et al. 1972; Paulson and Newman 1987), and adenosine (Rubio et al. 1975; Dirnagl et al. 1994). However, changes in the extracellular concentration of the two most thoroughly investigated ions, H^+ and K^+, apparently are not solely responsible for cerebrovascular coupling (Iadecola and Kraig 1991; Caesar et al. 1999). In addition, rCBF increases may exceed metabolic demands (as described above) and may change independently of energy metabolism (Vaucher et al. 1997a). Furthermore, the temporal resolution of the blood flow response may be too high (Lindauer et al. 1993) for the accumulation of metabolic end-products to induce vasodilation. Recently, several investigators have suggested that neurogenic mechanisms may account for the CBF increase during brain activation (Lou et al. 1987; Cohen et al. 1995, 1997; Krimer et al. 1998; Elhusseiny and Hamel 2000). The role of perivascular nerve endings in the control of the cerebrovasculature may have been underestimated for decades (Sandor 1999).

Several reviews have discussed the issue of mechanisms and chemical factors mediating the rCBF increase induced by cerebral activity (Goldman and Sapirstein 1973; Heistad and Kontos 1983; Lou et al. 1987; Iadecola 1993; Wahl and Schilling 1993; Siesjö 1994; Iadecola et al. 1994a; Villringer and Dirnagl 1995). Below we present a brief review, with special reference to new findings.

PROTONS

Recent evidence points to a transient increase in the tissue lactate concentration during neuronal activation (Ueki et al. 1988; Prichard et al. 1991; Fellows et al. 1993), reviving interest in the "oldest" of the chemical mediators. However, direct measurements of extracellular pH under physiological stimulation conditions are lacking. Decreases in the extracellular pH are to be expected as soon as lactate increases in brain tissue. Direct electrical stimulation of the cortical surface produces a slow acidification in the extracellular space of 0.2 pH units within 15 seconds of stimulation onset (Chesler and Kraig 1987). An extracellular pH change of this magnitude can increase CBF locally by about 20% (Niwa et al. 1993). However, the time course of the pH decrease due to such nonphysiological stimulation does not fit the time course of the rCBF response during physiological neuronal stimulation. In addition, the tissue acidosis observed during activation has been described as transient (Chesler and Kraig 1987). It is unlikely that the entire response can be explained by changes in pH because rCBF remains elevated during sustained activation. To resolve this issue, direct measurements of interstitial pH during neuronal activation, together with rCBF measurements, are needed to determine whether extracellular acidosis occurs and whether it could induce activity-dependent rCBF increases.

ADENOSINE AND ADENOSINE TRIPHOSPHATE

The "adenosine hypothesis" (Rubio et al. 1975) of metabolic coupling has been discussed for decades. A mismatch between energy and/or oxygen consumption and substrate delivery by a rise in tissue metabolism during neuronal stimulation would increase dephosphorylation of the energy-rich adenosine nucleotides. The resulting rise in adenosine concentrations within the cells and in the extracellular space would trigger adenosine-receptor-mediated vasodilatation. Specific blockade of adenosine receptors attenuates the blood flow responses to sensory stimulation (Ko et al. 1990; Dirnagl et al. 1994). However, it seems unlikely that a significant mismatch between energy metabolism and substrate delivery occurs during functional activation. Adenosine receptors are widely distributed in the CNS (Goodman and Snyder 1982) and can be found on neurons, astrocytes, and microvascular endothelial cells (Edvinsson and Fredholm 1983; Hösli et al. 1987). Such wide distribution points to a basic role of adenosine in physiological neurotransmission, so it is likely that adenosine has functions beyond being the end-product of energy-rich phosphate breakdown. Adenosine may be released in a transmitter/modulator fashion from neurons or astrocytes upon stimulation. However, the mechanisms of this process are not well characterized, and microdialysis studies in the sensory-motor cortex have yielded negative results during sciatic nerve stimulation (Northington et al. 1992). However, the latter findings may reflect the low spatial and temporal resolution of the method and the rapid biological turnover of adenosine.

ATP released by red blood cells during hypoxia has recently been implicated in the regulation of rCBF (Dietrich et al. 2000). Even small decreases in tissue oxygen concentration increase ATP release from erythrocytes (Ellsworth et al. 1995; Sprague et al. 1996; Dietrich et al. 2000). The released ATP may then diffuse to the vascular endothelium and bind to its receptors, resulting in vasodilation (Kelm et al. 1988). However, this mechanism would require a decrease in oxygen tension in the vascular environment during the whole period of increased neuronal activity, which seems unlikely to occur, at least during the period of hyperoxygenation at times of increased rCBF.

POTASSIUM

Potassium has been considered an ideal mediator of activation-dependent coupling for several decades (Kuschinsky et al. 1972). Paulson and Newman (1987) have promoted the K^+-siphoning hypothesis, where K^+ is released by neurons and then taken up by glial cells and transported to their endfeet, where it is released in the proximity of cerebral arterioles. There, K^+ hyperpolarizes smooth muscle cells. Finally, it is cleared from the brain via the increased blood flow. This hypothesis is based on computer simulations and on measurements of K^+ concentrations in retinal and hippocampal tissue (Paulson and Newman 1987; Emmi et al. 2000). However, potassium transport in cerebrocortical astrocytes has never been demonstrated experimentally, and so the hypothesis remains unproven. In addition, recent evidence indicates that changes in the extracellular K^+ concentration during increased neuronal activity cannot fully explain activity-dependent increases in CBF (Caesar et al. 1999).

ENERGY SUBSTRATES: OXYGEN/GLUCOSE

Hypoxia leads to vasodilatation, an effect that may be mediated via chemicals such as adenosine, ATP, or unknown endothelium-dependent vasodilators (Close et al. 1994) or may be directly mediated via oxygen-sensitive ion channels (Lopez-Barneo 1996; Lopez-Barneo et al. 1997). Evidence indicates prolonged hyperoxygenation during increased neuronal activity, so it is unlikely that local hypoxia is sustained during the period of activation. Local hypoxia may, however, occur at the very early phase of increased neuronal activity, and may provide the initial signal for the CBF response that is mediated by other factors during ongoing functional activation.

As discussed above, the local concentration of glucose decreases during cerebral stimulation. Hypoglycemia increases rCBF (Duckrow et al. 1985; Knudsen et al. 1992). However, after prolonged stimulation (>30 minutes), the local glucose concentration in the activated brain area returns to normal (Chen et al. 1994), whereas rCBF remains elevated. In addition, excessive glucose supply does not change the rCBF response to somatosensory stimulation in rats (Wolf et al. 1997). Therefore, we believe that hypoglycemia is not likely to be a relevant signal for the activation-dependent rise in rCBF.

NITRIC OXIDE

The bioradical nitric oxide (NO), a highly diffusible vasodilator, is widely agreed to be involved in the regulation of rCBF (Goadsby et al. 1992; Dirnagl et al. 1993; Irikura et al. 1994; Akgoeren et al. 1994). In fact, NO might be regarded as the ideal mediator for coupling, because (1) it is a potent vasodilator that is continually released from the cerebral endothelium and from neurons containing nitric oxide synthase (NOS), and as such provides a basal vasodilator tone; (2) it is produced locally by neurons and/or astrocytes via a glutamate-receptor-mediated mechanism; and (3) it is diffusible and has a short half-life (for review see Iadecola 1993). However, blockade of NOS, the enzyme responsible for producing NO, does not fully abolish the response to increased neuronal activity (Dirnagl et al. 1993; Irikura et al. 1994). Local application of NO donors or cyclic guanosine monophosphate (GMP) during NOS inhibition is capable of restoring the cortical rCBF response to somatosensory stimulation (Lindauer et al. 1999b) and to hypercapnia (Iadecola et al. 1994b) as well as the hyperperfusion due to increased extracellular potassium and cortical spreading depression (Dreier et al. 1995a,b). Stamler and colleagues (1997) suggested another mechanism by which NO could mediate neurovascular coupling, proposing that hemoglobin within erythrocytes binds and transports NO, which is co-released when oxygen is liberated in the microvasculature. Although substantial chemical evidence supports the ability of hemoglobin to bind and release NO together with oxygen, the experimental proof for its role in neurovascular coupling in vivo is still lacking.

In the cerebral cortex, NO acts as a modulator rather than as a mediator of vascular relaxation, i.e., it allows other agents to mediate vasodilation. Further experiments are needed to elucidate the nature of these mediators, which may include parenchymal factors such as potassium, protons, and adenosine. It seems unlikely that there is *one* major mediator of coupling. Rather, many different molecules that are produced by increased neuronal and glial metabolism are likely to interact and produce local vasodilatation in the cerebral cortex.

In contrast with findings within the cerebral cortex, in a cerebellar model of neurovascular coupling NO was shown convincingly to be a classical mediator of stimulation-induced vasodilation. The glutamate-receptor-mediated local vasodilation in the cerebellum can be attenuated by NOS inhibition and is not restored by NO donors or by cyclic GMP (Akgoeren et al. 1996; Yang and Iadecola 1997). NOS activity in the cerebral somatosensory cortex is significantly lower than in the cerebellum. Thus, profound neurochemical, neuroanatomical, and functional differences are possible between different stimulation paradigms in different brain regions. Differences in NOS levels may also account for discrepant findings concerning the role of NO in neurovascular coupling (Cholet et al. 1997). Taken together, the studies by Akgören et al. (1996), Yang and Iadecola (1997), and Lindauer et al. (1999b) suggest marked, region-specific differences in basic vascular functions of the brain.

ARACHIDONIC ACID METABOLITES

Arachidonic acid (AA) is synthesized by phospholipase A_2 from membrane phospholipids in a calcium-dependent fashion. AA is then metabolized via cyclooxygenases (COXs) to a number of prostaglandins with both vasoconstricting and vasodilating properties. Inhibition of the COX-2 isoform of the enzyme or targeted deletion of the COX-2 gene attenuates the blood flow response to somatosensory stimulation in mice (Niwa et al. 2000). COX-2 is constitutively expressed in postsynaptic elements of excitatory neurons. Thus, glutamatergic increases in intracellular calcium and in the phospholipase A_2/COX system may enable vasodilator prostaglandins to couple synaptic activity to cerebral blood flow. Astrocytes also release AA in response to stimulation with glutamate. In addition to COX, astrocytes express cytochrome p450 epoxygenase, which metabolizes AA to highly vasoactive epoxyeicosatrienoic acids (Harder et al. 1998).

NEUROGENIC MECHANISMS

Immunohistochemical and molecular studies have shown that the brain's macro- and microvasculature are innervated by a complex system of intrinsic axons containing acetylcholine, serotonin, norepinephrine, dopamine, nitric oxide, and several peptides (Lou et al. 1987; Cohen et al. 1995, 1997; Vaucher and Hamel 1995; Vaucher et al. 1997b; Krimer et al. 1998; Elhusseiny and Hamel 2000). This dense plexus of nerve fibers is connected to brainstem nuclei and, via interneurons, to local circuits. The interneurons could signal local neuronal activity to the nearby microvasculature, prompting the release of vasodilators from perivascular nerve terminals. Functional receptor subtypes for the relevant neurotransmitters and modulators have recently been identified on endothelial and smooth muscle cells and on perivascular astrocyte endfeet (Cohen et al. 1999; Abounader et al. 1999; Elhusseiny and Hamel 2000). Neurogenic stimuli via perivascular nerve endings may act as rapid initiators to induce and maintain a moment-to-moment dynamic adjustment of rCBF to locally increased neuronal activity. Whereas metabolites can only adjust rCBF post hoc during functional activation, regional neuronal circuits with perivascular connections could regulate rCBF in anticipation of, or in parallel with, metabolic activation.

CONCLUSIONS

The mechanisms of neurovascular coupling are evidently more complex than was previously thought. Strong evidence has shown that neurovascular coupling depends on numerous messenger molecules and on many factors that act in series as well as in parallel, some providing the basis for the vasodilation mediated by other agents. Clearly, drug treatments or pathology could easily disturb a highly complex mechanism such as rCBF regulation. Therefore, to properly interpret functional neuroimaging in health and disease, future research should include studies on the effects of aging, drug intake, and parenchymal and cerebrovascular diseases on the coupling of neuronal activity to rCBF.

ACKNOWLEDGMENTS

U. Lindauer and U. Dirnagl were supported by the Deutsche Forschungs-gemeinschaft, the German Israel Science Foundation, the Hermann and Lilly Schilling Foundation, and the Humboldt University Berlin (HSP III).

REFERENCES

Abounader R, Elhusseiny A, Cohen Z, et al. Expression of neuropeptide Y receptors mRNA and protein in human brain vessels and cerebromicrovascular cells in culture. *J Cereb Blood Flow Metab* 1999; 19:155–163.

Akgoeren N, Fabricius M, Lauritzen M. Importance of nitric oxide for local increases of blood flow in rat cerebellar cortex during electrical stimulation. *Proc Natl Acad Sci USA* 1994; 91:5903–5907.

Akgoeren N, Dalgaard P, Lauritzen M. Cerebral blood flow increases evoked by electrical stimulation of rat cerebellar cortex: relation to excitatory synaptic activity and nitric oxide synthesis. *Brain Res* 1996; 710:204–214.

Buxton RB, Frank LR. A model for the coupling between cerebral blood flow and oxygen metabolism during neural stimulation. *J Cereb Blood Flow Metab* 1997; 17:64–72.

Buxton RB, Wong EC, Frank LR. Dynamics of blood flow and oxygenation changes during brain activation: the balloon model. *Magn Reson Med* 1998; 39:855–864.

Caesar K, Akgoren N, Mathiesen C, Lauritzen M. Modification of activity-dependent increases in cerebellar blood flow by extracellular potassium in anaesthetized rats. *J Physiol (Lond)* 1999; 520(Part 1):281–292.

Chen W, Novotny EJ, Zhu X-H, et al. Localized 1 H NMR measurement of glucose consumption in the human brain during visual stimulation. *Proc Natl Acad Sci USA* 1994; 90:9896–9900.

Chesler M, Kraig RP. Intracellular pH of astrocytes increases rapidly with cortical stimulation. *Am J Physiol* 1987; 253:R666–R670.

Cholet N, Seylaz J, Lacombe P, Bonvento G. Local uncoupling of the cerebrovascular and metabolic responses to somatosensory stimulation after neuronal nitric oxide synthase inhibition. *J Cereb Blood Flow Metab* 1997; 17:1191–1201.

Close LA, Bowman PS, Paul RJ. Reoxygenation-induced relaxation of coronary arteries. A novel endothelium-dependent mechanism. *Circ Res* 1994; 74:870–881.

Cohen Z, Ehret M, Maitre M, Hamel E. Ultrastructural analysis of tryptophan hydroxylase immunoreactive nerve terminals in the rat cerebral cortex and hippocampus: their associations with local blood vessels. *Neuroscience* 1995; 66:555–569.

Cohen Z, Molinatti G, Hamel E. Astroglial and vascular interactions of noradrenaline terminals in the rat cerebral cortex. *J Cereb Blood Flow Metab* 1997; 17:894–904.

Cohen Z, Bouchelet I, Olivier A, et al. Multiple microvascular and astroglial 5-hydroxy-tryptamine receptor subtypes in human brain: molecular and pharmacologic characterization. *J Cereb Blood Flow Metab* 1999; 19:908–917.

Davis TL, Kwong KK, Weisskoff RM, Rosen BR. Calibrated functional MRI: mapping the dynamics of oxidative metabolism. *Proc Natl Acad Sci USA* 1998; 95:1834–1839.

Dietrich HH, Ellsworth ML, Sprague RS, Dacey RGJ. Red blood cell regulation of microvascular tone through adenosine triphosphate. *Am J Physiol Heart Circ Physiol* 2000; 278:H1294–H1298.

Dirnagl U, Lindauer U, Villringer A. Role of nitric oxide in the coupling of cerebral blood flow to neuronal activation in rats. *Neurosci Lett* 1993; 149:43–46.

Dirnagl U, Niwa K, Lindauer U, Villringer A. Coupling of cerebral blood flow to neuronal activation: role of adenosine and nitric oxide. *Am J Physiol* 1994; 267:H296–H301.

Dreier JP, Görner A, Körner K, et al. Nitric oxide modulates the CBF response to spreading depression. *J Cereb Blood Flow Metab* 1995a; 15:S155.

Dreier JP, Körner K, Görner A, et al. Nitric oxide modulates the CBF response to increased extracellular potassium. *J Cereb Blood Flow Metab* 1995b; 14:914–919.

Duckrow RB, Beard DC, Brennan RW. Regional cerebral blood flow decreases during hyperglycemia. *Ann Neurol* 1985; 17:267–272.

Edvinsson L, Fredholm BB. Characterization of adenosine receptors in isolated cerebral arteries of cat. *Br J Pharmacol* 1983; 80:631–637.

Elhusseiny A, Hamel E. Muscarinic—but not nicotinic—acetylcholine receptors mediate a nitric oxide-dependent dilation in brain cortical arterioles: a possible role for the M5 receptor subtype. *J Cereb Blood Flow Metab* 2000; 20:298–305.

Ellsworth ML, Forrester T, Ellis CG, Dietrich HH. The erythrocyte as a regulator of vascular tone. *Am J Physiol* 1995; 269:H2155–H2161.

Emmi A, Wenzel HJ, Schwartzkroin PA, et al. Do glia have heart? Expression and functional role for ether-a-go-go currents in hippocampal astrocytes. *J Neurosci* 2000; 20:3915–3925.

Ernst T, Hennig J. Observation of a fast response in functional MR. *Magn Reson Med* 1994; 32:146–149.

Fellows LK, Boutelle MG, Fillenz M. Physiological stimulation increases nonoxidative glucose metabolism in the brain of the freely moving rat. *J Neurochem* 1993; 60:1258–1263.

Fox PT, Raichle ME. Focal physiological uncoupling of cerebral blood flow and oxidative metabolism during somatosensory stimulation in human subjects. *Proc Natl Acad Sci USA* 1986; 83:1140–1144.

Fox PT, Raichle ME, Mintun MA, Dence C. Nonoxidative glucose consumption during focal physiologic neural activity. *Science* 1988; 241:462–464.

Fransson P, Kruger G, Merboldt KD, Frahm J. Temporal characteristics of oxygenation-sensitive MRI responses to visual activation in humans. *Magn Reson Med* 1998; 39:912–919.

Gjedde A, Ohta S, Kubawara H, Meyer E. Is oxygen diffusion limiting for blood-brain transfer of oxygen? In: Lassen NA, Ingvar DH, Raichle ME, Friberg L (Eds). *Brain Work and Mental Activity*. Alfred Benzon Symposium 31. Copenhagen: Munksgaard, 1991, pp 177–184.

Goadsby PJ, Kraube H, Hoskin KL. Nitric oxide synthesis couples cerebral blood flow and metabolism. *Brain Res* 1992; 595:167–170.

Goldman H, Sapirstein LA. Brain blood flow in the conscious and anesthetized rat. *Am J Physiol* 1973; 224:122–126.

Goodman RR, Snyder SH. Autoradiographic localization of adenosine receptors in rat brain using 3H-cyclohexyladenosine. *J Neurosci* 1982; 2:1230–1241.

Grinvald A, Slovin H, Vanzetta I. Non-invasive visualization of cortical columns by fMRI. *Nat Neurosci* 2000; 3:105–107.

Harder DR, Alkayed NJ, Lange AR, et al. Functional hyperemia in the brain: hypothesis for astrocyte-derived vasodilator metabolites. *Stroke* 1998; 29:229–234.

Heistad DD, Kontos, HA. Cerebral circulation. In: Shepherd JTA (Ed). *The Cardiovascular System* (5). Bethesda, MD: The American Physiological Society, 1983, pp 137–182.

Hoge RD, Atkinson J, Gill B, et al. Linear coupling between cerebral blood flow and oxygen consumption in activated human cortex. *Proc Natl Acad Sci USA* 1999; 96:9403–9408.

Hösli L, Hösli E, Uhr M, Della Briotta G. Electrophysiological evidence for adenosine receptors on astrocytes of cultured rat central nervous system. *Neurosci Lett* 1987; 79:108–112.

Hu X, Le TH, Ugurbil K. Evaluation of the early response in fMRI in individual subjects using short stimulus duration. *Magn Reson Med* 1997; 37:877–884.

Iadecola C. Regulation of the cerebral microcirculation during neural activity: is nitric oxide the missing link? *Trends Neurosci* 1993; 16:206–214.

Iadecola C, Kraig RP. Focal elevations in neocortical interstitial K+ produced by stimulation of the fastigial nucleus in rat. *Brain Res* 1991; 563:273–277.

Iadecola C, Pelligrino DA, Moskowitz MA, Lassen NA. Nitric oxide synthase inhibition and cerebrovascular regulation. *J Cereb Blood Flow Metab* 1994a; 14:175–192.

Iadecola C, Zhang F, Xu X. SIN-1 reverses attenuation of hypercapnic cerebrovasodilation by nitric oxide synthase inhibitors. *Am J Physiol* 1994b; 267:R228–R235.

Irikura K, Maynard KI, Moskowitz MA. The importance of nitric oxide synthase inhibition to the attenuated vascular responses induced by topical l-nitroarginine during vibrissae stimulation. *J Cereb Blood Flow Metab* 1994; 14:45–48.

Kelm M, Feelisch M, Spahr R, et al. Quantitative and kinetic characterization of nitric oxide and EDRF released from cultured endothelial cells. *Biochem Biophys Res Commun* 1988; 154:236–244.

Kim DS, Duong TQ, Kim SG. High-resolution mapping of iso-orientation columns by fMRI. *Nature* 2000; 3:164–169.

Knudsen GM, Tedeschi E, Jakobsen J. The influence of haematocrit and blood glucose on cerebral blood flow in normal and in diabetic rats. *Neuroreport* 1992; 3:987–989.

Ko KR, Ngai AC, Winn HR. Role of adenosine in regulation of regional cerebral blood flow in sensory cortex. *Am J Physiol* 1990; 259:H1703–H1708.

Krimer LS, Muly EC, Williams GV, Goldman-Rakic PS. Dopaminergic regulation of cerebral cortical microcirculation. *Nat Neurosci* 1998; 1:286–289.

Kuschinsky W, Wahl M, Bosse O, Thurau K. Perivascular potassium and pH as determinants of local pial arterial diameter in cats. A microapplication study. *Circ Res* 1972; 31:240–247.

Lassen N. Brain Extracellular pH: the main factor controlling cerebral blood flow. *Scand J Clin Lab Invest* 1968; 22:247–251.

Lindauer U, Villringer A, Dirnagl U. Characterization of CBF response to somatosensory stimulation: model and influence of anesthetics. *Am J Physiol* 1993; 264:H1223–H1228.

Lindauer U, Megow D, Schultze J, Weber JR, Dirnagl U. Nitric oxide synthase inhibition does not affect somatosensory evoked potentials in the rat. *Neurosci Lett* 1996; 216:207–210.

Lindauer U, Kohl M, Royl G, et al. Early deoxygenation ('dip') measured by optical methods during Whisker barrel cortex activation in rats? Use of a modified Lambert-Beer algorithm. *Soc Neurosci Abstr* 1999a, 25:1639.

Lindauer U, Megow D, Matsuda H, Dirnagl U. Nitric oxide: a modulator, but not a mediator, of neurovascular coupling in rat somatosensory cortex. *Am J Physiol* 1999b; 277:H799–H811.

Logothetis NK, Guggenberger H, Peled S, Pauls J. Functional imaging of the monkey brain. *Nat Neurosci* 1999; 2:555–562.

Lopez-Barneo J. Oxygen-sensing by ion channels and the regulation of cellular functions. *Trends Neurosci* 1996; 19:435–440.

Lopez-Barneo J, Ortega-Saenz P, Molina A, et al. Oxygen sensing by ion channels. *Kidney Int* 1997; 51:454–461.

Lou HC, Edvinsson L, MacKenzie ET. The concept of coupling blood flow to brain function: revision required? *Ann Neurol* 1987; 22:289–297.

Magistretti PJ, Pellerin L. Cellular mechanisms of brain energy metabolism. Relevance to functional brain imaging and to neurodegenerative disorders. *Ann NY Acad Sci* 1996; 777:380–387.

Magistretti PJ, Pellerin L, Rothman DL, Shulman RG. Energy on demand. *Science* 1999; 283:496–497.

Malonek D, Grinvald A. Interactions between electrical activity and cortical microcirculation revealed by imaging spectroscopy: implications for functional brain mapping. *Science* 1996; 272:551–554.

Malonek D, Dirnagl U, Lindauer U, et al. Vascular imprints of neuronal activity: relationships between the dynamics of cortical blood flow, oxygenation, and volume changes following sensory stimulation. *Proc Natl Acad Sci USA* 1997; 94:14826–14831.

Mandeville JB, Marota JJ, Ayata C, et al. MRI measurement of the temporal evolution of relative CMRO(2) during rat forepaw stimulation. *Magn Reson Med* 1999; 42:944–951.

Marota JJ, Ayata C, Moskowitz MA, et al. Investigation of the early response to rat forepaw stimulation. *Magn Reson Med* 1999; 41:247–252.

Mayhew J, Zheng Y, Hou Y, et al. Spectroscopic analysis of changes in remitted illumination: the response to increased neural activity in brain. *Neuroimage* 1999; 10:304–326.

Menon RS, Ogawa S, Hu X, et al. BOLD based functional MRI at 4 Tesla includes a capillary bed contribution: echo-planar imaging correlates with previous optical imaging using intrinsic signals. *Magn Reson Med* 1995; 33:453–459.

Merboldt KD, Bruhn H, Hänicke W, et al. Decrease of glucose in the human cerebral visual cortex during photic stimulation. *Magn Reson Med* 1992; 25:187–194.

Niwa K, Lindauer U, Villringer A, Dirnagl U. Blockade of nitric oxide synthesis in rats strongly attenuates the CBF response to extracellular acidosis. *J Cereb Blood Flow Metab* 1993; 13:535–539.

Niwa K, Araki E, Morham SG, et al. Cyclooxygenase-2 contributes to functional hyperemia in whisker-barrel cortex. *J Neurosci* 2000; 20:763–770.

Northington FJ, Matherne GP, Coleman SD, Berne RM. Sciatic nerve stimulation does not increase endogenous adenosine production in sensory-motor cortex. *J Cereb Blood Flow Metab* 1992; 12:835–843.

Paulson OB, Newman EA. Does the release of potassium from astrocyte endfeet regulate cerebral blood flow. *Science* 1987; 237:896–898.

Prichard J, Rothman D, Novotny E, et al. Lactate rise detected by 1H NMR in human visual cortex during physiologic activation. *Proc Natl Acad Sci USA* 1991; 88:5829–5831.

Roy C, Sherrington C. On the regulation of the blood supply of the brain. *J Physiol* 1890; 11:85–108.

Rubio R, Berne RM, Bockman EL, Curnish RR. Relationship between adenosine concentration and oxygen supply in rat brain. *Am J Physiol* 1975; 228:1896–1902.

Sandor P. Nervous control of the cerebrovascular system: doubts and facts. *Neurochem Int* 1999; 35:237–259.

Shen J, Petersen KF, Behar KL, et al. Determination of the rate of the glutamate/glutamine cycle in the human brain by in vivo 13C NMR. *Proc Natl Acad Sci USA* 1999; 96:8235–8240.

Siesjö BK. Cerebral circulation and metabolism. *J Neurosurg* 1994; 60:883–908.

Silva AC, Lee SP, Iadecola C, Kim SG. Early temporal characteristics of cerebral blood flow and deoxyhemoglobin changes during somatosensory stimulation. *J Cereb Blood Flow Metab* 2000; 20:201–206.

Silver I, Erecinska M. Extracellular glucose concentration in mammalian brain: continuous monitoring of changes during increased neuronal activity and upon limitation in oxygen supply in normo-, hypo-, and hyperglycemic animals. *J Neurosci* 1994; 14:5068–5076.

Sprague RS, Ellsworth ML, Stephenson AH, Lonigro AJ. ATP: the red blood cell link to NO and local control of the pulmonary circulation. *Am J Physiol* 1996; 271:H2717–H2722.

Stamler JS, Jia L, Eu JP, et al. Blood flow regulation by S-nitrosohemoglobin in the physiological oxygen gradient. *Science* 1997; 276:2034–2037.

Ueki M, Linn F, Hossmann KA. Functional activation of cerebral blood flow and metabolism before and after global ischemia of rat brain. *J Cereb Blood Flow Metab* 1988; 8:486–494.

Vaucher E, Hamel E. Cholinergic basal forebrain neurons project to cortical microvessels in the rat: electron microscopic study with anterogradely transported *Phaseolus vulgaris* leucoagglutinin and choline acetyltransferase immunocytochemistry. *J Neurosci* 1995; 15:7427–7441.

Vaucher E, Borredon J, Bonvento G, et al. Autoradiographic evidence for flow-metabolism uncoupling during stimulation of the nucleus basalis of Meynert in the conscious rat. *J Cereb Blood Flow Metab* 1997a; 17:686–694.

Vaucher E, Linville D, Hamel E. Cholinergic basal forebrain projections to nitric oxide synthase-containing neurons in the rat cerebral cortex. *Neuroscience* 1997b; 79:827–836.

Villringer A, Dirnagl U. Coupling of brain activity and cerebral blood flow: basis for functional neuroimaging. *Cerebrovasc Brain Metab Rev* 1995; 7:240–276.

Villringer A, Planck J, Hock C, et al. Near infrared spectroscopy (NIRS): a new tool to study hemodynamic changes during activation of brain function in human adults. *Neurosci Lett* 1993; 154:101–104.

Wahl M, Schilling L. Regulation of cerebral blood flow—a brief review. *Acta Neurochir* 1993; 59(Suppl):3–10.

Wolf T, Lindauer U, Villringer A, Dirnagl U. Excessive oxygen or glucose supply does not alter the blood flow response to somatosensory stimulation or spreading depression in rats. *Brain Res* 1997; 761:290–299.

Woolsey TA, Rovainen CM, Cox SB, et al. Neuronal units linked to microvascular modules in cerebral cortex: response elements for imaging the brain. *Cereb Cortex* 1996; 6:647–660.

Yang G, Iadecola C. Obligatory role of NO in glutamate-dependent hyperemia evoked from cerebellar parallel fibers. *Am J Physiol* 1997; 272:R1155–R1161.

Correspondence to: Ute Lindauer, DVM, Department of Experimental Neurology, Humboldt University, Charité Hospital, 10098 Berlin, Germany. Tel: 49-30-2802-5315; Fax: 49-30-2802-8756; email: ute.lindauer@charite.de.

Pain Imaging, Progress in Pain Research and
Management, Vol. 18, edited by Kenneth L.
Casey and M. Catherine Bushnell, IASP Press,
Seattle, © 2000.

3

The S1 Response to Noxious Skin Heating as Revealed by Optical Intrinsic Signal Imaging

Barry L. Whitsel,[a,b] Mark Tommerdahl,[b] Adam Kohn,[a]
Charles J. Vierck, Jr.,[c] and Oleg Favorov[b,d]

*Departments of [a]Cell and Molecular Physiology and [b]Biomedical
Engineering, University of North Carolina,
Chapel Hill, North Carolina, USA; [c]Department of Neuroscience, University
of Florida, Gainesville, Florida, USA; [d]Division of Computer Science,
University of Central Florida, Orlando, Florida, USA*

THE ROLE OF THE S1 CORTEX IN PAIN INFORMATION PROCESSING

THE PATH TO A CONSENSUS

The mechanisms and central neural pathways for pain and its modulation have been studied thoroughly over the last several decades, especially during the last 5–10 years (for review see Willis and Westlund 1997; also Willis 1995a,b). Despite this extensive body of work, remarkably little progress has been made toward understanding the role of the cerebral cortex in pain.

The pioneering single-neuron recording investigations of D.R. Kenshalo, Jr., and his colleagues yielded useful new information (Kenshalo et al. 1980, 1988; Kenshalo and Isensee 1983; for reviews see Mountcastle 1984; Kenshalo and Willis 1991; Roland 1992; Apkarian 1995a,b, 1996; Backonja 1996; Caselli 1996; Kenshalo 1996; Treede et al. 1999). Since 1988, however, the pain mechanisms of the cerebral cortex, and especially primary somatosensory (S1) cortex, have only rarely been studied using cellular neurophysiological approaches. While multiple factors undoubtedly explain why few cellular-level studies of the contributions of the S1 cortex to pain information processing have been conducted in the past decade, perhaps the most compelling reason is that Kenshalo and colleagues' microelectrode recording studies revealed so few nociceptive neurons in the S1 cortex that its role in pain was regarded as uncertain, at best. Indeed, some investigators viewed the apparent scarcity of S1 neurons sensitive to noxious stimulation as confirmation of the old idea (e.g., Head and Holmes 1911; Penfield and Boldrey 1937) that pain has little or no cortical representation. Most, however, continued to adhere to the more positive but minimalist view that the S1 cortex contributes to the clinical pain experience primarily through the localization and discrimination of noxious stimuli (Melzack and Casey 1968; Casey 1999).

Interest in experimental investigation of the role of the S1 cortex in pain was rekindled in the 1990s by newly available brain-imaging methodologies—positron emission tomography (PET), single photon emission computed tomography (SPECT), functional magnetic resonance imaging (fMRI), and magnetoencephalographic imaging (MEG). Unfortunately, concerning the role of the S1 cortex, the human imaging investigations conducted by different research groups have generated inconclusive and even contradictory results. For example, of the 33 studies reviewed by Bushnell and colleagues (1999), 19 (57.6%) reported S1 activation by stimulation reported as painful, while 14 (42.4%) reported that such stimulation did not significantly increase S1 activation or even inhibited S1 activity. This unresolved issue clearly merits further imaging studies, but Bushnell and colleagues interpreted the available evidence to indicate that the S1 cortex usually is activated during the pain experience. They attributed the failure of some studies to detect significant S1 activation during the delivery of painful stimuli either to cognitive factors such as inattention to the stimulus that might decrease the degree of S1 neuronal activity evoked by noxious stimulation, or to data grouping and analysis techniques that might have obscured a localized region of stimulus-evoked activation. Bushnell's team concluded that when these factors are taken into account, the available human brain-imaging findings "support the traditional view that SI is primarily involved in the discriminative aspects of somatic sensation and extend this view to include discriminative aspects of somatic stimulation that is potentially tissue-damaging" (Bushnell et al. 1999).

THE "TRADITIONAL" VIEW

The "traditional" view of the role of the S1 cortex has three major components.

1) The S1 cortex contributes to the sensory-discriminative aspects of nociception: This claim is directly supported by two lines of evidence:

(i) Neurons in cytoarchitectural areas 3b and 1 of the S1 cortex (Kenshalo et al. 1983) and also neurons in the ventrobasal thalamic nuclei that project to areas 3b and 1 (e.g., Kenshalo et al. 1980) have receptive field and response properties consistent with a role in processing of nociceptive information (for a review of the extensive literature on ventrobasal thalamic pain mechanisms, see Kenshalo and Willis 1991). (ii) Lesions of the S1 cortex interfere with subjects' capacity to detect and discriminate nociceptive stimuli (Kenshalo et al. 1989).

2) Regions of the nervous system other than the S1 cortex are responsible for the affective-motivational component of pain. This aspect of the traditional view appears to be based largely on the idea that the properties of S1 neurons are "static" (i.e., stable over time and relatively insensitive to the diverse factors that modify pain tolerance), whereas the activity evoked by a noxious stimulus in other regions of the central nervous system (CNS), such as the anterior cingulate cortex, corresponds to changes in the affective-motivational valence of noxious stimulation (e.g., Rainville et al. 1997).

3) The S1 cortex receives and processes nociceptor afferent drive in a manner parallel to the way in which it receives and processes mechanoreceptor afferent drive. Most investigators believe that the middle layers of areas 3b and 1, the subdivisions of S1 dominated by input from low-threshold cutaneous mechanoreceptors conveyed centrally via the dorsal column–medial lemniscal pathway (Mountcastle 1984), also are the S1 regions whose middle layer pyramidal neurons receive input from the spinothalamic pathways and respond with increased spike discharge activity to stimuli that activate skin nociceptors. Similarly, the S1 regions (areas 3a and 2) dominated by input to the middle layers from the "deep" mechanoreceptors in muscles, joints, and tendons are believed to be the regions in which spike discharge activity from pyramidal neurons increases in response to a stimulus that activates nociceptors in deep somatic tissues.

As this chapter will document, the first and third components of this "traditional" view of S1 in pain information processing are seriously flawed, and the second component may require significant modification.

RECENT NEUROANATOMICAL EVIDENCE

The validity of the traditional view of the role of S1 in pain has recently been called into question. Appreciable evidence has already accumulated to show that many, perhaps all, thalamic nuclei (regardless of their classification as sensory, motor, intralaminar, etc.) contain dual populations of cortically projecting neurons (Rausell and Jones 1991a,b; Rausell et al. 1992; for reviews see Jones 1994, 1998). For example, certain regions of somatosensory thalamus are dominated by input from skin receptors; these regions have been identified as the ventroposterior lateral (VPL) and ventroposterior medial (VPM) nuclei in both cats and monkeys. A population of small-diameter cells project from these regions to the upper layers of an extensive sector of the somatosensory cortex. These small thalamic neurons project principally to layer I, with fewer projections to layer II and almost none below upper layer III. They exhibit immunoreactivity for calbindin (an intracellular Ca^{2+} binding protein) and preferentially occupy a region (the "matrix" region) characterized by weak staining for the mitochondrial enzyme cytochrome oxidase. These small cells receive their major input from ascending brainstem or spinal axons that convey information about the status of skin nociceptors or thermoreceptors. In contrast, the large cells in the same thalamic nuclei project selectively to the middle layers of a restricted set of cell columns in area 3b and/or area 1. These cells exhibit immunoreactivity for a different Ca^{2+} binding protein (parvalbumin), are grouped into clusters ("rods") that stain strongly for cytochrome oxidase, and are completely embedded within the matrix region. They receive their major input from brainstem or spinal cord pathways occupied by the afferents that supply low-threshold, large-diameter skin mechanoreceptive afferents.

The ascending neural drive evoked by *non-noxious mechanical* skin stimulation activates a population of ventrobasal thalamic neurons that project to the middle layers of S1, and a second ventrobasal neuron population projects to the upper layers of S1 (Penny et al. 1982). A similar dual projection to S1 for the activity evoked by *noxious thermal* stimulation of a discrete skin site has recently been established. For example, in addition to their projection to the matrix region of the contralateral somatosensory thalamus and thence to the upper layers of S1, the axons of thermonociceptive dorsal horn neurons of lamina I also terminate synaptically in another small-celled, calbindin-positive region of the thalamus (Craig and Kniffki 1985; Craig 1991, 1995, 1996; Craig et al. 1994). This region has been identified as the ventromedial posterior nucleus (VMpo) in the monkey and the paralamellar ventrobasal nucleus (VB_{pl}) in the cat. Craig's team also demonstrated that VMpo or VB_{pl} nuclei not only project to neural targets such as the insular and anterior cingulate cortex, shown by human imaging studies to be activated during painful skin stimulation, (Craig et al. 1994, 1995), but also project topographically and selectively to the middle layers of area 3a (Craig and Kniffki 1985; Craig et al. 1995, 1996). An association between nociception and area 3a is supported by Craig and Kniffki's observation (1985) that in cats, the nociresponsive neurons in VB_{pl} that receive direct input from dorsal horn lamina I neurons project to area 3a.

The possibility of a link between area 3a in the S1 cortex and nociception was surprising because this area usually has been regarded as predominantly or exclusively devoted to the processing of information projected centrally by muscle and joint receptors (e.g., see Kaas et al. 1979; Jones and Porter 1980; Sur et al. 1982). However, such a link is consistent with studies of World War I and II patients who sustained localized cortical damage to a region in the depths of the posterior wall of the central sulcus (the position of most of area 3a in both humans and many nonhuman primates) (Kleist 1934; Russell 1945; Marshall 1951). These patients had a prominent and selective loss of cutaneous pain sensibility. Extensive parietal cortex lesions that spared this area caused no such deficits, but frequently caused hyperalgesia. Thus, these early clinical investigators suggested that activity of the areas posterior to area 3a (e.g., areas 3b, 1, and 2) inhibits area 3a. This early clinical literature has been comprehensively reviewed by Perl (1984) and more recently by Kenshalo and Willis (1991). Behavioral observations in monkeys also are compatible with a role for area 3a in pain. For example, Kenshalo et al. (1989) reported that after bilateral ablation of an extensive anterior parietal region that included area 3a (as well as areas 3b, 1, and 2), monkeys exhibited clear deficits in both the detection and discrimination of noxious thermal skin stimuli. Previously, Peele (1944) reported that 1 year following a large lesion involving areas 1, 2, 5, and 7 (thus sparing area 3a), he detected a hypersensitivity to pinprick suggestive of hyperalgesia.

AN INTRIGUING POSSIBILITY

The recent neuroanatomical literature described in the preceding section raises the possibility that S1 cortex responds differentially to noxious and non-noxious stimulation of the same skin site (i.e., the former activates area 3a, but the latter activates areas 3b and 1). This possibility is intriguing, as it would not only support the early clinical investigators' proposal that an anterior region in S1 (presumably area 3a) plays a leading role in pain processing, but would also explain the otherwise puzzling findings that relatively few middle-layer neurons in areas 3b and 1 receive selective input from skin nociceptors (Kenshalo et al. 1983), and that VPL and VPM thalamic nuclei contain a substantial number of nociceptive neurons (Kenshalo and Willis 1980, 1991; Bruggeman et al. 1997) that project to layers I–II of area 3b and/or area 1 (Rausell and Jones 1991a,b, 1992; Shi et al. 1993; Bruggeman et al. 1994). We decided that an efficient and direct way to evaluate this possibility would be to record the optical intrinsic response (OIS) of the S1 cortex to input drive evoked by natural skin stimuli.

Our findings using the OIS imaging method, both alone and in combination with neurophysiological recordings, suggest alternatives to the traditional view of the S1 cortex. Below we will suggest new interpretations of (1) the S1 response to the ascending afferent drive attributable to stimulus-evoked activation of cutaneous nociceptors, (2) the perceptual consequences of the S1 response to noxious skin stimulation, and (3) the connectional and cellular mechanisms that govern the S1 response to such stimulation.

BENCHMARKING THE OIS IMAGING METHOD

This section describes experimental findings obtained in "benchmarking" experiments conducted to obtain information that would allow mechanistic interpretation (explanation in terms of the responsible neural mechanisms) of the optical responses evoked in S1 by noxious stimulation of the skin.

IN VIVO STUDIES

Properties of the stimulus-evoked S1 intrinsic response. The sources of the optical intrinsic signal (OIS) recorded in vivo using near-infrared (near-IR) illumination are not completely understood, but this signal can plausibly can be regarded as a reflection ("trace") of a temporally delayed, cumulative process set up in the somatosensory cortex by the recent history of stimulation (Whitsel et al. 1989, 1991). In marked contrast to the signals detectable at shorter wavelengths (e.g., 650 nm), the intrinsic response recorded using near-IR illumination is substantially independent of hemodynamic effects such as cortical blood flow and hemoglobin oxidation state. Therefore, the OIS exhibits essentially the same properties and dynamics in the cortical slice preparation as it does in vivo (Kohn et al. 1997, 1999).

Several attributes of the OIS imaging method make it an effective and extremely efficient means of studying the cerebral cortical response to natural sensory stimulation. Most importantly, the intrinsic response is highly correlated with the spike discharge activity of cortical pyramidal neurons. For example, a stimulus-evoked *increase* in the average absorbance ($\Delta A/A$, a dimensionless quantity that indicates magnitude of optical change)[1] of a cortical region is accompanied by an *increase* in the average rate of spike discharge activity of the neurons that occupy that region (e.g., Grinvald 1985; Grinvald et al. 1991, 1994; Haglund at al. 1993; Tommerdahl and Whitsel 1996; Tommerdahl et al. 1998, 1999a). Conversely, in regions where stimulation leads to a *decrease* in absorbance, single-neuron discharge ac-

---

[1] $\Delta A/A$ is computed by dividing the difference between the prestimulus (reference) image and the poststimulus image by the reference image.

tivity typically *decreases* to a level below that observed in the absence of stimulation (Tommerdahl et al. 1999a). It is of great practical value to be able to obtain many images in the same subject of the intrinsic response of a given cortical region to the same or different stimulus conditions. With the OIS method, images can be acquired at relatively high spatial resolution (50–100 μm; Bonhoeffer and Grinvald 1996), and successive images can be acquired relatively rapidly—for example, our camera (Quantrix, Photometrics, Inc.) can capture three images per second. Importantly, the cortical intrinsic response detected under near-IR illumination is relatively independent of changes in blood flow (Haglund et al. 1993). This response reflects a variety of factors, of which the most significant is an alteration in the volume of the extracellular fluid compartment, presumably due to stimulus-evoked changes in the extracellular potassium concentration or to neurotransmitter release (Cohen 1973; Lieke et al. 1989; MacVicar and Hochman 1991). The increase in cortical absorbance evoked by sensory stimulation must reflect excitatory synaptic activity because it is attenuated dose-dependently by drugs that block glutamate receptors (MacVicar and Hochman 1991; Haglund et al. 1993). It derives mainly from the dendrites of cortical pyramidal neurons (Grinvald et al. 1994). Finally, the increase in cortical absorbance is not a "one-to-one" reflection of the stimulus-evoked elevation of neuronal spike discharge activity. We can assume that the increased absorbance does not result from the local cortical voltage change evoked by a sensory stimulus because of the much slower onset and decay of the absorbance increase compared with the neuroelectrical responses of single neurons or neuronal populations. Also, the increase in cortical absorbance is severely attenuated or even eliminated by drugs that exert relatively minor effects on the spike discharge activity of sensory cortical neurons that is evoked by direct, short-latency thalamocortical drive. Such drugs include selective NMDA-receptor blockers (Hagiwara et al. 1998; Armstrong-James 1995; Salt et al. 1995; Tommerdahl and Whitsel 1996; Kohn et al. 1997; Whitsel et al. 1999a) and selective blockers of astroglial potassium exchange, such as furosemide (MacVicar and Hochman 1991; Holthoff and Witte 1996).

Within-subject and between-subject variability; relationship to S1 topographical organization. Several additional properties of the OIS imaging method justify its use as a population-level neuroimaging tool. First, the method is *reliable,* in the sense that it generates imaging results that are highly repeatable both *within* and *between* subjects (Tommerdahl et al. 1999a; see Figs. 1 and 2). In fact, the within-subject reproducibility extends even to the single-trial level. Second, the method appears physiologically *valid,* in the sense that it yields results in substantial agreement with neurophysiological expectations and with the results delivered by other independent

Trials Averages Single Trials

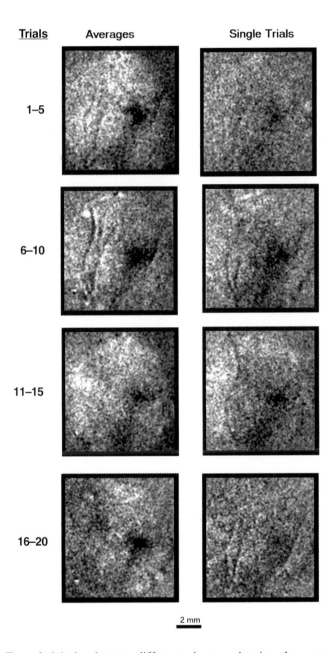

1–5

6–10

11–15

16–20

2 mm

Fig. 1. Top of right-hand page: difference images showing the average response evoked by 20 vibrotactile stimuli to the radial interdigital pad on the hand, with a stimulus duration of 8 seconds. The Run 2 response was obtained 1 hour after the Run 1 response. Images below the Run 1 and 2 responses show the surface vascular pattern (left) and locations of cytoarchitectonic boundaries (right; black region shows the locus of the absorbance increase in Run 1). Left-hand page: The column of images on the far

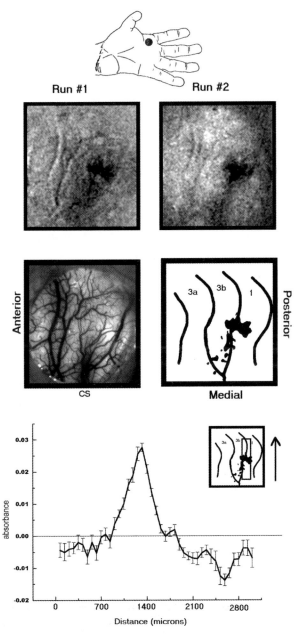

left ("Averages") demonstrates that the locus of the optical intrinsic signal (OIS) is reproducible even when an image is generated from the responses to few stimulus presentations. Each image in the left column was obtained by averaging the data from five successive stimuli. Good reproducibility of the OIS is evident, even for images generated from the data obtained during a single stimulus (column labeled "Single Trials"). *(Legend continues on next page.)*

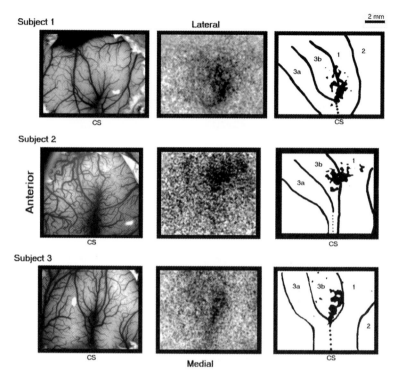

Fig. 2. Left-hand page: S1 responses to stimulation of the radial interdigital pad in three squirrel monkeys. Note that the locus of response is consistently at the area 3b/1 boundary. Right-hand page: responses to stimulation of the volar tip of the second digit in three subjects. This response consistently takes place at the boundary between area 3b and 3a. Both response locations are in accord with maps of squirrel monkey topographical organization provided by neurophysiological receptive-field-mapping studies. CS = central sulcus. From Tommerdahl et al. (1999a); reprinted with permission.

(Continued from previous page.) The image at the top was formed from the response to one trial out of trials 1–5, the next from the response to one trial out of trials 6–10, etc. Although trial-by-trial response variation is evident, the single-trial responses are relatively consistent. The plot at the bottom of the right-hand page shows (for the same subject and stimulus) how the magnitude of the stimulus-evoked change in absorbance varies with cortical distance (by convention, a positive *y*-value indicates an increase in absorbance). The vertical rectangle and arrow in inset show the region of the image that was analyzed using linear image segmentation. Note the negative *y*-values on both sides of the centrally located increase in absorbance (at the area 3b/1 boundary). From Tommerdahl et al. (1999a); reprinted with permission.

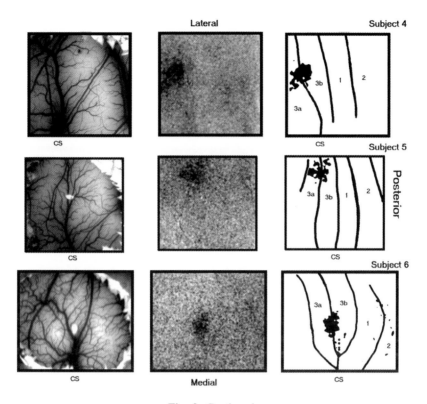

Fig. 2. Continued.

methods. A study using squirrel monkeys showed the clear correspondence between the locus in the anterior parietal cortex of the absorbance increase evoked by a 25-Hz vibrotactile stimulus and that of neurons whose receptive field includes the stimulated skin site (Tommerdahl and Whitsel 1996; see Fig. 2). This result is fully consistent with the idea that the region of S1 that increases in absorbance in response to skin stimulation corresponds to the region in which the stimulus evokes neuronal excitation. A similar correspondence between the locus of the OIS evoked by a stimulus and cortical topographical organization has been demonstrated in studies of other sensory cortical areas in cats, monkeys, and rodents (for the striate cortex in cats and monkeys see Grinvald et al. [1994] and for the barrel field cortex in rodents see Narayan et al. [1994]).

Correlation between the intrinsic response and S1 neuroelectrical activity. The properties of the intrinsic response evoked in the primary somatosensory or visual cortex by natural sensory stimulation accurately predict corresponding dimensions of the associated cortical neuroelectrical response. For example, it is widely accepted that the magnitude of a stimulus-evoked

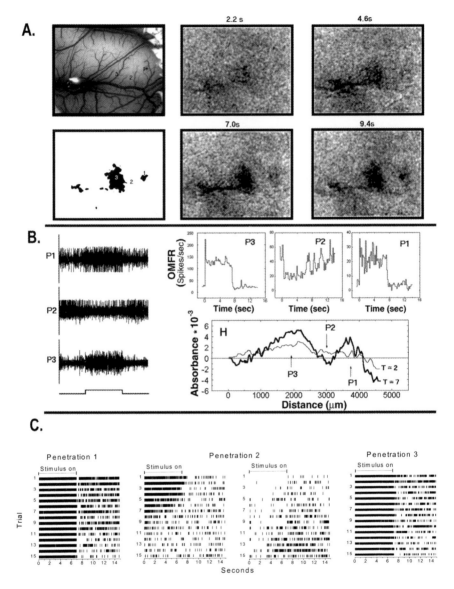

Fig. 3. (A) Top left: surface vascular pattern showing three microelectrode recording sites. Top middle and right: responses evoked in the squirrel monkey S1 by 25-Hz stimulation of the radial interdigital pad on the hand at 2.2, 4.6, 7.0, and 9.4 seconds after stimulus onset. Bottom left: thresholded image of the response at 9.4 seconds. (B) Spike trains (left) and PST histograms (top right) showing the activity of neurons studied in penetrations P1, P2, and P3. Plots show mean absorbance versus distance for the responses at 2.2 and 7.0 seconds after stimulus onset (0 on y-axis indicates the most medial location in the imaged region; arrows show locus of penetrations). (C) Spike trains for a neuron studied in P1, for two neurons studied in P2, and for a neuron studied in P3. Data are consistent with the idea that a stimulus-evoked change in absorbance is

increase in absorbance in either the striate (V-1) or the S1 cortex corresponds to the magnitude of stimulus-evoked *activation* measured in terms of neuron-firing rates (e.g., Grinvald et al. 1994; Narayan et al. 1994; Tommerdahl and Whitsel 1996; Tommerdahl et al. 1996a,b). Tommerdahl et al. (1999a) have extended this generalization symmetrically by showing that the spike discharge activity of S1 neurons sampled from regions in an OIS image characterized by *decreases* in absorbance are routinely *inhibited, often to below-background levels* (Fig. 3). In addition, S1 neurons sampled from those regions exhibiting the largest increase in absorbance in response to a pattern generated by a cutaneous flutter stimulus are systematically higher not only in their *responsivity* (response intensity), but also in their degree of *entrainment* to cutaneous flutter stimulation of the receptive field, than are neurons in regions in which the absorbance increase is smaller (B. Whitsel et al., unpublished manuscript).

IN VITRO STUDIES

Spatial properties. Imaging studies of the sensorimotor cortical slice (Kohn et al. 1997, 1999) have shown that a prominent optical intrinsic response (OIS) is evoked by electrical stimulation of thalamocortical afferents or corticocortical axons and that the magnitude of the intrinsic response and the stimulus-evoked cortical neuroelectrical response covary with stimulus intensity. The spatial properties of the OIS recorded from the sensorimotor cortical slice reflect the well-known spatial organization of radial and horizontal intrinsic connections in the somatosensory cortex (Fig. 4). The intrinsic response of the sensorimotor cortical slice to stimulus-evoked input does not result from stimulus-evoked hemodynamic changes.

Although the OIS evoked in the sensorimotor cortical slice by stimulation of thalamocortical afferents is stereotypical in that it remains column-shaped regardless of the stimulus intensity used to evoke it, the tangential width of the columnar response of the slice is shaped by synaptic inhibitory mechanisms mediated by γ-aminobutyric acid A ($GABA_A$) receptors (Kohn et al. 1999; see bottom images of Fig. 4).

Other properties. An interesting and potentially highly important property of the OIS evoked in the sensorimotor cortical slice by stimulation of thalamocortical afferents (but not observed with stimulation of corticocortical afferents) is that the optical response detected in the upper layers (layers I–II) is

---

correlated with a change in neuronal spike discharge activity, and the sign (increase versus decrease) and magnitude of the change in absorbance reflect the sign (excitation versus inhibition, respectively) and magnitude of the stimulus-evoked change in neuronal activity. From Tommerdahl et al. (1999a); reprinted with permission.

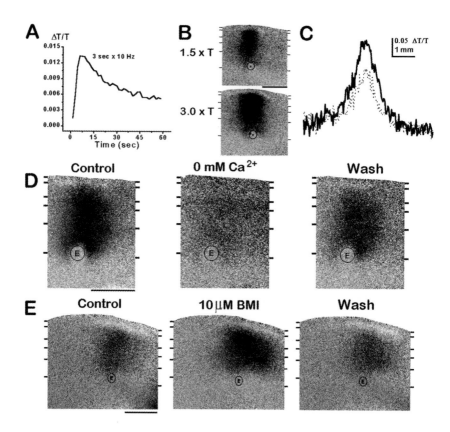

Fig. 4. (A) Time course and (B) column-like distribution of the OIS evoked in a sensorimotor cortical slice by a 3-second, 10-Hz stimulus to the white matter site (indicated by circle containing the letter "E"). The darker a region in an image, the larger the stimulus-evoked OIS. Stimulus intensity (constant current) was 1.5 times the threshold (*T*) for the top image in B, and three times the threshold for the bottom image. Horizontal ticks at the left and right edges of images indicate laminar boundaries in Nissl-stained sections cut from the same slice. (C) Plots show tangential spatial distribution of values of $\Delta T/T$ for the responses shown in panel B. (D) Images showing the OIS evoked by 10-Hz stimulation of thalamocortical afferents before (Control), during (0 mM Ca^{2+}), and after (Wash) removal of Ca^{2+} in the artificial cerebrospinal fluid that bathed the slice. Note that Ca^{2+} removal eliminated the OIS. (E) Images showing OIS before (Control), during (10 μM BMI), and after (Wash) treatment with bicuculline methiodide (BMI), a blocker of cortical inhibitory neurotransmission effected via GABA$_A$ receptors. Note the large increase in spatial extent and magnitude of stimulus-evoked OIS after BMI. Similar studies have shown that selective block of *N*-methyl D-aspartate (NMDA) or α-amino-3-hydroxy-5-methylisoxazole-4-propionic acid (AMPA) receptors decreases the stimulus-evoked OIS in a dose-dependent manner. From Kohn et al. (1999); reprinted with permission.

opposite to that observed in layers III–VI (e.g., see responses in layers I–II in images in the bottom row of Fig. 4). Moreover, this opposing response of layers I–II may reflect synaptic inhibition mediated by GABA$_A$ receptors because it is blocked by bicuculline methiodide, a relatively selective GABA$_A$-receptor blocker. Kohn et al. (1999) interpreted these in vitro observations to indicate that the most superficial layers (layers I–II) form a functionally distinct compartment within somatosensory cortical columns. This possibility will be reconsidered below in the context of S1 cortical pain information processing.

Implications for information processing. The implications of the intrinsic response for information processing at the cellular/biophysical level of analysis remain to be fully elucidated. Whole-cell, patch-clamp recording and OIS imaging methods, when used to study the same cortical slice, have yielded suggestive results (Kohn and Whitsel 1999; Kohn et al. 2000; see Fig. 5). (1) A brief, repetitive (10-Hz) electrical stimulus to the subjacent white matter evokes an OIS that occupies a column-shaped region in which the pyramidal neurons exhibit pronounced potentiation of the excitatory postsynaptic potentials (EPSPs) evoked by stimulation of corticocortical axons in layer III. (2) The degree to which the EPSPs evoked by stimulation of layer III corticocortical axons are potentiated is highly correlated with the increase in extracellular K$^+$ that accompanies repetitive thalamocortical afferent stimulation. (3) At the same time that the EPSPs evoked by stimulation of corticocortical axons in layer III are *potentiated,* the EPSPs evoked in the same neurons by stimulation of corticocortical axons in layers I–II are *inhibited.*

Collectively, the in vitro observations described above reveal that even a brief exposure to repetitive, direct thalamocortical drive facilitates the transfer of information to pyramidal neurons via layer III corticocortical axons arising from cells located in other columns, and simultaneously suppresses information transfer to the same neurons via the corticocortical axons in layers I–II. In other words, the set of corticocortical connections that can influence an individual somatosensory cortical pyramidal neuron appear to be rapidly, significantly, and selectively reshaped for periods as long as 30 seconds following even a 3-second exposure to repetitive 10-Hz, short-latency thalamocortical afferent drive. More generally, these in vitro observations establish that well-defined cellular processes triggered by thalamocortical drive effect short-term, reversible modifications of the functional and response properties of somatosensory pyramidal neurons. Findings consistent with this conclusion have been reported by investigators studying somatosensory cortical function at the cellular level (e.g., Larkum et al. 1999; Schiller et al. 2000).

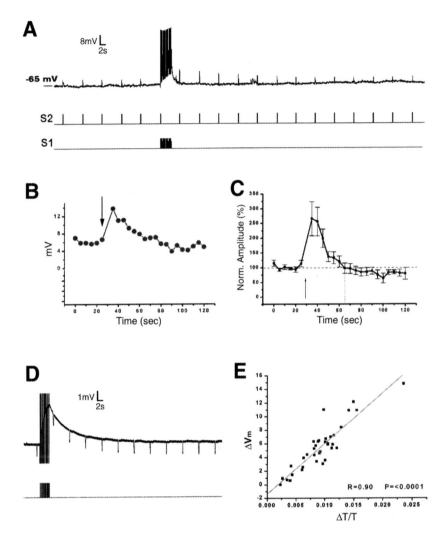

Fig. 5. (A) Current-clamp recording from S1 pyramidal cell in layer V in a sensorimotor cortical slice. Vertical ticks on the horizontal trace labeled "S1" indicate conditioning train of electrical stimuli applied to the white matter at a site directly below the cell column occupied by the neuron from which the recording was obtained. Vertical ticks on horizontal trace labeled "S2" indicate times at which a single electrical stimulus was delivered to corticocortical axons in layer III; each layer III stimulus evoked an excitatory postsynaptic potential (EPSP; small vertical deflection) in the layer V pyramidal neuron. Note the prominent EPSP potentiation that follows the thalamocortical conditioning train. (B) Plot of EPSP amplitude versus time for the same cell under identical conditions. The conditioning thalamocortical afferent drive was applied at the arrow (↓). (C) Average EPSP amplitude (data were obtained from 45 pyramidal cells) measured using protocol illustrated in panel A. (D) Current-clamp recording from a layer V astrocyte showing a 5-mV depolarization induced by the same thalamocortical conditioning train that potentiated the EPSP evoked by stimulation of layer III. Down-

THE S1 RESPONSE TO SKIN STIMULATION

S1 RESPONSE TO NOXIOUS SKIN HEATING
VERSUS CUTANEOUS FLUTTER STIMULATION

Tommerdahl and colleagues (1996a, 1998) have described the intrinsic responses evoked by two modes of precisely controlled stimulation to the same site on the radial interdigital pad of the contralateral hand: (1) a 7-second duration, 400-μm amplitude, 25-Hz sinusoidal vertical displacement (flutter) stimulus applied using a 2-mm diameter probe, with a static skin indentation of 500 μm; and (2) a triangular change in skin temperature (36°-52°-36°C, with a temperature increase and decrease of 19°C/second) applied using a 12.5-mm diameter contact thermode centered on the same site contacted by the flutter stimulus. These studies revealed a new and surprising finding highly relevant to cortical pain mechanisms: a skin-heating stimulus evoked little or no increase in absorbance in the same regions of areas 3b and 1 that responded with an increase in absorbance to cutaneous flutter. Instead, noxious skin heating substantially increased absorbance in a nearby part of area 3a (Fig. 6).

Tommerdahl et al. (1996a, 1998) also studied the responses of S1 using a protocol for skin stimulation (referred to as the *wind-up* protocol) virtually identical to an approach previously shown to elicit slow temporal summation of second pain in human subjects (Vierck et al. 1997; also Price et al. 1977, 1992). A series of brief skin taps (one every 3 seconds) was delivered to the skin using a probe maintained either at 52°C or at 36°C. Even though the mechanical component of the tapping stimulus was held constant (compare top right and bottom left images in Fig. 7), the area 3b/1 component of the intrinsic response was different at different probe temperatures. More specifically, with the probe at 52°C little or no absorbance increase was observed in areas 3b and 1, whereas at 36°C the absorbance increase in these areas was substantial (Fig. 7; see Tommerdahl et al. 1996a, and 1998 for details). This observation was interpreted to suggest (in the absence of confirmatory neurophysiological evidence) that the large-magnitude area 3a response that accompanied tapping with the 52°C thermode actively *suppressed* the response of areas 3b and 1 to the afferent drive triggered by the

---

ward deflections in this trace indicate the hyperpolarizing current injections used to estimate membrane resistance. (E) Plot showing a strong correlation between astrocyte membrane depolarization (ΔV_{m}) and the magnitude of the OIS ($\Delta T/T$) evoked by the train of stimuli applied to thalamocortical afferents. T = average intensity in the vicinity of the recording site 800 ms before the onset of the white matter stimulus; ΔT = average difference between prestimulus and poststimulus intensities in the same region. Reprinted with permission from Kohn and Whitsel (2000).

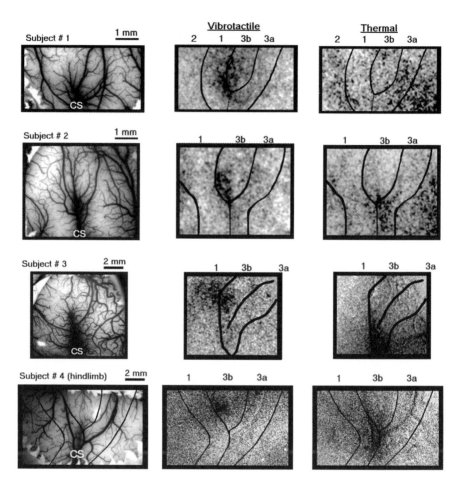

Fig. 6. S1 intrinsic responses to same-site cutaneous flutter versus noxious skin heating in four squirrel monkeys. Left: vascular patterns; CS = central sulcus. Middle: average poststimulus–prestimulus difference images obtained using a 7-second, 25-Hz, 400-μm cutaneous flutter stimulus. Right: average difference images obtained using a 36°-52°-36°C skin-heating stimulus applied to same skin site (at a rate of temperature change of 19°C/second). Solid lines on images indicate boundaries of areas 3a, 3b, 1, and 2. From Tommerdahl et al. (1996a); reprinted with permission.

mechanical component of the stimulus. The much stronger response in areas 3b and 1 and the weaker area 3a response observed when the thermode was at 36°C also were viewed as consistent with this interpretation, i.e., at 36°C the response of area 3a was relatively ineffective in suppressing areas 3b and 1.

The characteristic slow temporal summation (wind-up) of the intrinsic response evoked in area 3a of S1 by repetitive noxious skin heating suggests that the spike discharge activity of area 3a neurons might also exhibit this property under the same stimulus conditions. Tommerdahl et al. (1996a, 1998) examined this possibility in anesthetized squirrel monkeys in combined optical imaging and extracellular microelectrode recording experiments. The spike train data in Fig. 8 were obtained from a single neuron in the sector of area 3a that developed a prominent incremental increase in absorbance in response to repetitive noxious skin heating. As with most other area 3a neurons we have studied using this stimulus protocol, the spike train responses of this neuron to the skin-heating stimulus exhibited prominent slow temporal summation. In addition, the spike discharge response outlasted the stimulus (*response persistence*), and this characteristic of the response became increasingly prominent as the series of skin-heating stimuli progressed. The importance of such observations is in demonstrating that (1) the increasing area 3a OIS evoked by repetitive noxious skin heating is accompanied by increased spike discharge activity in area 3a neurons and (2) the temporal integrative properties exhibited by both the area 3a optical intrinsic response and the spike discharge response of neurons in the same region of area 3a closely approximate the slow temporal summation (wind-up and response persistence) characteristics of the *second pain* percept in human subjects. This led Tommerdahl et al. (1996a, 1998) to propose that area 3a might play an important and perhaps even a leading role in pain perception.

Other attributes of the spike discharge activity evoked in area 3a neurons by noxious skin heating appear consistent with neuroanatomical evidence (Craig 1995) that the middle layers of area 3a receive substantial input that originates in lamina I of the spinal dorsal horn. In particular, the poststimulus time (PST) histograms for the area 3a neurons shown in Fig. 9 (B. Whitsel, O. Favorov and M. Tommerdahl, unpublished observations; note vertical arrows) reveal an early decrease in mean firing rate, followed by a substantial increase in mean firing rate as the temperature of the skin-heating stimulus increased from a level that conscious subjects experience as painful. It seems likely that this behavior of area 3a neurons derives from the unique, nonmonotonic temperature–response relationship that Craig (1995) showed to be characteristic of heat-, cold-, and pain-responsive (HCP-type) cells in lamina I of the spinal cord dorsal horn. In squirrel monkeys, the activity of nociresponsive neurons in area 3a is lowest when the skin is exposed to a temperature perceived as thermoneutral or as non-noxious warming, and is greater at either lower or higher stimulus temperatures (as is evident in the PSTs of Fig. 9). This finding is consistent with the possibility that these cells receive a relatively untransformed copy of the output of the HCP-type cells in lamina I of the dorsal horn.

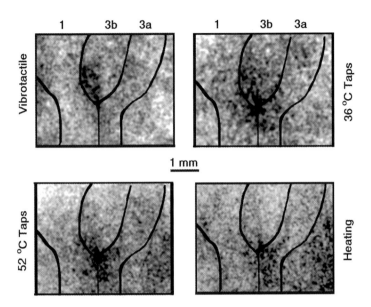

Fig. 7. OIS images showing the absorbance increase (indicated by dark region) evoked in S1 of the same subject by four different conditions of same-site skin stimulation. Top left: response to 25-Hz skin flutter with stimulator probe at 27°C. Top right: response to 1.2-second taps applied with probe at 36°C. Bottom left: response to 1.2-second taps applied with probe at 52°C. Bottom right: response to 1.2-second skin-heating ramps (36°-52°-36°C) with probe in stationary contact with the skin. From Tommerdahl et al. (1996a); reprinted with permission.

Tommerdahl et al. (1998) used two different OIS image analysis techniques to quantify the temporal changes in the somatosensory cortical intrinsic response to skin stimulation. The first method, paired boxel analysis (illustrated in Fig. 10), was used to compare and contrast the optical responses evoked in two regions of S1. These 1 × 1 mm regions (boxels) show differential activation by same-site cutaneous flutter and noxious skin-heating stimulation (in Fig. 10 one of the boxels is in area 3b and the other is in area 3a). The plots at the bottom of Fig. 10 show that during 25-Hz

Fig. 8. Spike train data recorded from a typical area 3a neuron during delivery of noxious skin-heating stimulation to the receptive field. The neuron was located in the middle layers in the area 3a region that increased in absorbance in response to stimulation of the radial interdigital pad on the hand. Top: OIS image showing area 3a response (dark region) to skin heating, and microelectrode recording site (white arrow = P1). Top panel: spike trains evoked by 10 successive skin-heating ramps (stimulus profile is shown below spike trains). Middle panel: PST histogram showing average firing-rate response of this neuron to the stimuli. Bottom panel: plot showing that average rate of spike discharge associated with each stimulus increased progressively (exhibited wind-up) with repeated skin heating. From Tommerdahl et al. (1996a); reprinted with permission. →

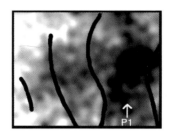

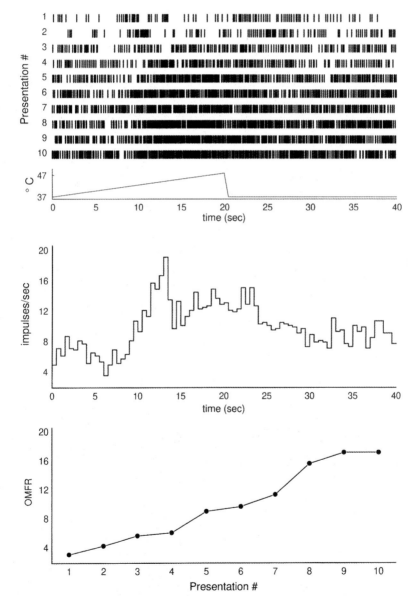

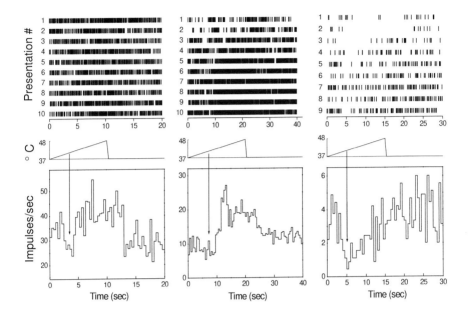

Fig. 9. Raster plots of spike trains (top) and PST histograms (bottom) for three squirrel monkey area 3a neurons studied using skin-heating stimulation. Vertical arrows between the stimulus profiles and the PSTs indicate the transient decrease in mean firing rate consistently observed when the thermode attained temperatures between 39° and 41°C.

cutaneous flutter stimulation, average absorbance in the area 3b boxel increases to a value greater than that attained at any other S1 locus, but does not increase in the area 3a boxel. In contrast, with same-site skin-heating stimulation in the same subject, average absorbance in the area 3a boxel increases to a value greater than that attained at any other S1 locus but simultaneously decreases in the area 3b boxel that was activated maximally during 25-Hz flutter. This outcome of the paired-boxel analysis strongly suggests that the sector of area 3b thus evaluated not only receives maximal excitatory drive from the mechanoreceptors in the stimulated skin site, but also receives a potent *inhibitory* influence from thermonociceptors in the same skin site.

A second image-analysis method demonstrates reciprocal inhibitory interactions between the two cytoarchitecturally distinct S1 territories that respond differentially to non-noxious mechanical versus skin-heating stimulation. Gross visual inspection of the "raw" images showing the stimulus–prestimulus difference obtained from S1 (Fig. 10) reveals that skin-heating stimulation causes maximal activation (increase in absorbance) in area 3a, and that 25-Hz cutaneous flutter causes maximal activation in area 3b and/ or area 1. The effects of skin stimulation on the territories adjacent to the

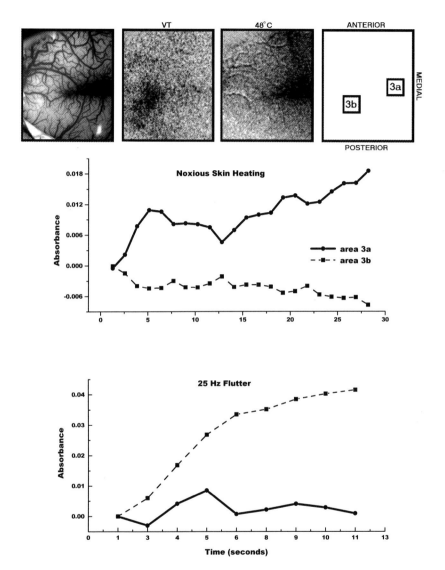

Fig. 10. Quantification of the temporal evolution of the S1 intrinsic response evoked by same-site thermal and mechanical skin stimuli. Top left: vascular pattern. Second image from left at top ("VT"): response to thermoneutral 25-Hz vibrotactile stimulus. Third image from left at top ("48°C"): response to same-site repetitive skin-heating stimulation. Top right: outline of imaged region containing two regions of the same size ("boxels," labeled 3a and 3b) within which the average absorbance change was determined for both conditions of skin stimulation as a function of time after stimulus onset. Boxel 3a lies within area 3a and exhibited the largest increase in absorbance (activation) in response to noxious skin heating; boxel 3b lies within area 3b and exhibited the most activation in response to the thermoneutral 25-Hz stimulus. Graphs at the bottom show the time course of the responses of areas 3b and 3a detected in the boxels during same-site noxious skin heating (48°C) versus 25-Hz flutter. From Tommerdahl et al. (1998); reprinted with permission.

maximally activated region typically are neither large nor obviously consistent from one subject to the next. Thus, it is not clear whether the smaller and more variable changes in absorbance (usually small decreases in absorbance) at such "off-focus" sites are meaningful, or are due to random variation ("noise"). The need to resolve this issue prompted Tommerdahl et al. (1998) to use a more powerful and comprehensive image analysis method—correlation mapping (Plate 1; p. 82). This method allowed us to put a functionally important hypothesis to a rigorous test. We confirmed that the changes in absorbance evoked in areas 3a and in areas 3b and 1 by noxious skin heating versus 25-Hz flutter skin stimulation not only are *different*, but are *opposing*—that is, the changes in absorbance evoked in areas 3a, 3b, and 1 by each mode of skin stimulation not only follow approximately the same time course, but are negatively correlated.

The main strengths of correlation mapping are that (1) it uses *all* the information in an image, (2) it provides objective measures (correlation values) of the associations between the time-dependent absorbance changes at loci within the region of maximal activity and at all other loci within the imaged field, and (3) it enables objective delineation of anterior parietal regions functionally related to each stimulus mode based on the value and sign of the correlation with the time course of the absorbance change in the region activated maximally by skin stimulation. Stated more formally, a correlation map is made by choosing a reference region within the imaged field and then computing the correlation r_{ij} between the absorbance values of each pixel (i, j) and the absorbance values within the reference region over time after stimulus onset. The region selected as the reference is that defined by the boxel (usually a 1×1 mm area) for which average absorbance underwent the largest increase during stimulation. Each pixel (i, j) on the correlation map is represented by a correlation value r_{ij} ($-1 < r < +1$), where -1 indicates negative correlation and $+1$ indicates positive correlation.

Application of the method to the S1 intrinsic responses evoked by a repetitive skin-heating stimulus (Tommerdahl et al. 1998) showed that absorbance in an extensive region of S1 changes with a time course similar to that measured in the region of area 3a that responded maximally to the skin-heating stimulus. Plate 1 shows results of four subjects studied using virtually identical conditions of skin-heating stimulation. The time course of the changes in average absorbance observed at every locus within a large, mostly continuous, anterior parietal zone (red coding in each panel in the middle column showing anterior parietal loci with correlation values between +0.5 and +0.8) was positively correlated with the time course of the response of the localized region that responded with the maximal absorbance increase (designated with black code in each panel on the right). In other words, at all locations within the red zone in each middle panel, average absorbance increased after onset of skin heating with a time course very similar to that observed in the 1 × 1 mm region of maximal activation in area 3a. Also evident in the correlation maps of Plate 1 are extensive, largely continuous regions comprising loci whose average absorbance *decreased* at the same time that absorbance *increased* in the maximally activated region (blue regions in the middle panels showing loci with correlation values between –0.5 and –0.8).

Each correlation map in the middle panels of Plate 1 demonstrates a spatially extensive region of the anterior parietal cortex (red-yellow region) within which the change in average absorbance correlates positively with the absorbance change measured in the 1 × 1 mm region of area 3a that responded maximally to skin heating. Similarly, in each subject the change in absorbance within an extensive region correlates positively with the absorbance change measured in the area 3b region that responded maximally to 25-Hz flutter. With either skin-heating or cutaneous flutter stimulation, the region of correlated response is clearly much larger than the area of maximal stimulus-evoked absorbance increase. Each middle panel in Plate 1 reveals the region (shown in blue) in which the change in average absorbance correlates *negatively* with the change in absorbance measured in the area that responded maximally to skin heating. The region of negative correlation only partially approximates the location of the region that responded maximally to 25-Hz flutter. The former region typically is much larger than the latter, and in three of the four subjects shown in Plate 1, it is almost exclusively located within area 1.

In conclusion, the results obtained with the correlation mapping method are consistent with the idea that spatially extensive regions in areas 3b, 1, and 3a in the hindlimb or forelimb region of the S1 cortex participate *simultaneously* in the global S1 response to repetitive delivery of either a 25-Hz or a noxious skin-heating stimulus. More specifically, the results indicate that the spatiotemporal distribution of influences evoked within S1 by skin heating versus 25-Hz flutter stimulation are systematically opposed—i.e., noxious skin heating evokes strong activation of area 3a and simultaneous suppression of extensive anterior parietal regions located posterior to area 3a, whereas 25-Hz flutter evokes vigorous activation of areas 3b and 1 and weak suppression of area 3a.

S1 RESPONSE TO SAME-SITE FLUTTER VERSUS VIBRATION

Our interest in comparing the intrinsic responses to same-site flutter versus vibration was motivated by the literature on vibratory analgesia. Both clinical and experimental pain can be significantly reduced by a concurrent vibrotactile stimulus, and the effect is largest and most robust if the frequency of stimulation is 100 Hz or higher and if the stimulus is applied at or very close to the site of pain (Pertovaara 1979; Ekblom and Hansson 1982, 1985; Lundeberg 1984; Lundeberg et al. 1984). Accordingly, we investigated the responses of S1 in anesthetized squirrel monkeys to same-site 25-Hz as compared to 200-Hz sinusoidal stimulation to determine whether these two frequencies of vibrotactile stimulation might have different effects on area 3a, as is predicted if area 3a is involved in pain information processing (Tommerdahl et al. 1999a). Although 25-Hz stimulation (200-µm peak-to-peak amplitude) produced a prominent *increase* in absorbance within the regions of areas 3b and 1 known to be occupied by neurons whose receptive field includes the site of stimulation, 200-Hz stimulation (50-µm peak-to-peak amplitude) produced a prominent *decrease* in absorbance over a much larger S1 territory, most frequently involving areas 3b, 1, *and 3a,* but sometimes area 2 as well. Furthermore, while the response to flutter developed quickly in areas 3b and 1 and remained nearly constant for the duration of stimulation, the response to 200 Hz was biphasic and consisted of an initial absorbance increase within the same topographically appropriate region, which was replaced after 4–6 seconds by a prominent decrease in absorbance.

We also evaluated the effects on S1 of a "compound vibrotactile" stimulus consisting of 25-Hz (200-µm peak-to-peak amplitude) flutter with a superimposed 200-Hz component (50-µm peak-to-peak) (Tommerdahl et al. 1999a). With this stimulus an early increase in absorbance again occurred in areas 3b and 1, but its magnitude was much smaller than was observed with a "pure" flutter stimulus to the same skin site. This result suggests that after a transient period of excitation, the 200-Hz stimulus mobilizes a process that suppresses the normal responsivity of areas 3b and 1 and of area 3a.

Others have suggested that S2 neurons are more responsive than S1 neurons to high-frequency sinusoidal skin stimulation (Bennett et al. 1980; Rowe et al. 1985; Ferrington et al. 1988). Thus, S2 was an obvious candidate as the source, via corticocortical connections, of the observed suppression of S1 (and especially area 3a) during 200-Hz skin stimulation. This possibility was investigated in cats (Tommerdahl et al. 1999b), where it is possible to image simultaneously the intrinsic responses of both S1 and S2 in the same subject. These experiments demonstrated that a 25-Hz flutter stimulus evokes a prominent and well-maintained increase in absorbance in *both* the contralateral S1 and S2, whereas 200-Hz vibration evokes a strong and well-maintained absorbance increase *only* in S2. As had been observed in squirrel monkeys (Tommerdahl et al. 1999a), the response to 200-Hz stimulation of the contralateral S1 in cats also was biphasic—that is, the region of S1 that in the same subject had responded to same-site 25-Hz flutter initially increased slightly in absorbance; but within 1–2 seconds of the onset of the 200-Hz stimulus this response was replaced by a large-magnitude and more spatially extensive decrease in absorbance involving area 3a. These S1/S2 spatiotemporal patterns (S1/S2 response congruence during and throughout flutter stimulation and S1/S2 response divergence during same-site vibration) were captured quantitatively using the paired boxel and correlation-mapping procedures described above (see Tommerdahl et al. 1999b for details).

TIME COURSE OF S1 RESPONSES TO FLUTTER VERSUS VIBRATION VERSUS HEAT

Another experiment carried our understanding of the stimulus- and time-dependency of the S1 intrinsic response one stage further. Fig. 11 shows the *time course* of the S1 intrinsic responses in the same squirrel monkey to three different modes (25-Hz, 200-Hz, and noxious skin heating) of same-site skin stimulation. With the 25-Hz stimulus (left column) the S1 intrinsic response appears shortly after stimulus onset (1.2 seconds) in areas 3b and 1, and is already maximal by the time the second image is acquired at 2.4 seconds. In addition, continuation of the 25-Hz stimulus leads to only a slight though significant decline in the magnitude and spatial extent of the intrinsic response in areas 3b and 1. The repetitive noxious skin-heating stimulus produces a very different S1 response pattern (six temperature ramps at 3-second intervals, with each ramp at 36°-50°-36°C). With this stimulus the response is concentrated in area 3a, its onset is delayed relative to that of the response to 25-Hz stimulation, and it not only continues to increase in both intensity and spatial extent throughout the period of stimulus delivery, but persists for at least 15–30 seconds after stimulus termination (not shown in Fig. 11). The time course of the S1 intrinsic response to 200-Hz vibration in the same subject exhibits a third distinct pattern. Under this condition the response is biphasic, beginning with a small focal increase in absorbance in areas 3b and 1 at about the same time and in the same locus as the response to same-site cutaneous flutter, followed by a progressively larger and more widespread decrease in absorbance as 200-Hz stimulation continues. Two further properties of the S1 response to 200-Hz stimulation are especially intriguing. First, the region of the maximal absorbance decrease (inhibition) is virtually coincident with the region—predominantly area 3a—activated by noxious skin-heating stimulation of the same skin site. Second, like the response to noxious skin heating, the decrease in absorbance evoked by 200-Hz vibration persists for at least 15–30 seconds following stimulus termination.

Considered collectively, the results in Fig. 11 suggest a possible basis for the differential effectiveness of vibratory versus flutter stimuli in producing analgesia. Specifically, high-frequency vibration, but apparently not flutter, evokes a strong decrease in absorbance in the subregion of area 3a that is activated by noxious heating of the same skin site (this is most evident after 2.4 seconds of continuous stimulation). Although the evidence is incomplete, it already appears certain that high-frequency vibration produces a similarly long-lasting suppression of both the optical and single-neuron neurophysiological responses to cutaneous flutter in areas 3b and 1 of monkey subjects, and that in normal human subjects it interferes with the perception of frequency evoked by cutaneous flutter (K.D. Hester et al., unpublished observation). The responses of S1 neurons to high-frequency skin stimuli remain to be investigated in detail. However, the prediction that such stimulation will inhibit area 3b/1 neurons seems compatible with reports (first noted by Mountcastle et al. 1969) that only the "fast-spiking" neurons in areas 3b and 1 entrain[2] to vibrotactile stimulation at the high frequencies at which Pacinian receptors are known to be exquisitely sensitive. Such neurons are widely believed to be GABAergic, inhibitory neurons in the upper layers, such as the double bouquet cells that inhibit most other neurons in the same macrocolumn.

EFFECTS OF MANIPULATIONS

Spinal dorsal column transection. The OIS imaging method might be a useful way to study the contributions of different somatosensory pathways of the spinal cord to the S1 response to natural skin stimuli. To investigate the feasibility of this application, imaging experiments were conducted in squirrel monkeys whose fasciculus gracilis had been cut at midthoracic level 6 months earlier (bottom panel on right in Fig. 12; Tommerdahl and Whitsel 1996). This tract is principally composed of fibers that innervate rapidly adapting hindlimb cutaneous mechanoreceptors (Whitsel et al. 1969, 1971; Dreyer et al. 1974). Thus, we anticipated that a complete midthoracic dorsal column lesion would selectively deprive the contralateral hindlimb area in S1 (and especially areas 3b and 1) of its major source of low-threshold rapidly adapting mechanoreceptive afferent drive, but at the same time would spare the afferent drive that ascends via other spinal cord pathways and reaches more anterior and posterior regions of S1 (i.e., areas 3a and 2) during non-noxious mechanical skin stimulation.

---

[2] i.e., exhibit precise phase locking of spike discharge to the stimulus waveform.

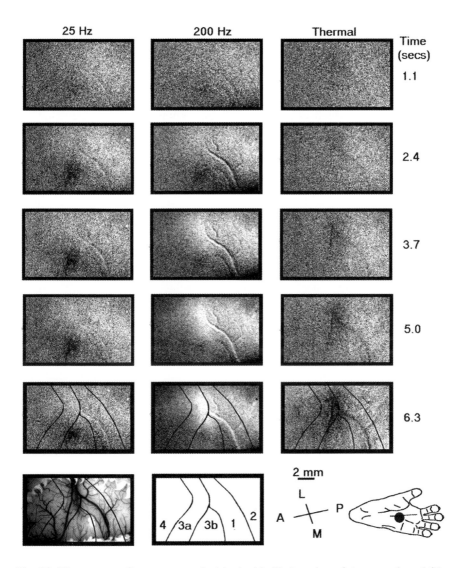

Fig. 11. Time course of responses evoked in the hindlimb region of the contralateral S1 of a squirrel monkey by same-site 25-Hz flutter (images in left column) versus 200-Hz vibration (middle column) versus noxious skin heating ("Thermal"; right column). Vascular pattern, cytoarchitectural boundaries, and stimulus site are shown at the bottom.

Fig. 12 shows OIS imaging results obtained in an experiment in which same-site thermal (42°C and 51°C skin-heating) and vibrotactile (25-Hz flutter) stimuli were applied independently in interleaved trials to a discrete region on the contralateral volar foot of a squirrel monkey with a dorsal column lesion (Tommerdahl and Whitsel 1996). In the absence of input from the dorsal column, the optical sign of area 3b/1 neuronal activation (an absorbance increase) in response to 25-Hz vibrotactile stimulation is virtually absent. We expected that the spinal dorsal column lesion would not affect the intrinsic response of area 3a to noxious skin heating (51°C) because the afferent drive evoked by skin heating is conveyed via the spinothalamic pathways, which in this subject were assumed to be intact. (This assumption was confirmed by histological examination of the spinal cord.) While absorbance did increase in S1 with noxious skin heating, we were surprised to find that the increase was abnormally large in both intensity and extent relative to the response evoked by the same stimulus in intact subjects. Fig. 12 shows that the absorbance increase evoked in the lesioned subject by skin heating extended across areas 1, 3b, 3a, and 4. Our working hypothesis is that such an abnormally *exaggerated response* of the dorsal-column-deprived S1 to noxious skin heating is due to a "release" of the upper layer area 3b and 1 nociresponsive neurons from a normally present, tonic inhibitory influence. Particularly intriguing in this regard is the well-documented but only rarely cited clinical neurological evidence that "in man, lesions of the dorsal columns cause an *increase* in pain, tickle, warmth and cold" (Nathan et al. 1986, p. 1003).

Several published findings suggest plausible cellular/connectional mechanisms for the abnormally intense and widespread activation of S1 after spinal dorsal column interruption. First, the enzyme (glutamic acid decarboxylase) required for intraneuronal synthesis of the inhibitory neurotransmitter GABA is present at abnormally low levels in the inhibitory neurons located in cortical regions chronically deprived of their afferent innervation (Liang et al. 1996; also Hendry and Jones 1988). Second, areas 3b and 1 are the main regions of anterior parietal cortex deprived of their principal source of thalamocortical input by interruption of the contralateral spinal dorsal column (Dreyer et al. 1974; Jain et al. 1997; also Vierck et al. 1985, 1990a,b). As a result, corticocortical interactions that allow area 3a to inhibit areas 3b and 1 in normal subjects might be deficient in subjects with lesions of the spinal dorsal columns.

Expression in normal, intact subjects of a strong, tonic inhibition on the nociresponsive neurons that occupy the upper layers of areas 3b and 1 could explain why previous microelectrode recording studies (e.g., Kenshalo and Willis 1991) did not find large numbers of upper layer nociresponsive S1 neurons, even though the thalamocortical pathways that receive their principal input from the spinothalamic and trigeminothalamic pathways project to layers I–II in areas 3b and 1 (e.g., Rausell and Jones 1991a,b, 1994; Rausell et al. 1992).

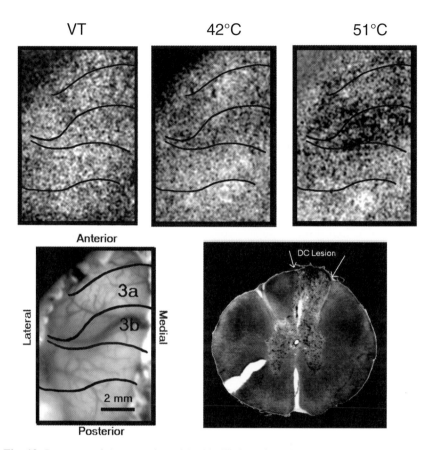

Fig. 12. Response of the contralateral S1 hindlimb region of a squirrel monkey to 25-Hz cutaneous flutter (image labeled "VT") and two conditions of skin-heating stimulation (36°-42°-36°C, "42°C"; and 36°-51°-36°C, "51°C"). Bottom left: vascular pattern and cytoarchitectonic boundaries. Bottom right: spinal cord lesion; note that the lesion is unilateral, and that there is little involvement of either the spinal dorsal horn or tracts other than the dorsal column.

NMDA-receptor block. If we are correct in assuming that the area 3a intrinsic response to noxious skin heating is attributable to afferent drive conveyed via the spinothalamic pathway, then that response should be eliminated or at least attenuated by a manipulation that lowers input via the spinothalamic tract. The most direct demonstration of this mechanism would be to surgically interrupt the spinothalamic tract, but we have yet to attempt this manipulation. Instead, we performed a manipulation that we anticipated might *reversibly and selectively* reduce the contribution of activity in the spinothalamic pathway to the S1 response to skin stimulation.

To this end, we studied the effects of intravenous administration of 5 mg/kg of ketamine (a selective, noncompetitive NMDA-receptor blocker)

on the responses of the contralateral S1 (the forelimb region of an anesthetized squirrel monkey) to repetitive tapping of a skin region with a probe at
36°C (Fig. 13; top right image) or at 52°C (Fig. 13; third image from left at
top). The overlap of the S1 response patterns evoked in this subject by the
36°C and the 52°C tapping stimuli is appreciable (and understandable, given
the fact that both stimulus conditions involved the same substantial mechanical component—a 750-ms duration skin indentation or "tap"). However, with 52°C tapping the focus of the response is located anteriorly (mainly
in area 3a), whereas with 36°C tapping the maximal increase in absorbance
is located in area 1. (Much of area 3b could not be imaged in this subject
because it was buried in the posterior bank of the central sulcus.) The
thresholded "raw" images shown at the bottom of Fig. 13 show the major
differences between the responses evoked by the 36°C and the 52°C tapping
stimuli.

After ketamine administration, the dominant component of the S1 response evoked by the 52°C stimulus does not occupy area 3a (as it did prior
to ketamine; Fig. 13), but mainly occupies area 1. Thus, the post-ketamine
response to 52°C tapping resembles the response to 36°C skin tapping prior
to ketamine administration. This result suggests that ketamine eliminates the
normally differential response of S1 to non-noxious mechanical versus noxious skin heating. This outcome is consistent with the hypothesis that motivated the experiment: we anticipated that low-dose ketamine administration
would selectively reduce the nociceptive afferent drive conveyed to S1 via
the spinothalamic tract because NMDA-receptor block reduces the response
of the WDR spinal dorsal horn neurons that contribute axons to the spinothalamic tract. We also assumed that the drug would spare the mechanoreceptive afferent drive conveyed to S1 via the dorsal column–medial lemniscal
pathway. These expectations and the OIS imaging results shown in Fig. 13
are consistent with reports that low-dose administration of an NMDA-receptor blocker significantly reduces the sensitivity of human subjects to noxious stimulation, but spares (and frequently enhances) subjects' sensitivity
to non-noxious mechanical skin stimulation (Eide et al. 1994; Felsby et al.
1996; Dray and Urban 1996; Nikolajsen et al. 1996; also Morgenstern et al.
1962; for related actions of ketamine on S1 neurons, see Roppolo et al.
1973; Duncan et al. 1982; Whitsel et al. 1999a).

HUMAN PSYCHOPHYSICAL CORRELATES

We attempted to identify perceptual correlates for our finding that high-
frequency skin vibration suppresses the optical response of areas 3b and 1
in cats and squirrel monkeys. The first of these studies of human subjects

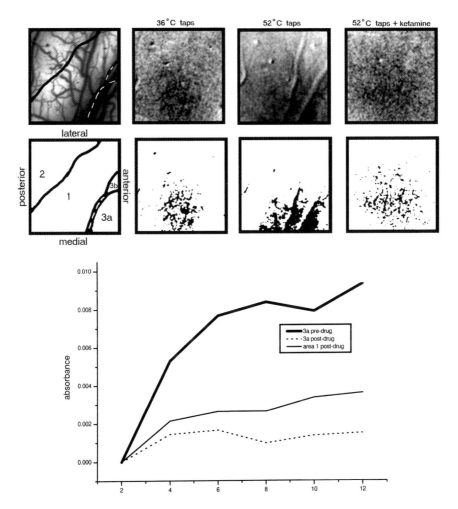

Fig. 13. Top left: surface vascular pattern and cytoarchitectural boundaries. Second–fourth panels from left: stimulus-prestimulus difference images showing intrinsic responses of S1 forelimb region to different conditions of repetitive skin-heating stimulation. Each response was evoked by six taps (each 750 ms in duration) to the same site on the hand. Second image from left: response to the stimulator probe at 36°C. Third image from left: response to the stimulator probe at 52°C. Fourth image from left: response to the 52°C probe 7 minutes after intravenous administration of 5 mg/kg of ketamine. Middle left: location of cytoarchitectural boundaries. Second–fourth images from left: thresholded images showing for each condition the location of pixels with the highest (upper 5%) absorbance values in the response pattern. Bottom: plots of absorbance versus time after stimulus onset for the different conditions. Note that after low-dose ketamine administration (i.e., after NMDA-receptor block) the absorbance increase in area 3a to the repetitive noxious skin-heating stimulus is smaller than the absorbance increase in area 1. The normal pattern of S1 response to noxious skin heating (the absorbance increase in area 3a exceeds that in areas 3b/1) is thus reversed under ketamine, and resembles the normal S1 response pattern evoked by non-noxious mechanical skin stimulation.

used rapidly repeated, brief thermal taps, which elicited clear second pain sensations that summated temporally, or in other words, produced wind-up (Vierck et al. 1997). We found that (1) with intervals between taps equal to or less than 3 seconds, delivery of a series of 700-ms taps ($n = 20$) leads in most subjects to a progressive increase in the intensity of the second pain sensation evoked by each tap ("slow temporal summation"); (2) slow temporal summation of the second pain percept becomes increasingly prominent with increasing thermode temperature over the range 45°–53°C; (3) the slow temporal summation cannot be accounted for by stimulus-evoked alterations in skin temperature (determined in a separate series of experiments by direct measurements of subepidermal skin temperature during delivery of the same thermomechanical stimulus patterns used to obtain the psychophysical observations); and (4) the slow temporal summation is significantly attenuated by prior administration of dextromethorphan, an NMDA-receptor antagonist. These results lend additional support to the idea that the prominent slow temporal summation of pain intensity (wind-up) achieved by repetitive thermomechanical skin tapping is mostly attributable to CNS mechanisms that modify the response of central somatosensory neurons to C-fiber-mediated afferent drive (Vierck et al. 1997).

In another study, Hester et al. (1999) assessed the effects of a relatively brief (15-second) pre-exposure to vibration on human frequency discriminatory capacity. The stimuli were applied to the thenar eminence of the hand. In three subjects, vibrotactile frequency thresholds for 25-Hz and 200-Hz standard stimuli (matched in intensity to eliminate intensity cues) were measured both before and after exposure of the same site to a 15-second, 25-Hz or 200-Hz adapting stimulus. When the frequency of the standard and adapting stimuli was the same, adaptation led in each subject to a small, but significant, improvement in frequency discrimination relative to the frequency threshold measured in the absence of adaptation. In contrast, when the frequency of the standard and adapting stimuli was different, adaptation led in each subject to a substantial elevation of the frequency threshold. The finding most relevant to the role of S1 in pain was that exposure to high-frequency skin stimulation (200 Hz) led to a decline in subjects' capacity to discriminate frequency in the flutter range. This outcome, like the results we obtained in OIS imaging and neurophysiological recording studies in animal subjects, is consistent with the idea that even a relatively brief exposure to high-frequency skin stimulation exerts an inhibitory influence on area 3b/1 neurons that degrades their capacity to encode the frequency of cutaneous flutter stimulation.

A third human psychophysical study (Y. Li, M. Tommerdahl, and B. Whitsel, unpublished manuscript) was conducted to obtain information more directly relevant to the phenomenon of vibratory analgesia. A run of 20 brief skin-heating stimuli were applied to the right thenar eminence of two subjects, who reported the magnitude of the second pain experience evoked by each stimulus. Stimuli were applied with a vibrotactile/thermal stimulator (CS-540T; Cantek Metatron Corp.) with a cylindrical (5-mm diameter) probe. Each stimulus consisted of a step-like, vertical skin displacement ("tap," producing a 0.5-mm skin indentation) with the probe maintained at a specified temperature (56.0°C for subject 1; 57.5°C for subject 2). Three different conditions of repetitive tapping stimulation were studied in each subject: (1) heated taps without superimposed sinusoidal axial motion; (2) heated taps with superimposed 25-Hz/200-μm amplitude axial motion; and (3) heated taps with superimposed 150-Hz/50-μm amplitude sinusoidal axial motion. Subjects rated the magnitude of the second pain sensation evoked by each tap according to a continuous scale anchored by the following points: 0 = no sensation; 20 = threshold for second pain; 100 = intolerable pain.

The data shown in Fig. 14 reveal a sizable effect on subjects' report of the magnitude of second pain of sinusoidal vertical axial motion at 150 Hz, but not at 25 Hz. Whereas 25-Hz/200-μm amplitude sinusoidal axial motion exerted little or no influence on the magnitude of second pain at any time during the series of stimuli, repetitive taps that included 150-Hz/50-μm amplitude sinusoidal motion were accompanied by reports of substantially reduced second pain. This effect in the averaged data from both subjects (Fig. 14) is very prominent. In fact, under the condition of tapping with superimposed 150-Hz/50-μm sinusoidal motion, the average magnitude of the second pain evoked by taps 13–20 approximates the magnitude that subjects were instructed to regard as the minimally detectable experience of second pain (Fig. 14). This result indicates that under this condition the subjects experienced little or no pain during repetitive skin-heating stimulation. We tentatively attribute the observed selectivity and large magnitude (relative to the complete lack of effect of superimposed 25-Hz flutter) of the suppressive influence of 150-Hz vibration on the subjects' report of second pain to an inhibitory influence of high-frequency skin vibration on the mechanisms (presumably located in area 3a) that support slow temporal summation of neuronal activity in area 3a during repetitive noxious skin-heating stimulation.

THE ROLE OF S1 IN PAIN INFORMATION PROCESSING

AN ALTERNATIVE VIEW

The cortical neural mechanisms that subserve the sensation evoked by high-frequency (>50-Hz) vibration (i.e., attributable to Pacinian corpuscle

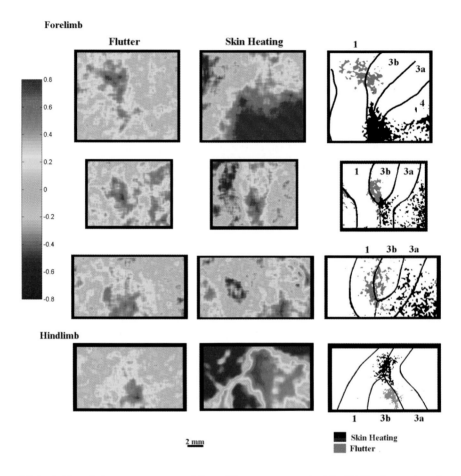

Plate 1. Correlation maps generated from S1 responses evoked by 25-Hz flutter (panels in left column) versus skin heating (middle column). Each row of maps was obtained from a different squirrel monkey ($n = 4$). Maps in the top three rows were obtained from three subjects stimulated on a forelimb skin site; maps in the bottom row are from a single subject stimulated on a hindlimb site. Panels at right show thresholded responses to both modes of same-site stimulation (gray shading = region of maximal response to 25-Hz flutter; black shading = region of maximal response to skin heating). Color scale at left indicates the value of the correlation coefficient (r). For each map the correlation was computed between the changes in absorbance over time at each pixel and the time course of the average absorbance decrease within the region of maximal response for each stimulus condition. The regions of maximal response were 1×1 mm regions within areas 3b and 3a). From Tommerdahl et al. (1998); reprinted with permission.

[PC] activation) or the sensation of pain are poorly understood. For example, like previous studies that found very few nociresponsive neurons in areas 3b and 1, neurophysiological studies of areas 3b and 1 have identified relatively few neurons with properties consistent with those of PC receptors (Lebedev et al. 1996). Moreover, the incidence of such neurons in S1 may

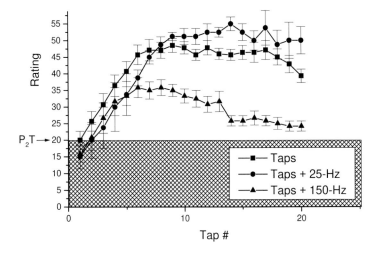

Fig. 14. Magnitude estimation data obtained from two human subjects studied using three conditions of repetitive skin-tapping stimulation (taps with no superimposed sinusoidal axial motion, taps with superimposed 25-Hz axial motion, and taps with superimposed 150-Hz axial motion. All stimuli were delivered to the right thenar eminence. P_2T indicates the rating level (20) at which subjects first reported the evoked sensation as painful.

be lower than Lebedev's estimate of 1–4% because at least some of the area 3b/1 recordings described as exhibiting PC-like properties had characteristics (e.g., short action potential duration and/or the ability to discharge action potential at high rates) typical of either thalamocortical fibers or local inhibitory neurons, rather than of pyramidal neurons.

Other observations indicate that the neural mechanisms that encode information about high-frequency skin stimulation and those that encode pain may differ fundamentally from the mechanisms that subserve cutaneous flutter sensation. First, like the thalamic neurons that receive nociceptive and/or thermal input from the spinothalamic and trigeminothalamic pathways, the axons of the dorsal thalamic neurons dominated by input arising in PC afferents (e.g., the ventroposterior inferior nucleus [VPI]; Dykes et al. 1981) project to the most superficial layers of areas 3b and 1 (layers I–II; Jones 1991; 1998; Rausell and Jones 1991a,b; Rausell et al. 1992). Thus, the thalamocortical input to areas 3b and 1 that results from either PC afferent or skin nociceptor activation can directly access only the most distal and synaptically insecure portion of a pyramidal neuron's apical dendrite. Second, observations obtained in both metabolic (2-DG) and OIS imaging studies indicate that areas 3b and 1 *do not* undergo sustained activation during either sustained high-frequency vibrotactile or noxious skin-heating stimulation. For example, during either type of stimulation 2-DG uptake in areas

3b and 1 is reduced to below-background levels in the regions occupied by neurons with receptive fields that include the stimulus site (Tommerdahl et al. 1999a,b). Similarly, the optical intrinsic response of the topographically appropriate regions of areas 3b and 1 to either 200-Hz vibration or noxious skin heating is a *decrease* in absorbance, in contrast to the *increase* in absorbance widely believed to be the hallmark of cortical neuronal activation (Tommerdahl et al. 1999a,b).

In summary, four observations appear incompatible with the "traditional" view that areas 3b and 1 are the major S1 regions involved in processing the afferent drive evoked by noxious skin heating: (1) the virtual absence of either PC-type or nociresponsive neurons in the middle layers of areas 3b and 1; (2) the lack of thalamocortical connections that could convey a high-fidelity and secure signal of either high-frequency mechanical or noxious skin stimulation to area 3b/1 pyramidal neurons; (3) the failure of high-frequency mechanical stimulation of the skin to increase 2-DG uptake; and (4) the observation that the optical response of areas 3b and 1 to noxious skin heating is inconsistent with neuronal activation. Collectively, these factors strongly imply that it is not areas 3b and 1, but area 3a that plays the leading role in the cortical processing of the afferent drive evoked by noxious skin heating.

MECHANISMS OF AREA 3B/1 SUPPRESSION BY NOXIOUS SKIN HEATING

It is conceivable that the reason why low-frequency skin stimuli that primarily activate rapidly adapting mechanoreceptors have excitatory influences on areas 3b and 1, whereas stimuli that activate skin nociceptors exert an inhibitory influence on these cortical areas, is because these two modes of skin stimulation differentially activate the dual thalamocortical projection systems (described in the previous section) that terminate in areas 3b and 1. The problem with this explanation is that both the projection to the middle layers of areas 3b and 1 (from the rod domains of VPL and VPM, conveying stimulus-evoked mechanoreceptor afferent drive) and the projection to layers I–II of areas 3b and 1 (from the matrix domain of the dorsal thalamus, conveying nociceptive afferent drive) are excitatory. Also, both projections target pyramidal cell dendrites. Thus, the vigorous activation of the projection to the upper layers, which according to recent neuroanatomical evidence should be evoked by noxious skin heating, does not, at first glance, fit with the decrease in area 3b/1 absorbance that our OIS imaging studies detected routinely in response to noxious skin heating.

A deeper consideration of cortical intrinsic circuitry, however, reveals a possible explanation. The axons of the two major types of local inhibitory cells in the upper layers of the somatosensory cortex terminate on the cell bodies and initial segments of pyramidal cells. Axons of these cells, known as basket and chandelier cells (Jones 1975), either have no synaptic contacts with other inhibitory cells (as is the case for chandelier cells) or terminate only on the dendrites of inhibitory neurons (as is characteristic of basket cells). This differential pattern of local intracortical synaptic termination could enable the strong and sustained excitatory thalamocortical input to the upper layers evoked by repetitive noxious skin heating to vigorously activate the highly responsive inhibitory cells in the upper layers. If this were so, the result would be a suppression of neuronal activity in areas 3b and 1. Unfortunately, there is no direct evidence for this or any other explanation of how the activity of these areas is supported during noxious skin heating.

CONCLUSIONS

The evidence obtained in experiments that have used the OIS imaging method, either alone or in combination with neurophysiological recording approaches, conflicts fundamentally with the long-held idea that activity in areas 3b and 1 subserves the sensory-discriminative aspects of cutaneous pain perception. Instead, this new evidence, together with recent neuroanatomical observations, strongly implies that it is area 3a (or at least a subregion of area 3a), and not areas 3b and 1, that plays the major role in the S1 signaling of the intensity and spatial attributes of a noxious skin-heating stimulus.

A study of the effects of intracortical microstimulation (Yezierski et al. 1983; see Figs. 8 and 9 in their paper) foreshadowed the recent OIS imaging and neurophysiological observations in suggesting the outlines of a pain information processing system to which areas 3a, 3b, and 1 each make an important but very different contribution. Consistent with our OIS imaging studies, Yezierski and colleagues detected a prominent functional discontinuity in the monkey S1 cortex. In particular, their 1983 study demonstrated that intracortical microstimulation at loci posterior to the transition between areas 3b and area 3a exerts predominantly *inhibitory* effects on WDR-type neurons of the dorsal horn spinothalamic tract that exhibit response wind-up during repetitive noxious skin stimulation. Microstimulation anterior to this transition (in areas 3a and 4) has the opposite effect—it *facilitates* the responses of the WDR-type dorsal horn neurons to nociceptive stimuli.

This finding of Yezierski et al. (1983), together with both the neuroanatomical tracing evidence of A.D. Craig, Jr., and coworkers and the OIS imaging evidence of Tommerdahl and colleagues (1996a, 1998), suggests that the natural activation of area 3a by noxious skin heating, like direct activation of area 3a by electrical microstimulation, enhances the excitability of the cells of origin of the major projection pathways that subserve pain and temperature sensibility (i.e., the trigemino- and spinothalamic tracts). We propose that a positive feedback loop exists between area 3a and the WDR-type neurons in the spinal dorsal horn. If so, whenever area 3a neurons are activated by input from skin noci-thermoreceptors (as indicated by the data of A.D. Craig, Jr., and coworkers as well as the OIS imaging and neurophysiological observations of Tommerdahl et al. 1996a, 1998), operation of this loop would have the following consequences. First, the corticofugal influences of area 3a activity would enhance the response of the WDR-type dorsal horn neurons to subsequent noxious skin stimulation. Second, the corticopetal influences of the facilitated nociceptive dorsal horn neuron activity would further increase the already elevated activity of the contralateral area 3a. Consistent with such a positive feedback loop, Tommerdahl et al. (1996a, 1998) reported prominent temporal summation in area 3a of the optical and single-neuron response to repetitive skin heating. A mechanism of this type would have obvious and important survival value if we are correct in assuming that it is the magnitude of the response in the part of area 3a that responds during noxious stimulation that encodes the intensity of the pain (second pain?) experience. By this mechanism, the initial response that signals the presence of environmental stimuli that may cause skin damage could rapidly, but reversibly, increase the system's sensitivity to subsequent noxious stimulation.

The inhibitory effect of area 3b/1 microstimulation on nociceptive spinal dorsal horn neurons (Yezierski et al. 1983) predicts that skin stimuli that preferentially activate areas 3b and 1 (e.g., flutter-vibratory stimuli) should have corticofugal influences that would actively inhibit the responses of the WDR-type nociceptive dorsal horn neurons. This inhibitory effect would reduce the input to area 3a neurons that is evoked by noxious skin stimulation. The effect of 200-Hz skin vibration on area 3a optical activity (a decrease in absorbance) that Tommerdahl et al. (1998, 1999a,b) demonstrated with the OIS imaging method appears compatible with this prediction. The effects of such stimulation on spike discharge activity of neurons of area 3a remain to be demonstrated. To this end, we are conducting combined single-neuron and OIS imaging studies. In addition, OIS imaging evidence indicates a symmetrical interaction pattern in response to noxious skin heating: Tommerdahl et al. (1996a, 1998) have shown that areas 3b and 1 are suppressed, while area 3a is activated, by noxious skin heating. This interaction is predicted to influence the capacity to detect vibrotactile stimuli in a manner comparable to that achieved by operation of the "touch gate" demonstrated by Apkarian et al. (1994). Experiments designed to obtain direct neurophysiological evidence for this possibility also are underway in our laboratory.

Fig. 15 schematically summarizes the major peripheral and central neuroanatomical ingredients of the pain-information-processing system suggested by the evidence described above. The figure identifies the different modulatory influences exerted on the spinal dorsal horn by the differential corticofugal activities that may accompany non-noxious mechanical and noxious skin-heating stimulation.

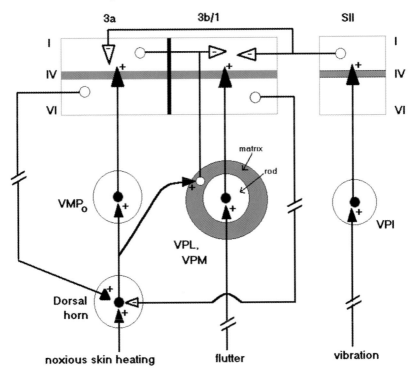

Fig. 15. Schematic summary of connectional mechanisms proposed to underlie (1) the differential responses of contralateral S1 to same-site, non-noxious vibrotactile stimulation (flutter or vibration) versus noxious skin heating, and (2) the centrifugal effects of those responses on spinothalamic tract (WDR) neurons in the spinal dorsal horn. A plus or minus sign associated with an arrow indicates the effect (increase, decrease) of that input on the level of activity in and/or on the responsivity of the targeted structure (e.g., on area 3a cell columns). The ventroposterior lateral (VPL) and medial (VPM) thalamic nuclei consist of "matrix" (gray shading) and "rod" domains (no shading); cortical layer 4 also is indicated by shading.

None of the OIS imaging and single-neuron recording evidence substantiates the widely held idea that S1 does *not* contribute to the affective/motivational aspects of pain. However, given the extensive system of corticocortical connections that arise in and return to area 3a (e.g., DeFelipe et al. 1986; Burton and Fabri 1995), it seems plausible that alterations in the activity of area 3a might have considerable impact on the activity of multiple cortical regions known to be important to both affect and motivation. From this perspective, it seems possible that this component of the "traditional" view of S1 in pain information processing also may require significant revision or perhaps even outright rejection. At the very least, this component of the "traditional view" of S1 in pain processing needs to be evaluated more directly and objectively, given the newly available information about thalamocortical and corticocortical connectivity and about how the S1 response to noxious stimulation is altered by selective interruption of the dorsal column or spinothalamic tracts. High-resolution imaging and neurophysiological studies in conscious, behaving subjects also are needed to demonstrate the simultaneous responses of S1 and other regions in the same hemisphere to noxious stimulation. Until such results are available, it would be premature to reject the possibility that S1 activity may contribute significantly to the affective-motivational aspects of pain.

ACKNOWLEDGMENTS

We gratefully acknowledge the technical contributions of Mrs. Carol B. Metz and Mr. Calvin Wong. Dr. E.F. Kelly of the University of North Carolina School of Dentistry provided valuable discussion of the ideas and experimental observations and contributed importantly to their presentation in this chapter. Partial support to B.L. Whitsel was provided by NIH grant RO1 NS34979; M. Tommerdahl was supported in part by NIH First Investigator Award R29 NS32358.

REFERENCES

Apkarian AV. Functional imaging of pain: new insights regarding the role of the cerebral cortex in human pain perception. *Semin Neurosci* 1995a; 7:279–293.

Apkarian AV. Thalamic anatomy and physiology of pain perception: connectivity, somatovisceral convergence, and spatiotemporal dynamics of nociceptive information coding. In: Besson JM (Ed). *Forebrain Mechanisms of Pain*. New York: John Libby, 1995b, pp 93–118.

Apkarian AV. Primary somatosensory cortex and pain. *Pain Forum* 1996; 5:188–191.

Apkarian AV, Stea RA, Bolanowski SJ. Heat-induced pain diminishes vibrotactile perception: a touch gate. *Somatosens Mot Res* 1994; 11:259–267.

Armstrong-James M. The nature and plasticity of sensory processing within adult rat barrel cortex. In: Jones EG, Diamond IT (Eds). *The Barrel Cortex in Rodents,* Cerebral Cortex, Vol. 11. New York: Plenum Press, 1995, pp 333–373.

Backonja MM. Primary somatosensory cortex and pain perception. *Pain Forum* 1996; 5:174–180.

Bonhoeffer T, Grinvald A. Optical imaging based on intrinsic signals: the methodology. In: Toga AW, Mazziotta JC (Eds). *Brain Mapping: The Methods.* New York: Academic Press, Inc., 1996, pp 55–97.

Bruggemann J, Shi T, Apkarian AV. Squirrel monkey lateral thalamus. II. Viscero-somatic convergent representation of urinary bladder, colon, and esophagus. *J Neurosci* 1994; 14:6796–6814.

Bruggemann J, Shi T, Apkarian AV. Viscero-somatic neurons in the primary somatosensory cortex (SI) of the squirrel monkey. *Brain Res* 1997; 756:297–300.

Burton H, Fabri M. Ipsilateral intracortical connections of physiologically defined cutaneous representations in areas 3b and 1 of macaque monkeys: projections in the vicinity of the central sulcus. *J Comp Neurol* 1995; 355:508–538.

Bushnell MC, Duncan GH, Hofbauer RK, et al. Pain perception: is there a role for primary somatosensory cortex? *Proc Natl Acad Sci USA* 1999; 96:7705–7709.

Caselli RJ. Primary somatosensory cortex, cortical somatosensory networks, and cortical somatosensory functions. *Pain Forum* 1996; 5:184–187.

Casey KL. Forebrain mechanisms of nociception and pain: analysis through imaging. *Proc Natl Acad Sci* 1999; 96:7668–7674.

Clements JA, Nimmo WS. Pharmacokinetics and analgesic effect of ketamine in man. *Br J Anaesth* 1991; 53:805–810.

Cohen LB. Changes in neuron structure during action potential propagation and synaptic transmission. *Physiol Rev* 1973; 53:373–418.

Craig AD Jr. Supraspinal pathways and mechanisms relevant to central pain. In: Casey K (Ed). *Pain and Central Nervous System Disease: The Central Pain Syndromes.* New York: Raven Press, 1991, pp 157–170.

Craig AD Jr. Supraspinal projections of lamina I neurons. In: Besson JM (Ed). *Forebrain Processing of Pain.* New York: Libby, 1995, pp 16–36.

Craig AD Jr. Pain, temperature and the sense of the body. In: Franzen O, Johansson R, Terenius L (Eds). *Somesthesis and the Neurobiology of Somatosensory Cortex.* Basel: Birkhauser Verlag, 1996, pp 27–39.

Craig AD Jr, Kniffki KD. Spino-thalamo-cortical mechanisms of nociception. In: Sharma KN, Nayar U (Eds). *Current Trends in Pain Research and Therapy,* Vol. 1. New Delhi: Indian Society for Pain Research and Therapy, 1996.

Craig AD Jr, Bushnell MC, Zhang E-T, Blomqvist A. A thalamic nucleus specific for pain and temperature sensation. *Nature* 1994; 372:770–773.

DeFelipe J, Conley M, Jones EG. Long-range focal collateralization of axons arising from corticocortical cells in monkey sensory-motor cortex. *J Neurosci* 1986; 6:3749–3766.

Dray A, Urban L. New pharmacological strategies for pain relief. *Annu Rev Pharmacol Toxicol* 1996; 36:253–280.

Dreyer DA, Metz C, Schneider R, Whitsel BL. Differential contributions of spinal pathways to the body representation in the postcentral gyrus of *Macaca mulatta. J Neurophysiol* 1974; 37:119–145.

Duncan GH, Dreyer DA, McKenna TM, Whitsel BL. Dose- and time-dependent effects of ketamine on SI neurons with cutaneous receptive fields. *J Neurophysiol* 1982; 47:677–699.

Duncan GH, Kupers RC, Marchland S, et al. Stimulation of human thalamus for pain relief: possible modulatory circuits revealed by positron emission tomography. *J Neurophysiol* 1998; 80:3326–3330.

Dykes RW, Sur M, Merzenich MM, Kaas JH, Nelson RJ. Regional segregation of neurons responding to quickly adapting, slowly adapting, deep and Pacinian receptors within thalamic ventroposterior lateral and ventroposterior inferior nuclei in the squirrel monkey (*Saimiri sciureus*). *Neuroscience* 1981; 6:1687–1692.

Eide PK, Jorum E, Stubhaug A, Bremnes J, Breivik H. Relief of post-herpetic neuralgia with the N-methyl-D-aspartic acid receptor antagonist ketamine: a double-blind, cross-over comparison with morphine and placebo. *Pain* 1994; 58:347–354.

Ekblom A, Hansson P. Effects of conditioning vibratory stimulation on pain threshold of the human tooth. *Acta Physiol Scand* 1982; 114:601–604.

Ekblom A, Hansson P. Extrasegmental transcutaneous electrical nerve stimulation and mechanical vibratory stimulation as compared to placebo for the relief of acute orofacial pain. *Pain* 1985; 23:223–229.

Felsby S, Nielsen J, Arendt-Nielsen L, Jensen TS. Effect of NMDA receptor antagonism with ketamine and magnesium chloride in chronic neuropathic pain. *Pain* 1996; 64:283–291.

Grinvald A. Real-time optical mapping of neuronal activity: from single growth cones to the intact mammalian brain. *Annu Rev Neurosci* 1985; 8:263–305.

Grinvald A, Frostig RD, Lieke E, Hildesheim R. Optical imaging of neuronal activity. *Physiol Rev* 1988; 68:1285–1366.

Grinvald A, Bonhoeffer T, Malonek D, et al. Optical imaging of architecture and function in the living brain. In: Squire L, Weinberger N, Lynch G, McGaugh J (Eds). *Memory Organization and Locus of Change*. New York: Oxford University Press, 1991, pp 49–85.

Grinvald A, Lieke EE, Frostig RD, Hildesheim R. Cortical spread-point function and long-range lateral interactions revealed by real-time optical imaging of macaque monkey primary visual cortex. *J Neurosci* 1994; 14:2545–2568.

Hagiwara K, Tsmuoto T, Sato H, Hata Y. Actions of amino acid antagonists on geniculo-cortical transmission in the cat's visual cortex. *Brain Res* 1988; 69:407–416.

Haglund MM, Ojemann GA, Blasdel GG. Optical imaging of bipolar cortical stimulation. *J Neurosurg* 1993; 78:785–793.

Head H, Holmes G. Sensory disturbances from cerebral lesions. *Brain* 1911; 34:102–254.

Hendry SHC, Jones EG. Activity dependent regulation of GABA expression in the visual cortex of adult monkeys. *Neuron* 1988; 1:701–712.

Holthoff K, Witte OW. Intrinsic optical signals measured with near-infrared dark-field microscopy reveals changes in extracellular space. *J Neurosci* 1996; 16:2740–2749.

Jain N, Catania KC, Kaas JH. Deactivation and reactivation of somatosensory cortex after dorsal spinal cord injury. *Nature* 1997; 386:495–498.

Jones EG. Varieties and distribution of non-pyramidal cells in the somatosensory cortex of the squirrel monkey. *J Comp Neurol* 1975; 16:205–267.

Jones EG. Transmitter chemistry in the somatosensory thalamus. In: Casey KL (Ed). *Pain and Central Nervous System Disease: The Central Pain Syndromes*. New York: Raven Press, 1991, pp 201–218.

Jones EG. Viewpoint: the core and matrix of thalamic organization. *Neuroscience* 1998; 85:331–345.

Jones EG, Porter R. What is area 3a? *Brain Res Rev* 1980; 2:1–43.

Kaas JH, Nelson RJ, Sur M, Lin CS, Merzenich MM. Multiple representations of the body within the primary somatosensory cortex of primates. *Science* 1979; 204:521–523.

Kenshalo DR Jr. Pain and the primary somatosensory cortex. *Pain Forum* 1996; 5:181–183.

Kenshalo DR Jr, Giesler GJ, Leonard RB, Willis WD. Responses of neurons in primate ventral posterior lateral nucleus to noxious stimuli. *J Neurophysiol* 1980; 43:1594–1614.

Kenshalo DR Jr, Isensee O. Responses of primate SI cortical neurons to noxious stimuli. *J Neurophysiol* 1983; 50:1479–1496.

Kenshalo DR Jr, Chudler EH, Anton F, Dubner R. SI cortical nociceptive neurons participate in the encoding process by which monkeys perceive the intensity of noxious thermal stimulation. *Brain Res* 1988; 460:281–296.

Kenshalo DR Jr, Thomas DA, Dubner R. Somatosensory cortex lesions change the monkey's reaction to noxious stimulation. *J Dent Res Abstr* 1989; 68:649–661.

Kenshalo DR Jr, Willis WD Jr. The role of the cerebral cortex in pain sensation. In: Peters A, Jones EG (Eds). *Normal and Altered States of Function, Cerebral Cortex*, Vol. 9. New York: Plenum Press, 1991, pp 153–212.

Kleist K. Kreigsverletzungen des Gehirns in ihrer Bedeutung fur die Hirnlokalisation und Hirnpathologie. In: von Schjerning O (Ed). *Handbuch der ärztlichen Erfahrungen im Weltkriege 1914–1918.* Geiste und Nervenkrankheiten, Vol. 4. Leipzig: Barth, 1934, pp 343–1393.

Kohn A, Whitsel BL. Dynamic, stimulus-driven changes in functional cortical connectivity: a mechanism for the temporal integration of sensory information. In: Franzen O (Ed). *Brain Mechanisms of Tactile Perception,* Wenner-Gren International Symposium Series. Basel: Birkhauser Verlag, 2000, in press.

Kohn A, Pinheiro A, Tommerdahl MA, Whitsel BL. Optical imaging *in vitro* provides evidence for the minicolumnar nature of cortical response. *Neuroreport* 1997; 8:3513–3518.

Kohn A, Metz C, Quibrera M, Tommerdahl M, Whitsel BL. Functional neocortical circuitry recorded with intrinsic signal optical imaging *in vitro. Neuroscience* 1999; 95:51–62.

Kohn A, Whitsel BL, Metz CB. Stimulus-evoked modulation of sensorimotor pyramidal neuron EPSPs. *Neuron* 2000; in press.

Larkum ME, Zhu JJ, Sakmann B. A new cellular mechanism for coupling inputs arriving at different cortical layers. *Nature* 1999; 398:338–341.

Lebedev MA, Nelson RJ. High-frequency vibratory sensory neurons in monkey primary somatosensory cortex: entrained and non-entrained responses to vibration during the performance of vibratory-cued hand movements. *Exp Brain Res* 1996; 111:313–325.

Lieke EE, Frostig RD, Arieli A, et al. Optical imaging of cortical activity: real-time imaging using extrinsic dye-signals and high resolution imaging based on slow intrinsic signals. *Annu Rev Physiol* 1989; 51:543–559.

Liang F, Isackson PJ, Jones EG. Stimulus-dependent, reciprocal up- and down-regulation of glutamic acid decarboxylase and Ca^{++}/calmodulin-dependent protein kinase II expression in rat cerebral cortex. *Exp Brain Res* 1996; 110:163–174.

Lundeberg, T. The pain suppressive effect of vibratory stimulation and transcutaneous electrical nerve stimulation (TENS) as compared to aspirin. *Brain Res* 1984; 294:201–209.

Lundeberg T, Nordemar R, Ottoson D. Pain alleviation by vibratory stimulation. *Pain* 1984; 20:25–44.

MacVicar BA, Hochman D. Imaging of synaptically evoked intrinsic signals in hippocampal slices. *J Neurosci* 1991; 11:1458–1469.

Marshall J. Sensory disturbances in cortical wounds with special reference to pain. *J Neurol Neurosurg Psychiatr* 1951; 14:187–204.

Melzack R, Casey KL. Sensory, motivational and central control determinants of pain: a new conceptual model. In: Kenshalo DR (Ed). *The Skin Senses.* Springfield, IL: C.C. Thomas, 1968, pp 423–443.

Morgenstern FS, Beech HR, Davies BM. An investigation of drug induced sensory disturbances. *Psychopharmacologica* 1962; 3:193–201.

Mountcastle VB. Central nervous mechanisms in mechanoreceptive sensibility. In: *The Nervous System: Sensory Processes,* Handbook of Physiology, Vol. III. Bethesda, MD: American Physiological Association, 1984, pp 789–878.

Mountcastle VB, Talbot WH, Sakata H, Hyvarinen H. Cortical neuronal mechanisms in flutter vibration studied in unanesthetized monkeys: neuronal periodicity and frequency discrimination. *J Neurophysiol* 1969; 32:452–484.

Narayan SM, Santori EM, Toga AW. Mapping functional activity in rodent cortex using optical intrinsic signals. *Cereb Cortex* 1994; 4:195–204.

Nathan PW, Smith MC, Cook AW. Sensory effects in man of lesions of the posterior columns and of some other afferent pathways. *Brain* 1986; 109:1003–1041.

Nikolajsen L, Hansen CL, Nielsen J, et al. The effect of ketamine on phantom pain: a central neuropathic disorder maintained by peripheral input. *Pain* 1996; 67:69–77.

Peele TL. Acute and chronic parietal lobe ablations in monkeys. *J Neurophysiol* 1944; 7:269–286.

Penfield W, Boldrey E. Somatic motor and sensory representation in the cerebral cortex of man as studied by electrical stimulation. *Brain* 1937; 60:389–443.

Penny R, Itoh K, Diamond IT. Cell size in the ventral nuclei and layers of the somatic cortex in the cat. *Brain Res* 1982; 242:55–65.

Perl ER. Pain and nociception. In: *The Nervous System: Sensory Processes,* Handbook of Physiology, Vol. III. Washington, DC: American Physiological Society, 1984, pp 915–975.

Pertovaara A. Modification of human pain threshold by specific tactile receptors. *Acta Physiol Scand* 1979; 107:339–341.

Price DD, Hu JW, Dubner R, Gracely RH. Peripheral suppression of first pain and central summation of second pain evoked by noxious heat pulses. *Pain* 1977; 3:57–68.

Price DD, McHaffie JG, Stein BE. The psychophysical attributes of heat-induced pain and their relationships to neural mechanisms. *J Cogn Neurosci* 1992; 4:1–14.

Rainville P, Duncan GH, Price DD, Carrier B, Bushnell MC. Pain affect encoded in human anterior cingulate but not somatosensory cortex. *Science* 1997; 277:968–971.

Rausell E, Jones EG. Histochemical and immunocytochemical compartments of the thalamic VPM nucleus in monkeys and their relationship to the representational map. *J Neurosci* 1991a; 11:210–225.

Rausell E, Jones EG. Chemically distinct compartments of the thalamic VPM nucleus in monkeys relay principal and spinal trigeminal pathways to different layers of the somatosensory cortex. *J Neurosci* 1991b; 11:226–237.

Rausell E, Bae CS, Vinuela A, Huntley GW, Jones EG. Calbindin and parvalbumin cells in monkey VPL nucleus: distribution, laminar cortical projections, and relations to spinothalamic terminations. *J Neurosci* 1992; 12:4088–4111.

Roland P. Cortical representation of pain. *Trends Neurosci* 1992; 15:3–5.

Roppolo JR, Werner G, Whitsel BL, Dreyer DA, Petrucelli LM. Phencyclidine (PCP) actions on neural mechanisms of somesthesis. *Neuropharmacology* 1973; 12:417–431.

Russell WR. Transient disturbances following gunshot wounds of the head. *Brain* 1945; 68:79–97.

Salt TE, Meier CL, Seno N, Krucker T, Heerling PL. Thalamocortical and corticocortical excitatory postsynaptic potentials mediated by excitatory amino acid receptors in the cat motor cortex *in vivo. Neuroscience* 1995; 64:433–442.

Schiller J, Major G, Koester HJ, Schiller Y. NMDA spikes in basal dendrites of cortical pyramidal neurons. *Nature* 2000; 404:285–289.

Shi T, Stevens RT, Tessier J, Apkarian AV. Spinothalamocortical inputs nonpreferentially innervate the superficial and deep cortical layers of SI. *Neurosci Lett* 1993; 160:209–213.

Sur M, Nelson RJ, Kaas JH. Representations of the body surface in cortical areas 3b and 1 of squirrel monkeys: comparisons with other primates. *J Comp Neurology* 1982; 211:177–192.

Tommerdahl M, Whitsel BL. Optical imaging of intrinsic signals in somatosensory cortex. In: Franzen O, Johansson R, Terenius L (Eds). *Somesthesis and the Neurobiology of Somatosensory Cortex.* Basel: Birkhauser Verlag, 1996, pp 369–384.

Tommerdahl M, Delemos KD, Vierck CJ Jr, Favorov OV, Whitsel BL. Anterior parietal cortical response to tactile and skin-heating stimuli applied to the same skin site. *J Neurophysiol* 1996a; 75:2662–2670.

Tommerdahl M, Whitsel BL, Vierck CJ Jr. Effects of spinal dorsal column transection on the response of monkey anterior parietal cortex to repetitive skin stimulation. *Cereb Cortex* 1996b; 6:131–155.

Tommerdahl M, Delemos KA, Favorov OV. Response of anterior parietal cortex to different modes of same-site skin stimulation. *J Neurophysiol* 1998; 80:3272–3283.

Tommerdahl M, Delemos KD, Whitsel BL, Favorov OV, Metz CB. Response of anterior parietal cortex to cutaneous flutter versus vibration. *J Neurophysiol* 1999a; 82:1982–1992.

Tommerdahl M, Whitsel BL, Favorov OV, Metz CB, O'Quinn BL. Responses of contralateral SI and SII in cat to same-site cutaneous flutter vs. vibration. *J Neurophysiol* 1999b; 82:1982–1992.

Treede R-D, Kenshalo DR, Gracely RH, Jones AKP. The cortical representation of pain. *Pain* 1999; 79:105–111.

Vierck C J Jr, Cohn RH, Cooper B. Effects of spinal lesions on temporal resolution of cutaneous sensations. *Somatosens Mot Res* 1985; 3:45–56.

Vierck CJ Jr, Whitsel BL, Kulics A, Cooper B. Alterations of a cortical network of neurons following interruption of the dorsal spinal columns. In: Seil F (Ed). *Advances in Neural Regeneration Research,* Proceedings of the 3rd International Symposium, Neurology and Neurobiology. New York: Wiley-Liss, 1990a, pp 335–368.

Vierck CJ Jr, Whitsel BL, Makous J, Friedman R. Effects of a dorsal spinal lesion on temporal discriminations and on physiological responses of primate S-I cortex. *Neurosci Abstracts* 1990b; 16:1081.

Vierck CJ Jr, Cannon RI, Fry G, Maixner W, Whitsel B. Characteristics of temporal summation of second pain sensations elicited by brief contact of glabrous skin by a preheated thermode. *J Neurophysiol* 1997; 78:992–1002.

Vnek N, Ramsden BM, Hung CP, Goldman-Rakic PS, Roe AW. Optical imaging of functional domains in the cortex of the awake and behaving monkey. *Proc Natl Acad Sci* 1999; 96:4057–4060.

Willis WD. From nociceptor to cortical activity. In: Bromm B, Desmedt JE (Eds). *Pain and the Brain: From Nociception to Cognition,* Advances in Pain Research and Therapy, Vol. 22. New York: Raven Press, 1995a, pp 1–19.

Willis WD. Cold, pain and the brain. *Nature* 1995b; 373:19–20.

Willis WD, Westland KN. Neuroanatomy of the pain system and of the pathways that modulate pain. *J Clin Neurophysiol* 1997; 14(1):2–31.

Whitsel BL, Petrucelli LM, Sapiro G. Modality representation in the fasciculus gracilis of the squirrel monkey. *Brain Res* 1969; 15:67–78.

Whitsel BL, Dreyer DA, Roppolo JR. Determinants of body representation in the postcentral gyrus of macaques. *J Neurophysiol* 1971; 34:1018–1034.

Whitsel BL, Favorov O, Tommerdahl M, et al. Dynamic processes govern the somatosensory cortical response to natural stimulation. In: Lund LS (Ed) *Sensory Processing in the Mammalian Brain: Neural Substrates and Experimental Strategies.* New York: Oxford University Press, 1989, pp 84–116.

Whitsel BL, Favorov O, Kelly DG, Tommerdahl M. Mechanisms of dynamic peri- and intra-columnar interactions in somatosensory cortex: Stimulus-specific contrast enhancement by NMDA receptor activation. In: Franzen O, Westman J (Eds). *Information Processing in the Somatosensory System.* New York: Stockton Press, 1991, pp 353–369.

Whitsel BL, Favorov OV, Delemos KD. SI neuron response variability is stimulus tuned and NMDA receptor dependent. *J Neurophysiol* 1999a; 81:2988–3006.

Whitsel BL, Kelly EF, Delemos KD, Xu M, Quibrera PM. Entrainment and responsivity of cat and monkey rapidly adapting (RA) skin afferents. *Somatosens Mot Res* 1999b; 17:13–31.

Yezierski RP, Gerhart KD, Schrock BJ, Willis WD. A further examination of effects of cortical stimulation on primate spinothalamic tract cells. *J Neurophysiol* 1983; 49:424–441.

Correspondence to: Barry L. Whitsel, PhD, CB7545, School of Medicine, University of North Carolina, Chapel Hill, NC 27599-7545, USA. Tel: 919-966-1291; Fax: 919-966-6927; email: bwhitsel@med.unc.edu.

Pain Imaging, Progress in Pain Research and
Management, Vol. 18, edited by Kenneth L.
Casey and M. Catherine Bushnell, IASP Press,
Seattle, © 2000.

4

Brain Activation Studies Using PET and SPECT: Execution and Analysis

Satoshi Minoshima,[a,b] Donna J. Cross,[a,b] Robert A. Koeppe,[a] and Kenneth L. Casey[b,c,d]

[a]Department of Internal Medicine, [b]Neuroscience Program, and Departments of [c]Neurology and [d]Physiology, The University of Michigan Medical School, Ann Arbor, Michigan, USA

Positron emission tomography (PET) and single photon emission computed tomography (SPECT) can measure various physiological and neurochemical indices of brain function. In the early 1980s, PET and ^{18}F-fluorodeoxyglucose (FDG) studies demonstrated an increased cerebral metabolic rate of glucose (CMRglc) in the occipital cortex of awake humans in response to visual stimulation (Phelps et al. 1981). Tomographic imaging permitted visualization of cerebral activities in three dimensions and provided a new exciting research tool to investigate human brain activity. The FDG method has two major limitations, however. The use of a radioisotope that has a relatively long half-life (^{18}F, 110 minutes) does not permit repeated scanning of the same subject within a short time interval. Thus, it is difficult to obtain repeat scans under different stimulus or task conditions on the same day. In addition, the fixation of radiotracer uptake within the brain takes at least 10 minutes, during which time the stimulation or task must be constant. The use of a radiotracer with a shorter half-life, such as ^{15}O-labeled water or gas, overcomes these limitations (Fox et al. 1984). The use of radiolabeled water is based on the assumption that changes in regional neuronal activities are tightly coupled with those in regional cerebral blood flow (rCBF) and CMRglc under physiological conditions (Sokoloff 1978; Tsubokawa et al. 1980; Collins et al. 1986; Frostig et al. 1990; Narayan et al. 1995) (Plate 1; see also Chapter 2). Thus, the detection of changes in rCBF can localize changes in neuronal activities associated with stimuli or tasks given to the subject during imaging. In fact, this approach, commonly

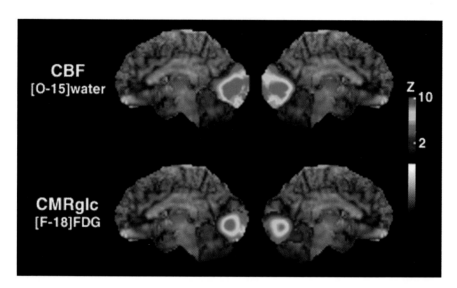

Plate 1. Coupling between regional glucose metabolism and blood flow responding to neuronal excitation. Visual stimulation (reversing checkerboard) was administered to subjects by a computer screen placed in the PET scanner gantry. Cerebral blood flow (CBF) was measured using ^{15}O-water, and cerebral glucose metabolism (CMRglc) was measured using ^{18}F-fluorodeoxyglucose (FDG). Data were analyzed stereotactically, and subtraction images (visual stimulation minus baseline) were averaged over four subjects. Both CMRglc and CBF images (medial views of the brain) demonstrate similar activation in the primary visual cortex of the occipital lobe, although CBF changes appear to be more extensive. Stereotactic coordinates of peak CMRglc and CBF changes were $(-6, -78, 2)$ and $(-6, -80, 0)$, respectively (millimetric coordinates, x, y, and z represent right-to-left, posterior-to-anterior, and inferior-to-posterior of the brain with positive coordinates for left, anterior, and superior). Magnitudes of peak CMRglc and CBF changes were 34.8% and 31.2%, respectively, relative to the global activity. These findings support coupling of increased neuronal activity, CMRglc, and CBF in human brains under physiological conditions.

known as a "brain activation study," was reported long before PET techniques became available (Ingvar and Risberg 1967). Because of the shorter half-life of [15]O (124 seconds), rCBF imaging can be repeated after an interval of several minutes. Image acquisition lasts from 40 to 90 seconds depending on the protocol. Investigators can perform various control and stimulus/task conditions within the same subject to test research hypotheses. Brain activation studies using ^{15}O-labeled radiotracers and PET imaging became one of the most widely applied techniques for the investigation of human brain physiology and pathophysiology prior to the emergence of functional magnetic resonance imaging (fMRI). The advantages of PET, such as non-invasiveness, known relation between signals and physiological mechanisms, uniform sensitivity throughout the brain, and established methodology, outweigh certain methodological limitations. The use of brain activation techniques has significantly advanced our understanding of the cerebral processing of pain in humans (Jones et al. 1991; Talbot et al. 1991; Casey et al. 1994).

Image analysis techniques for functional brain imaging have evolved significantly with the widespread use of PET in activation studies. When activation studies were initially developed, early-generation PET scanners were capable of acquiring data in only two dimensions, and their sensitivity and spatial resolution were limited. It was impossible to consistently identify brain activities responding to stimuli or tasks within a single subject. To overcome this problem, researchers developed stereotactic image registration techniques (Fox et al. 1985; Friston et al. 1989; Minoshima et al. 1993b; Woods et al. 1998). In this approach, PET image sets from different subjects are transformed to a common coordinate system, and the image sets are averaged across subjects to increase signal-to-noise ratios. These methods have significantly advanced the field of tomographic brain image analysis.

This chapter will review the methodology and execution of brain activation studies involving PET and SPECT. However, we emphasize that PET instrumentation, experimental design, image acquisition, and data analysis and interpretation are all critical for optimal specificity and sensitivity in detecting and localizing task- or stimulus-specific rCBF and rCMRglc changes in humans.

OVERVIEW OF IMAGE ACQUISITION AND ANALYSIS

In general, brain activation studies employ experimental protocols that are optimized for subtraction analysis (task/stimulus minus baseline/control). The goal of the subtraction technique is to separate neuronal activities of interest from other activities associated with a task or stimulus condition. For example, if investigators are interested in the neuronal response to pain administered by a contact heat thermode, they can remove the tactile component by subtracting values from a control condition using the same thermode without the painful heat. Multiple image sets under task/stimulus or baseline conditions can be obtained in the same subject. Cerebral blood flow (CBF) typically is measured using diffusible agents for PET (e.g., ^{15}O-water, $C^{15}O_2$ gas, or ^{15}O-butanol) or trapping agents for SPECT (technetium-99m-d,l-hexamethylpropyleneamine oxime [^{99m}Tc-HMPAO] or technetium-99m-L,L-ethyl cysteinate dimer [^{99m}Tc-ECD]). The radiotracer is administered intravenously while a subject is performing a task or being stimulated, and images are acquired subsequently. Use of shorter-lived radiotracers such as ^{15}O-labeled compounds allows investigators to perform repeat scans within a short interval (several minutes) in the same subject. This technique allows the acquisition of multiple image sets under either replicated or different physiological conditions in a single experimental session. Alternatively, CMRglc can be measured by PET using longer-lived radiotracers such as FDG; however, image sets under different conditions may need to be obtained on different days.

Following image acquisition, data are analyzed to detect changes in brain activities associated with stimuli or tasks given to the subject. A typical subtraction analysis of stimulus minus control conditions involves several steps (Fig. 1). *Intrasubject* image coregistration is done to correct for head motion across multiple image sets obtained within the same subject. Image sets are then transformed to a stereotactic coordinate system, and individual anatomical differences are minimized by an *intersubject* image registration technique. Following normalization of pixel values for each image set, a paired subtraction (stimulus minus control) is performed within each subject. Subtracted image sets from different subjects are averaged and converted to a statistical parametric map using estimated mean differences and variances for each pixel. An estimated statistical threshold defines areas of significant change in rCBF (activation) within the brain. Selection of a particular data analysis method depends on the experimental design and hypotheses. There are many variations in the specific implementation of the data analysis routines for activation studies, but many techniques depend on the procedures outlined in Fig. 1. Because of the improved spatial resolution and sensitivity of a modern SPECT scanner, sets of paired images (task/stimulus and control/baseline) from both PET and SPECT scanners can be analyzed in a similar manner. However, PET ^{15}O-water studies generally

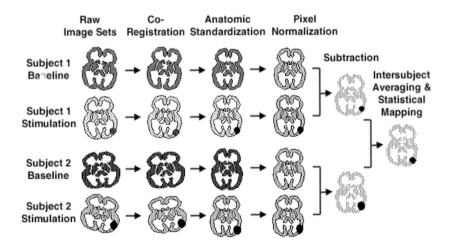

Fig. 1. General scheme of image analysis for PET activation studies.

allow more repetitions within each subject, and thus provide more statistically robust results.

RADIOTRACERS AND IMAGE ACQUISITION

The aim of an activation study is to identify and localize regional neuronal activities that respond to a particular task or stimulus. PET and SPECT imaging is based on an assumption of general coupling of neuronal activity, CBF, and CMRglc (Chapter 2) (Sokoloff 1978). When selecting a radiotracer or imaging modality, researchers should validate to what extent CBF and CMRglc will reflect neuronal activity within the planned experimental design. Certain pharmacological interventions used in activation studies may alter or even abolish coupling between neuronal activity and rCBF through direct effects on cerebral vasculature or modulatory mechanisms (Tsukada et al. 1997). Researchers thus should consider using a standard stimulus or task with a known activation response to estimate the extent of such uncoupling.

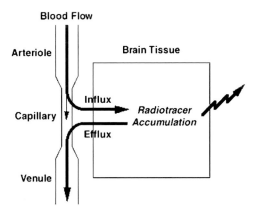

Fig. 2. Radiotracer accumulation in the brain. Under physiological conditions, regional blood flow is coupled with neuronal activities. Trapping-type radiotracers, such as ^{99m}Tc-HMPAO and ^{99m}Tc-ECD, have low efflux from the brain, so their accumulation in the brain is determined by the amount of influx that is proportional to regional blood flow. The longer accumulation of tracer in the brain permits imaging long after injection. Diffusible tracers, such as ^{15}O-water, have both influx to and efflux from the brain. The amount of radiotracer accumulation on PET images is determined by the overall influx and efflux during an imaging period. A complication occurs if regional blood flow changes during the imaging period. For example, if blood flow decreases during the imaging period, initial influx of a large amount of tracer stays within the brain because of decreased efflux. In contrast, an increase in blood flow during the imaging period decreases tracer accumulation due to greater efflux. The maintenance of stable neuronal activities (and stable regional blood flow) are essential for proper interpretation of results.

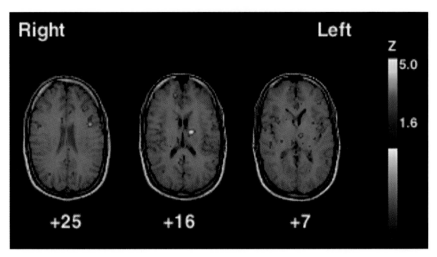

Plate 2. Pain activation localized with coregistered magnetic resonance images in a single subject. Tonic heat pain was given to the subject's right arm. PET images were obtained in 3-D data acquisition mode. Two pairs of baseline and tonic heat pain scans were obtained, and paired t statistical values (converted to Z values) were calculated on a pixel-by-pixel basis using a pooled variance. Significant focal activation ($P < 0.05$ corrected for multiple pixel comparisons) is seen in the region of the left anterior insula (slice 25 mm above the bicommissural line) and the anterolateral aspect of the left thalamus (16 mm above the bicommissural line).

Alternatively, glucose metabolic imaging may be used for a measurement of brain activities that is independent of blood flow changes. Researchers should also consider altered vascular responsiveness when comparing subjects with different age groups or patients with pathological cerebral vessels.

The technetium radiotracers used in SPECT imaging are considered trapping agents (agents that are trapped in capillaries relative to blood flow) (Fig. 2), although their kinetic behaviors differ from those of true microsphere-type agents (agents that accumulate in tissue "linearly" to blood flow) in the strictest sense. In general, these tracers enter the brain through cerebral capillaries during the first pass (when the initial bolus activity passes through the capillaries) and accumulate in proportion to regional blood flow. Once in the brain, their relative stability for a certain period means that SPECT imaging can be performed subsequently in a resting state. Thus, the task or stimulation can be given to a subject outside the SPECT scanner, and

Plate 3. Subtraction artifacts introduced by small head motions of approximately 2 mm between baseline scans (top row) and stimulation scans (tactile stimulus to the left arm, second row). Subtraction images without head motion correction (third row) show "rimlike" subtraction artifacts at the edge of the brain. After head motion correction (bottom row), the artifacts have disappeared, and activation in the right primary somatosensory cortex is detected (arrow). →

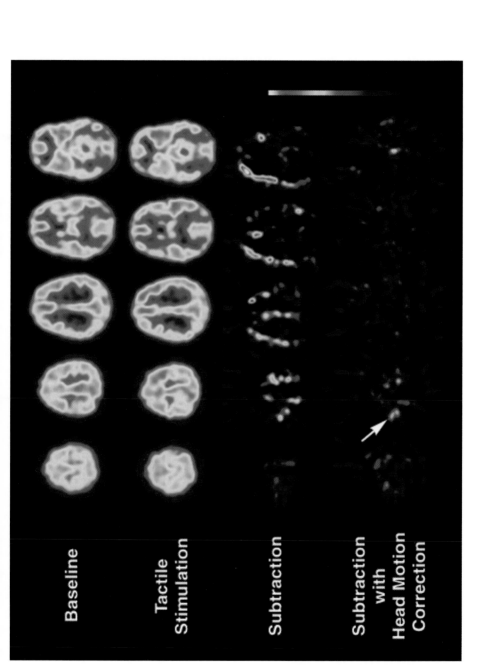

tracers can be injected under various physiological conditions. The resulting "snapshot" of neuronal activities at the time of injection permits a unique
experimental design. However, SPECT tracers have certain drawbacks. First,
because of a longer radionuclide half-life, only one scan, or two with dose
differentiation, can be obtained in a single day. Thus, task/baseline paired
scanning may require separate days. Second, limitations inherent in SPECT
imaging include lower sensitivity and spatial resolution compared to PET.
Third, the accumulation of ^{99m}Tc-HMPAO and ^{99m}Tc-ECD within the brain
does not correspond in a strictly linear fashion to rCBF. Radiotracer accumulation becomes attenuated in a high-flow area due to limited first pass
extraction and increased back-diffusion, leading to underestimates of the
magnitude of brain activation and limited sensitivity. Finally, although the
localization of these radiotracers is relatively stable after reaching the brain,
regional clearance of the tracer from the brain is not necessarily uniform
(Ishizu et al. 1996), and the timing of imaging after tracer accumulation
needs to be consistent from scan to scan and from subject to subject.

Diffusible radiotracers such as ^{15}O-water are used most commonly to
measure CBF in PET and in activation studies (Fig. 2). The tracer's shorter
half-life permits repeated administration within several minutes, allowing
multiple image acquisitions under different task/stimulus conditions in a
single experimental session—a significant advantage in comparison to SPECT
tracers or FDG. However, this diffusible nature creates additional complexity in data acquisition and interpretation, which is often overlooked in the
experimental design. In general, acquisition of each image for an ^{15}O-water
activation study takes approximately 1 minute. During this period, ^{15}O-wa-
ter diffuses into the brain tissue in proportion to regional blood flow (and
thus to regional neuronal activity), but then washes back out of the brain to
the blood. Overall summation of these activities for 1 minute determines the
pixel counts on a resultant PET image set. Problems can occur when the
neuronal activities associated with a task or stimulus are unstable within the
imaging period. For example, suppose that neurons in "structure A" are very
active at the beginning of image acquisition due to attention to the onset of
painful stimuli, but are less active toward the end. Within this region, blood
flow will be high at the beginning (coupled with neuronal activities), but
will decrease toward the end of the scanning. This instability results in
greater influx of the radiotracer from blood to brain at the beginning of
image acquisition when the plasma concentration of ^{15}O-water is still high.
Washout of radioactivity (back-diffusion from brain to blood), however,
decreases because of the attenuated blood flow toward the end of imaging.
Thus, more radioactivity stays in the brain tissue, resulting in higher pixel
counts on acquired PET images. In extreme cases, when stimulation is termi-

nated in the middle of image acquisition, PET activation signals may be enhanced significantly in this structure because reduced blood flow in the later part of image acquisition decreases the washout of radioactivity from the brain (Cherry et al. 1995). In contrast, if neuronal activities in "structure B" are increasing with time during image acquisition due to spatial and temporal summation of pain, there is a slower influx of radioactivity at the beginning and greater washout toward the end of scanning. The result is relatively lower pixel counts for "structure B" compared to "structure A," even when total neuronal activities are equal over the period of image acquisition. Consequently, "structure A" appears more active than "structure B" on resultant PET images, which can bias the interpretation of results, particularly in comparisons of multiple regions within the brain. This problem can be partly overcome by shortening the duration of imaging, but this will reduce image counts and thus diminish sensitivity. It is often difficult to assume a true physiological "steady" state throughout the brain during an image acquisition period. Task or stimulation paradigms must be designed carefully to minimize temporal changes in neuronal activities over the period of PET image acquisition. Even then, potential changes in neuronal activities during the image acquisition period must be considered when interpreting results. The finer temporal resolution of fMRI has a potential advantage in this regard, although it is still limited by the relatively slow hemodynamic responses to neuronal activation.

With ^{15}O-water activation studies, image acquisition begins approximately at the time the injected radiotracer arrives at the brain. By delaying the start of image acquisition several seconds after the arrival of radiotracer at the brain, investigators can avoid a large signal from initial radioactivity within the intravascular blood volume. Using a semi-bolus intravenous injection technique (injection of radiotracer over several seconds), the time lag between injection and arrival of radioactivity to the brain is approximately 20–30 seconds; this lag should be considered when timing the task or stimulation. As described previously, neuronal activities should be at steady state upon the arrival of radioactivity to the brain. Thus, the task or stimulation generally begins shortly after radiotracer injection and before image acquisition. When more precise timing is required, the time interval between injection and arrival at the brain can be determined using a small trial injection before starting experimental imaging.

Optimal image acquisition for ^{15}O-water PET activation studies is approximately 1 minute. Given the tradeoff between physical and physiological signals, different investigators have found slightly different optimal times (Kanno et al. 1991). A longer scanning time improves image quality by increasing cumulative counts, but physiological information is lost because

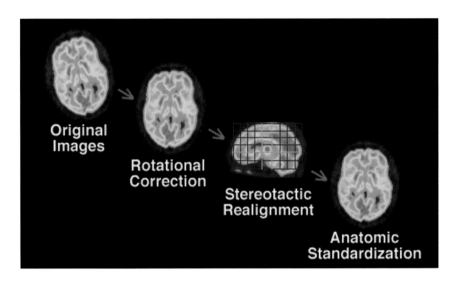

Plate 4. Stereotactic reorientation (reorienting the brain into a symmetrical position about the midsagittal plane and then into the orientation parallel to the bicommissural line) and anatomical standardization (minimizing individual anatomical differences by matching the shape of the brain to the standard atlas brain, while preserving functional information). Once the image set is standardized, image sets from different subjects can be analyzed consistently in the standard stereotactic space, and functional changes can be localized using stereotactic coordinates.

the radioactivity initially accumulated within the brain in proportion to neuronal activities is washed out and becomes more evenly distributed. For ^{99m}Tc-HMPAO and ^{99m}Tc-ECD, image acquisition typically begins several minutes to half an hour after radiotracer administration. Since these agents are trapped within the brain much longer than ^{15}O-water, the timing of imaging is less critical, but it should be consistent from scan to scan and from subject to subject because of slightly different regional washout ratios. Image acquisition typically takes 15–30 minutes depending on the sensitivity of the SPECT camera. With ^{18}F-FDG, image acquisition typically starts 30 minutes to 1 hour after radiotracer administration. However, physiological information obtained by this method is weighted toward the initial 10 minutes after radiotracer injection (Sokoloff et al. 1977; Ginsberg et al. 1988). Thus, it is critical to maintain the task or stimulation during this period. For ^{15}O-water and ^{18}F-FDG, CBF and CMRglc can be measured quantitatively using arterial blood sampling with or without serial dynamic imaging. This technique, particularly quantitative rCBF measurement, is not commonly used in brain activation studies because absolute CBF levels are modulated not only by neuronal activities but also by other physiological factors (see "Pixel (Data) Normalization," below).

Modern PET scanners can acquire images in three dimensions. In this mode, annihilating gamma rays emitted from positrons can be detected in all directions within the PET gantry, resulting in a significantly improved signal-to-noise ratio. This technique permits many repeat scans with a smaller dose of ^{15}O-water injection, which allows a single-subject statistical analysis (Plate 2). Due to an increase in scattered photons and in scanner "dead time" for a given dose, the estimated optimal amount of ^{15}O-water was estimated at approximately 10 mCi per injection for a common commercial PET scanner (Sadato et al. 1997). The use of 3-D PET can also reduce radiation exposure to subjects because of generally smaller total doses of ^{15}O-water injection. If the maximum allowable amount of ^{15}O-water administration is 400 mCi per subject per year, repeat PET scans can be obtained up to 40 times within a subject. However, the approximately 8–10 minutes required between scans to allow for radioactive decay would translate into 320–400 minutes for the entire experiment, a time frame that most subjects would find intolerable. The maximum number of scans per subject using 3-D PET must be determined by subject tolerance and other practical factors.

INTRASUBJECT IMAGE REGISTRATION

The first step in image analysis is the coregistration of all image sets from the same subject to remove any differences in head orientation between scans. If task/stimulus and control/baseline scans were obtained on different days for SPECT or FDG PET imaging, registration of these image sets into the same orientation is an essential step in subtraction analysis. Even when multiple image sets are obtained on the same day with ^{15}O-water, small head motions (on the order of a few millimeters) from scan to scan can produce large subtraction artifacts (Plate 3). Fortunately, most modern image registration techniques are fully automated and work extremely well. *Intrasubject intramodality* registration (e.g., PET to PET or SPECT to SPECT) can be performed using a multidimensional search algorithm combined with the proper cost function to estimate similarity between two scans within the image matrix. Various cost functions have been proposed, such as sum of absolute difference, standard deviation, and stochastic criteria (Woods et al. 1992; Hoh et al. 1993; Minoshima et al. 1993a), which have resulted in similar accuracy with better than 1 mm for translations and 1° rotations.

In single-subject analysis, activation foci can be localized by use of a structural image set (such as magnetic resonance imaging [MRI]) obtained from the same subject (Plate 2). In this approach, PET/SPECT image sets are "coregistered" with the magnetic resonance (MR) image set into the same

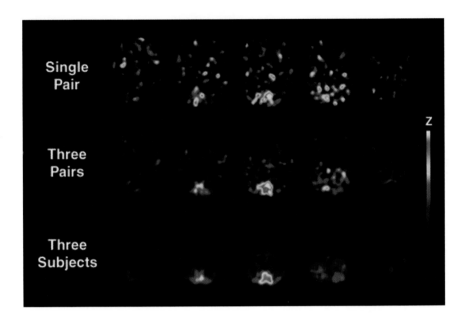

Plate 5. Improved signal-to-noise ratios for PET activation study by repeat scans within the subject and by intersubject averaging in stereotactic coordinates in a visual stimulation study using a reversing checkerboard. The top row represents subtraction results of a single pair of visual stimulation/baseline scans obtained in a single subject. Brain activation is noted in the occipital cortex, but it is obscured by high background noise. The second row represents averaged subtraction images of three pairs of visual stimulation/baseline scans obtained in a single subject. Reduction in background noise is noticeable. The bottom row represents averaged subtraction images of three pairs of visual stimulation/baseline scans obtained in three different subjects. There is clearly a further reduction in background noise and an improvement in signal-to-noise ratios.

Plate 6. Changes in regional pixel variances by anatomical standardization. The top row represents the levels of brain sections. The second through the bottom rows represent pixel standard deviations calculated from 16 normal subjects. Greater standard deviations indicate greater mismatches of gray matter activities. Stereotactic reorientation without brain size correction or anatomical standardization creates large mismatches of cortical activities. Brain size correction using linear scaling reduces mismatches substantially. However, residual mismatches still occur outside the structures that are used to measure the size of the brain (i.e., fronto-occipital and bitemporal poles). Residual mismatches just above the pyramidal bones are also apparent. A combination of linear scaling and nonlinear warping (bottom row) reduces further individual anatomical variation and creates uniform pixel variances throughout the brain. This enhancement is important for detection of brain activation with a uniform sensitivity throughout the brain, particularly when pixel variances are used to form a statistical map. ⟶

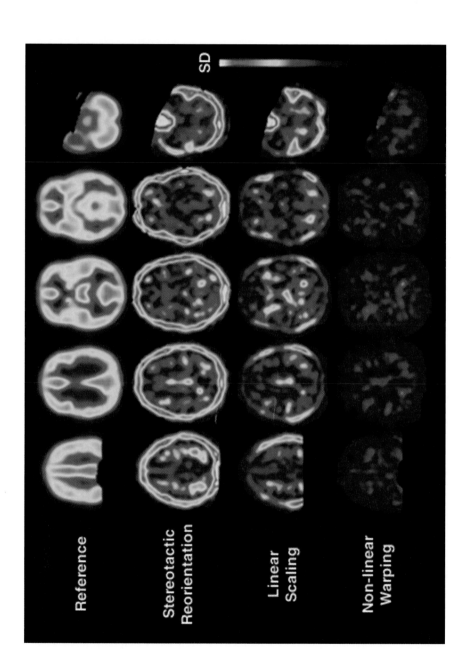

Reference

Stereotactic Reorientation

Linear Scaling

Non-linear Warping

SD

orientation. *Intrasubject intermodality* registration (e.g., PET to MRI) is performed using a similar algorithm but different cost functions to measure image matching (Pelizzari et al. 1989; Woods et al. 1993; Mangin et al. 1994; Ardekani et al. 1995). Distances of contours or equivalent landmarks, tissue homogeneity, and mutual information are examples of such cost functions. *Intermodality* image registration is accurate within a few millimeters, although it is generally less accurate than *intramodality* registration (Strother et al. 1994). This error range limits accuracy in the localization of activation foci using MR images in an individual subject analysis.

INTERSUBJECT IMAGE REGISTRATION

Intersubject image registration consists of image realignment to a common brain orientation (stereotaxy) and minimization of differences in individual brain shape (anatomical standardization) (Plate 4). When PET activation techniques were first developed, scanner sensitivity was limited. Intersubject summation analysis increases the signal-to-noise ratio of activation signals by averaging data obtained from multiple subjects (Plate 5). The same brain structure (or functional architecture) in different subjects must be mapped to a common location or coordinates. Image analysis using a common stereotactic system also permits the localization of activation foci by coordinates and allows objective comparisons across different studies from different institutions.

The concept of stereotaxy of the brain was proposed originally by Horsley and Clark (1908). A bicommissural stereotactic coordinate system, defined by the line passing through anterior (AC) and posterior (PC) commissures (the bicommissural line), is used most widely for human activation studies (Talairach and Tournoux 1988). Once the brain is reoriented parallel to the bicommissural line, cortical and subcortical structures can be mapped in consistent stereotactic coordinates. The bicommissural line can be determined visually on MR or PET images (Friston et al. 1989), or estimated automatically (Minoshima et al. 1993b; Friston et al. 1995). A major source of registration error arises from the anatomical variation of individual brains in the stereotactic coordinate system. The variance of major telencephalic structures in the bicommissural stereotactic system ranges from several millimeters to a centimeter (standard deviation across different subjects) (Talairach and Tournoux 1988; Steinmetz et al. 1990), although mean locations are fairly consistent across different groups of subjects. This uncertainty translates into potential error in the localization of individual PET activation foci using the stereotactic approach. Moreover, a small site of activation may be overlooked if its location is too variable. For consistent accuracy in stereotactic localization of cerebral structures for group analysis, the number of subjects must be adequate. Otherwise, peak locations of brain activation group analysis will be unstable and may be unreliable for comparisons across different studies. Standardization techniques have been developed to further reduce individual anatomical variance (Friston et al. 1991b; Collins et al. 1994; Minoshima et al. 1994b). In a general anatomical standardization approach, the size and skewness of the individual brain are matched linearly to the standard brain. Subsequently, local anatomical differences between the individual brain and the standard brain are minimized using a nonlinear warping algorithm. The proposed methods include matching an individual brain image set to a standard brain using a mathematically defined transformation function or matching corresponding landmarks or control points. Most proposed methods are automated and thus are completely user-independent.

Estimation of the accuracy of anatomical standardization is not always straightforward, partly because the consistent identification of exact structural landmarks or features across subjects is difficult, especially in cerebral cortices. In addition, a small number of landmarks or features may be insufficient to evaluate the accuracy of anatomical standardization of the whole brain (Sugiura et al. 1999). A fundamental argument remains about the elements that are to be standardized. Are they cortical surfaces, cortical gyri, cytoarchitectural territories, cortical layers, cortical columns, or areas defined by specific functions? Anatomical standardization is used not only to match certain structures of the brain across subjects, but also to reduce residual regional anatomical variation evenly throughout the brain (Plate 6). For example, extensive residual anatomical variation in "structure A" across subjects after anatomical standardization will blur brain activation signals at this site in group summation analysis and reduce the sensitivity of the procedure. If "structure B" has the same amount of activation, but less anatomical variation across subjects, this site will show greater activation in group summation analysis. Therefore, heterogeneous regional anatomical variation results in inconsistent sensitivity in the detection of regional activation and interferes with the physiological interpretation of results.

PIXEL (DATA) NORMALIZATION

In the reconstructed PET image sets obtained in activation studies, the pixel count represents the amount of radioactivity accumulated within a pixel for a given scan. Pixel counts can be influenced by multiple factors, including the level of global and local CBF. In addition, although similar doses of radiotracer are administered for repeat scans within a subject or from subject to subject, slight differences in the injection dose and changes in the fraction of cardiac output to the brain result in variability of pixel counts not attributable to regional neuronal activities. Measuring absolute CBF is not a sensitive way to detect regional brain activation because the level of absolute flow can be influenced independently from neuronal activities by other physiological factors, such as changes in plasma carbon dioxide level or the activation of certain cerebellar nuclei that modulate global CBF (Chida et al. 1989) (Plate 7). In addition, quantitative flow measurement typically is two to three times less precise than relative flow measurement due to various technical and physical factors. Normalization to remove confounding global factors permits the detection of regional blood flow changes associated with changes in neuronal activities. Two different data normalization approaches have been proposed for brain activation studies. One is a proportional model (linear scaling with zero intercept) (Fox et al. 1984). This model assumes that the magnitudes of regional brain activities are proportional to the global activity. The other approach uses an analysis of covariance (Friston et al. 1990), in which the relationship between regional and global activities are not only proportional, but also can be additive (linear scaling with non-zero intercept). In addition to these models, a nonlinear stochastic model may also be applied (Venot et al. 1986). Data normalization directly affects the magnitude of flow/metabolic changes seen on subtraction images. For example, some of these approaches may exaggerate regional "deactivation" (Plate 8). Further investigation is needed to validate these methods in terms of the physiological relationship between global and regional flow/metabolic changes during neuronal activation (Ramsay et al. 1993; Shimosegawa et al. 1995) and to confirm the statistical robustness of each model (Clark and Carson 1993).

Plate 7. Pixel normalization. Quantitative measurement (QUANT) of cerebral blood flow (CBF) was performed during voluntary hyperventilation (VENT) and was compared to resting CBF (REST). During hyperventilation, there is a global decrease in CBF due to a decreased plasma CO_2 level. Subtraction of VENT – REST (QUANT – Z) demonstrates no brain activation due to global CBF reduction. This is also evident with all negative values on the subtracted images by the pixel distribution histogram (QUANT – DIST). Once the same image sets are normalized to the global activity and are analyzed in the same manner (NORM), the subtraction Z map (NORM – Z) demonstrates bilateral activation of primary motor cortices. The pixel distribution histogram (NORM – DIST) demonstrates an approximate Gaussian distribution of pixel values with a mean value of 0. This example indicates that normalized CBF is a sensitive marker of neuronal activity. Quantitative CBF measurement is often confounded by physiological factors other than neuronal activity such as changes in respiratory rates (and thus plasma CO_2 levels) or physical factors such as accuracy of blood sampling and cross-calibration factors. ⟶

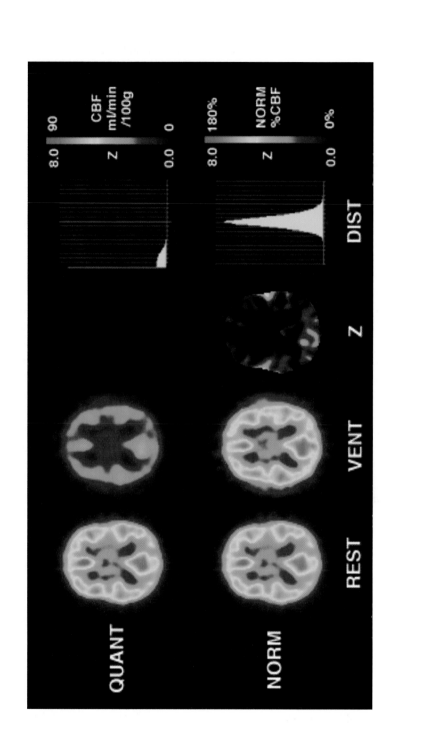

FORMATION OF STATISTICAL SUBTRACTION MAPS

Individual paired subtraction image sets (task/stimulus minus baseline/control) are averaged across different subjects to produce statistical parametric maps. Statistical parametric mapping is a powerful alternative to conventional, hypothesis-driven, region-of-interest analysis. Statistical parametric maps require an estimate of mean regional flow/metabolism changes and the associated variances. The variance can be estimated on a pixel-by-pixel basis (Friston et al. 1991a) or can be pooled for the entire brain (Worsley et al. 1992). Since regional physical factors (e.g., high versus low image counts) and physiological factors (e.g., CBF variation in the primary versus association cortices) may vary within the brain, the use of pixel-by-pixel variance may be desirable theoretically. However, when the number of subjects in the analysis is small, resultant statistical maps can be dominated by unstable pixel variance estimates. In such cases, the use of pooled variance may be more robust (Plate 9), reducing the chance of false positives and stabilizing the peak localization of brain activation (Taylor et al. 1993). Empirically, when the number of subjects or repeat scans becomes sufficiently large, the two approaches generally yield similar patterns of results, but the use of pixel variances becomes more appropriate. Resultant t maps can be transformed to Z maps for further statistical assessment using probability integral transformation.

More complex experimental designs require more elaborate statistical analyses. For example, investigators may wish to compare more than two conditions or may decide to perform correlation analysis with external variables. To accommodate a wide range of statistical analyses in a relatively common analytical format, the use of a *general linear model* for functional brain image analysis has been proposed (Friston et al. 1995). This approach is based on the fact that most conventional statistical analyses can be described as a linear combination of variables. Several commercially available statistical software packages use this algorithm internally to calculate Student's t values, analysis of variance (ANOVA), analysis of covariance (ANCOVA), correlation, and other statistical values. The resultant F maps can be transformed to Z maps for further statistical assessment.

STATISTICAL ASSESSMENT

In order to determine areas with significant flow/metabolism changes on statistical parametric maps, a proper statistical threshold must be estimated. A statistical map typically contains 60–100 thousand pixels that are

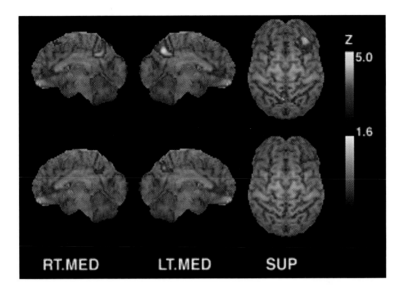

Plate 8. Deactivation exaggerated by pixel normalization. Brain activation PET scans with phasic heat pain to the left forearm were analyzed with two different pixel normalization methods. Commonly used "proportional" normalization uses global activity as a denominator. Calculations of global activity include areas of brain activation. Thus, extensive activation increases estimates of global activity. This increase, in turn, exaggerates areas of relatively silent or mildly decreased activity as significant "deactivation" (top row, showing significant deactivation in the precuneus and right prefrontal cortex). When stochastic correction is made for pixel normalization that is insensitive to local activation, the above areas of deactivation do not reach statistical significance (bottom row). Although pixel normalization methods should be validated physiologically, clearly differences in normalization methods can result in different magnitude estimates of brain activation.

intercorrelated among adjacent pixels. Statistical models for parametric images must control Type I error rates at desirable levels (e.g., $P = 0.05$) while taking multiple comparisons of intercorrelated pixels into account. The popular models consider statistical maps a stationary Gaussian process and determine thresholds as a function of search volume, image smoothness, and desirable error rates (Friston et al. 1991a; Worsley et al. 1992). Each model assumes certain conditions such as a stationary process, normal pixel distribution, and a relatively large process compared to image smoothness. Violations in these conditions result in false positive or negative results (Fig. 3). Statistical models are available for not only Z, but also t and F fields, allowing for more complex experimental designs and analyses (Worsley 1994), although the sensitivity of such analyses may be inadequate with too few subjects or scans. In contrast to threshold determination based on the magnitude of activation, the extent of activation is also subject to statistical modeling (Poline and Mazoyer 1993; Friston et al. 1994). An alternative to the above *parametric* approaches is a *nonparametric* test without any assumption of underlying pixel distribution (Holmes et al. 1996). Other statistical tests also can be applied to PET activation studies. Correlation analysis between external indices and intracranial pixel values during activation permits experimental designs without the need for two-state subtraction paradigms. In contrast to univariate analysis, multivariate analysis, such as principal components analysis, is applicable to PET data sets and can reveal potentially latent regional correlation patterns during functional brain activation (Friston et al. 1993; Strother et al. 1995). Although such multivariate analysis is commonly exploratory, confirmatory multivariate analysis has also been attempted (McIntosh et al. 1994). The variety of options for statistical analysis reveals the richness of functional information embodied in data sets produced by PET brain activation.

APPLICATIONS TO OTHER PET IMAGING STUDIES

Investigators have applied the methodology established in brain activation studies to intergroup comparisons or "disease" mapping using flow/metabolic or neurochemical PET and SPECT imaging (Minoshima et al. 1994b; Frey et al. 1996) (Plate 10). This type of image analysis can be used, for example, when comparing resting metabolic or blood flow image sets between normal controls and patients with chronic pain. Certain precautions must be taken when applying the above techniques to intergroup comparisons. Unlike the paired subtraction employed in activation analysis, individual anatomical differences cannot be canceled out in an intergroup analysis. Insufficient anatomical standardization may cause large false signals on intergroup subtraction images and may increase false positive rates. This flaw is in contrast to increased false negative rates in a paired activation analysis, in which mismatches of individual brain anatomy often reduce focal activation signals on the resultant map. The same consideration must be given to the comparison of brain activation results from different groups. Statistical modeling must be adequate for the underlying pixel distribution of intergroup subtracted maps, which may differ from the averaged paired subtraction results of activation data. The application of statistical mapping to intergroup comparisons requires further technical development and validation. The use of intergroup subtraction techniques can reveal regional functional changes without a regional a priori hypothesis; this method thus can generate further research hypotheses (Minoshima et al. 1994a). The exploratory nature of this approach is also useful when testing a new neuro-

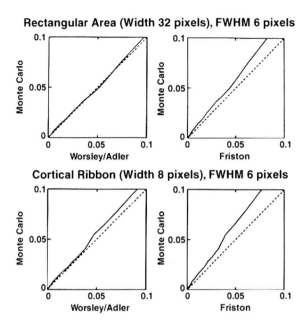

Fig. 3. Increased false positive rates within a narrow cortical ribbon. The determination of appropriate statistical thresholds involves several assumptions. One such assumption is that the stochastic process is "large" compared to the resolution of images. In the analysis of a large rectangular region (32-pixel width as compared to image resolution of 6 pixels full-width-at-half-maximum [FWHM]), Worsley and Adler's equation more precisely controls false positive rates as compared to the results of Monte Carlo simulation (Worsley et al. 1992) (upper left graph). (A dotted line represents the line of identity. A solid line represents actual estimation by simulation. A deviation of the solid line from the dotted line indicates increased false positive rates). Friston's equation also yields approximately the same result (Friston et al. 1991a), but underestimates the threshold, causing increased false positive rates (upper right graph, upward deviation from the line of identity). In the analysis of a narrow cortical ribbon, which is a common practice in activation analysis, the process is no longer large relative to the image resolution (8-pixel width as compared to 6-pixel FWHM). This violation in the assumption causes increased false positive rates in both statistical threshold estimates (lower graphs). This violation has been overlooked in many applications of statistical mapping. A method has been proposed to address this issue (Worsley et al. 1996).

chemical radiotracer such as opioid receptor ligands whose regional distribution has yet to be characterized in humans. Intergroup comparison, when used with a normal reference database, is also beneficial when interpreting clinical diagnostic cases in which the locations of functional abnormalities are not known in advance (Burdette et al. 1996). These approaches may permit researchers to examine functional image data sets from individuals suffering from pain disorders.

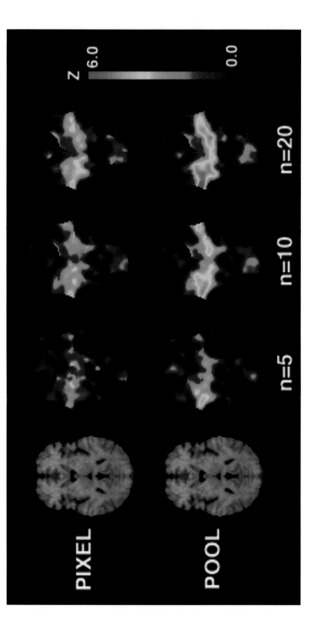

Plate 9. Formation of statistical maps using pixel versus pooled variances. Brain activation PET scans (5 to 20 subjects) with phasic heat pain to the left forearm were analyzed using pixel variances versus a pooled variance when calculating statistical values. When the number of subjects is relatively small ($n = 5$), a statistical map generated with pixel variances is dominated by unstable estimates of pixel variance (top left). Generally, pooled variance gives more robust results. Analysis of 10 subjects with pooled variance gives results similar to or more robust than that of 20 subjects with pixel variances. Despite physiological and physical limitations in the assumption of "uniformity" in a pooled variance approach, the technique is useful when the number of subjects involved in the experiment is small and pixel variance estimates are unreliable.

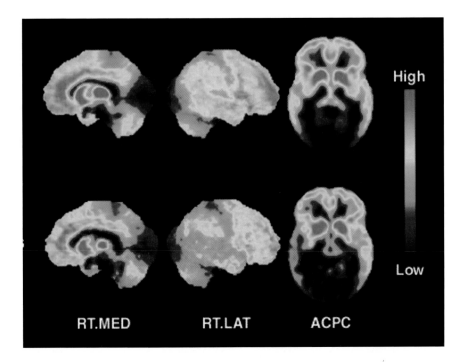

Plate 10. ^{11}C-diprenorphine imaging analyzed using stereotactic methods (Willoch et al. 1999). The top row represents averaged ^{11}C-diprenorphine binding in 14 normal controls. The bottom row represents ^{11}C-diprenorphine images of five patients with central poststroke pain. The right medial (MED) and lateral (LAT) hemispheres contralateral to the pain and a transaxial slice at the level of the bicommissural (AC–PC) line are presented. Decreased binding in the right thalamus, anterior cingulate cortex, posterior insula, and temporal cortex is noted in patients with central poststroke pain. Neuroreceptor PET data were analyzed using stereotactic brain-mapping techniques (Minoshima et al. 1994b, 1995).

CONCLUSIONS

PET and SPECT brain activation methods have generated exciting new findings about cerebral pain mechanisms in humans. Methodologies for PET and SPECT activation studies have been investigated extensively over the past decade by multidisciplinary groups of researchers including physicists, statisticians, anatomists, physiologists, nuclear medicine physicians, radiologists, neurologists, psychiatrists, neurosurgeons, and psychologists. Some of these techniques and concepts have been transferred to brain activation studies using fMRI. An understanding of the basic concepts and techniques of these methods is necessary for appropriate experimental designs and proper interpretation of results. Advances in emission computed tomography and radiochemistry promise to improve these methods regarding spatial and temporal resolution, signal-to-noise level of images, and specificity of signal changes in relationship to populations of active neurons.

ACKNOWLEDGMENTS

The authors thank David E. Kuhl, MD, for his continuing support for the project; Frode Willoch, MD, for his contribution of opioid imaging data; and Pamela Paulson, PhD, and Thomas J. Morrow, PhD, for their critical discussions. This project is funded in part by the Department of Veterans Affairs (Merit Review, to K.L. Casey) and by grants DE-FG02-87-ER60561 from the Department of Energy and PO1 HD33986-04 from the National Institutes of Health.

REFERENCES

Ardekani BA, Braun M, Hutton BF, Kanno I, Iida H. A fully automatic multimodality image registration algorithm. *J Comput Assist Tomogr* 1995; 19:615–623.

Burdette JH, Minoshima S, Vander Borght T, Tran DD, Kuhl DE. Alzheimer disease: improved visual interpretation of PET images by using three-dimensional stereotaxic surface projections. *Radiology* 1996; 198:837–843.

Casey KL, Minoshima S, Berger KL, et al. Positron emission tomographic analysis of cerebral structures activated specifically by repetitive noxious heat stimuli. *J Neurophysiol* 1994; 71:802–807.

Cherry SR, Woods RP, Doshi NK, Banerjee PK, Mazziotta JC. Improved signal-to-noise in PET activation studies using switched paradigms. *J Nucl Med* 1995; 36:307–314.

Chida K, Iadecola C, Reis DJ. Global reduction in cerebral blood flow and metabolism elicited from intrinsic neurons of fastigial nucleus. *Brain Res* 1989; 500:177–192.

Clark C, Carson R. Analysis of covariance in statistical parametric mapping. *J Cereb Blood Flow Metab* 1993; 13:1038–1040.

Collins DL, Neelin P, Peters TM, Evans AC. Automatic 3D intersubject registration of MR volumetric data in standardized Talairach space. *J Comput Assist Tomogr* 1994; 18:192–205.

Collins RC, Santori EM, Der T, Toga AW, Lothman EW. Functional metabolic mapping during forelimb movement in rat. I. Stimulation of motor cortex. *J Neurosci* 1986; 6:448–462.

Fox PT, Mintun MA, Raichle ME, Herscovitch P. A noninvasive approach to quantitative functional brain mapping with $H_2^{(15)}O$ and positron emission tomography. *J Cereb Blood Flow Metab* 1984; 4:329–333.

Fox PT, Perlmutter JS, Raichle ME. A stereotactic method of anatomical localization for positron emission tomography. *J Comput Assist Tomogr* 1985; 9:141–153.

Frey KA, Minoshima S, Koeppe RA, et al. Stereotaxic summation analysis of human cerebral benzodiazepine binding maps. *J Cereb Blood Flow Metab* 1996; 16:409–417.

Friston KJ, Passingham RE, Nutt JG, et al. Localisation in PET images: direct fitting of the intercommissural (AC–PC) line. *J Cereb Blood Flow Metab* 1989; 9:690–695.

Friston KJ, Frith CD, Liddle PF, et al. The relationship between global and local changes in PET scans. *J Cereb Blood Flow Metab* 1990; 10:458–466.

Friston KJ, Frith CD, Liddle PF, Frackowiak RS. Comparing functional (PET) images: the assessment of significant change. *J Cereb Blood Flow Metab* 1991a; 11:690–699.

Friston KJ, Frith CD, Liddle PF, Frackowiak RS. Plastic transformation of PET images. *J Comput Assist Tomogr* 1991b; 15:634–639.

Friston KJ, Frith CD, Liddle PF, Frackowiak RS. Functional connectivity: the principal-component analysis of large (PET) data sets. *J Cereb Blood Flow Metab* 1993; 13:5–14.

Friston KJ, Worsley KJ, Frackowiak RSJ, Mazziotta JC, Evans AC. Assessing the significance of focal activations using their spatial extent. *Hum Brain Mapp* 1994; 1:214–220.

Friston KJ, Holmes AP, Worsley KJ, et al. Statistical parametric maps in functional imaging: a general approach. *Hum Brain Mapp* 1995; 2:189–210.

Frostig RD, Lieke EE, Ts'o DY, Grinvald A. Cortical functional architecture and local coupling between neuronal activity and the microcirculation revealed by in vivo high-resolution optical imaging of intrinsic signals. *Proc Natl Acad Sci USA* 1990; 87:6082–6086.

Ginsberg MD, Chang JY, Kelley RE, et al. Increases in both cerebral glucose utilization and blood flow during execution of a somatosensory task. *Ann Neurol* 1988; 23:152–160.

Hoh CK, Dahlbom M, Harris G, et al. Automated iterative three-dimensional registration of positron emission tomography images. *J Nucl Med* 1993; 34:2009–2018.

Holmes AP, Blair RC, Watson JD, Ford I. Nonparametric analysis of statistic images from functional mapping experiments. *J Cereb Blood Flow Metab* 1996; 16:7–22.

Horsley V, Clark RH. The structure and functions of cerebellum examined by a new method. *Brain* 1908; 31:45–124.

Ingvar DH, Risberg J. Increase of regional cerebral blood flow during mental effort in normals and in patients with focal brain disorders. *Exp Brain Res* 1967; 3:195–211.

Ishizu K, Yonekura Y, Magata Y, et al. Extraction and retention of technetium-99m-ECD in human brain: dynamic SPECT and oxygen-15-water PET studies. *J Nucl Med* 1996; 37:1600–1604.

Jones AK, Brown WD, Friston KJ, Qi LY, Frackowiak RS. Cortical and subcortical localization of response to pain in man using positron emission tomography. *Proc R Soc Lond B Biol Sci* 1991; 244:39–44.

Kanno I, Iida H, Miura S, Murakami M. Optimal scan time of oxygen-15-labeled water injection method for measurement of cerebral blood flow. *J Nucl Med* 1991; 32:1931–1934.

Mangin JF, Frouin V, Bloch I, Bendriem B, Lopez-Krahe J. Fast nonsupervised 3D registration of PET and MR images of the brain. *J Cereb Blood Flow Metab* 1994; 14:749–762.

McIntosh AR, Grady CL, Ungerleider LG, et al. Network analysis of cortical visual pathways mapped with PET. *J Neurosci* 1994; 14:655–666.

Minoshima S, Koeppe RA, Fessler JA, et al. Integrated and automated data analysis method for neuronal activation studies using [O-15]water PET. In: Uemura K, Lassen NA, Jones T, Kanno I (Eds). *Quantification of Brain Function, Tracer Kinetics and Image Analysis in Brain PET*. Amsterdam: Excerpta Medica, 1993a, pp 409–415.

Minoshima S, Koeppe RA, Mintun MA, et al. Automated detection of the intercommissural line for stereotactic localization of functional brain images. *J Nucl Med* 1993b; 34:322–329.

Minoshima S, Foster NL, Kuhl DE. Posterior cingulate cortex in Alzheimer's disease. *Lancet* 1994a; 344:895.

Minoshima S, Koeppe RA, Frey KA, Kuhl DE. Anatomic standardization: linear scaling and nonlinear warping of functional brain images. *J Nucl Med* 1994b; 35:1528–1537.

Minoshima S, Frey KA, Koeppe RA, Foster NL, Kuhl DE. A diagnostic approach in Alzheimer's disease using three-dimensional stereotactic surface projections of fluorine-18-FDG PET. *J Nucl Med* 1995; 36:1238–1248.

Narayan SM, Esfahani P, Blood AJ, Sikkens L, Toga AW. Functional increases in cerebral blood volume over somatosensory cortex. *J Cereb Blood Flow Metab* 1995; 15:754–765.

Pelizzari CA, Chen GT, Spelbring DR, Weichselbaum RR, Chen CT. Accurate three-dimensional registration of CT, PET, and/or MR images of the brain. *J Comput Assist Tomogr* 1989; 13:20–26.

Phelps ME, Kuhl DE, Mazziota JC. Metabolic mapping of the brain's response to visual stimulation: studies in humans. *Science* 1981; 211:1445–1448.

Poline JB, Mazoyer BM. Analysis of individual positron emission tomography activation maps by detection of high signal-to-noise-ratio pixel clusters. *J Cereb Blood Flow Metab* 1993; 13:425–437.

Ramsay SC, Murphy K, Shea SA, et al. Changes in global cerebral blood flow in humans: effect on regional cerebral blood flow during a neural activation task. *J Physiol (Lond)* 1993; 471:521–534.

Sadato N, Carson RE, Daube-Witherspoon ME, et al. Optimization of noninvasive activation studies with ^{15}O-water and three-dimensional positron emission tomography. *J Cereb Blood Flow Metab* 1997; 17:732–739.

Shimosegawa E, Kanno I, Hatazawa J, et al. Photic stimulation study of changing the arterial partial pressure level of carbon dioxide. *J Cereb Blood Flow Metab* 1995; 15:111–114.

Sokoloff L. Local cerebral energy metabolism: its relationships to local functional activity and blood flow. *Ciba Found Symp* 1978:171–197.

Sokoloff L, Reivich M, Kennedy C, et al. The [^{14}C]deoxyglucose method for the measurement of local cerebral glucose utilization: theory, procedure, and normal values in the conscious and anesthetized albino rat. *J Neurochem* 1977; 28:897–916.

Steinmetz H, Furst G, Freund HJ. Variation of perisylvian and calcarine anatomic landmarks within stereotaxic proportional coordinates. *Am J Neuroradiol* 1990; 11:1123–1130.

Strother SC, Anderson JR, Xu XL, et al. Quantitative comparisons of image registration techniques based on high-resolution MRI of the brain. *J Comput Assist Tomogr* 1994; 18:954–962.

Strother SC, Anderson JR, Schaper KA, et al. Principal component analysis and the scaled subprofile model compared to intersubject averaging and statistical parametric mapping: I. "Functional connectivity" of the human motor system studied with [^{15}O]water PET. *J Cereb Blood Flow Metab* 1995; 15:738–753.

Sugiura M, Kawashima R, Sadato N, et al. Anatomic validation of spatial normalization methods for PET. *J Nucl Med* 1999; 40:317–322.

Talairach J, Tournoux P. *Co-planar Stereotaxic Atlas of the Human Brain*. New York: Thieme, 1988.

Talbot JD, Marrett S, Evans AC, et al. Multiple representations of pain in human cerebral cortex. *Science* 1991; 251:1355–1358.

Taylor SF, Minoshima S, Koeppe RA. Instability of localization of cerebral blood flow activation foci with parametric maps. *J Cereb Blood Flow Metab* 1993; 13:1040–1042.

Tsubokawa T, Katayama Y, Kondo T, et al. Changes in local cerebral blood flow and neuronal activity during sensory stimulation in normal and sympathectomized cats. *Brain Res* 1980; 190:51–64.

Tsukada H, Kakiuchi T, Ando I, Ouchi Y. Functional activation of cerebral blood flow abolished by scopolamine is reversed by cognitive enhancers associated with cholinesterase inhibition: a positron emission tomography study in unanesthetized monkeys. *J Pharmacol Exp Ther* 1997; 281:1408–1414.

Venot A, Liehn JC, Lebruchec JF, Roucayrol JC. Automated comparison of scintigraphic images. *J Nucl Med* 1986; 27:1337–1342.

Willoch F, Tolle TR, Wester HJ, et al. Central pain after pontine infarction is associated with changes in opioid receptor binding: a PET study with ^{11}C-diprenorphine. *Am J Neuroradiol* 1999; 20:686–690.

Woods RP, Cherry SR, Mazziotta JC. Rapid automated algorithm for aligning and reslicing PET images. *J Comput Assist Tomogr* 1992; 16:620–633.

Woods RP, Mazziotta JC, Cherry SR. MRI-PET registration with automated algorithm. *J Comput Assist Tomogr* 1993; 17:536–546.

Woods RP, Grafton ST, Watson JD, Sicotte NL, Mazziotta JC. Automated image registration: II. Intersubject validation of linear and nonlinear models. *J Comp Assist Tomogr* 1998; 22:153–165.

Worsley KJ. Local maxima and the expected Euler characteristics of excursion sets of chi-square, F and t fields. *Adv Appl Prob* 1994; 26:13–42.

Worsley KJ, Evans AC, Marrett S, Neelin P. A three-dimensional statistical analysis for CBF activation studies in human brain. *J Cereb Blood Flow Metab* 1992; 12:900–918.

Worsley KJ, Marrett S, Neelin P, Evans AC. A unified statistical approach for determining significant signals in location and scale space images of cerebral activation. In: Myers R, Cunningham V, Bailey D, Jones T (Eds). *Quantification of Brain Function using PET*. San Diego: Academic Press, 1996, pp 327–333.

Correspondence to: Satoshi Minoshima, MD, PhD, University of Washington Medical School, 1959 NE Pacific Street, Box 356004, Seattle, WA 98195-6004, USA. Tel: 206-598-2707; email: minoshim@u.washington.edu.

Pain Imaging, Progress in Pain Research and Management, Vol. 18, edited by Kenneth L. Casey and M. Catherine Bushnell, IASP Press, Seattle, © 2000.

5

PET Studies of the Subjective Experience of Pain

Pierre Rainville,[a] M. Catherine Bushnell,[b] and Gary H. Duncan[c]

[a]Department of Neurology, University of Iowa Hospitals and Clinics, Iowa City, Iowa, USA; [b]Departments of Anesthesia, Dentistry, and Physiology, McGill University, Montreal, Quebec, Canada; [c]Faculty of Dental Medicine, University of Montreal, Montreal, Quebec, Canada

THE POTENTIAL OF PET IMAGING

During the 1990s, modern brain-imaging techniques added an important perspective to the field of pain research. Previous studies, mostly in animals, had yielded increasingly detailed knowledge of the electrophysiological and molecular mechanisms involved in both the transduction of noxious stimulation into neuronal activity and the modulation of this activity by endogenous and exogenous factors. These nociceptive processes in the peripheral nervous system and spinal cord underlie an organism's reflexive reactions to tissue-damaging stimuli and initiate its adaptive (and maladaptive) responses to those stimuli. Classical methods, such as neuroanatomical tracing techniques, single-unit neurophysiological recordings, direct electrical stimulation, and analysis of cortical lesions, have yielded further tantalizing details about the processing of nociceptive information within the brain. However, as important as these discoveries have been in advancing our knowledge of nociception, they fall short of providing a comprehensive understanding of the process we call *pain.* Ultimately, peripheral nociceptive signals must transform into a pattern of central nervous activity that underlies the conscious experience of pain in humans. The ideal approach to this problem would reveal "pain-related" neuronal activity, recorded simultaneously across the entire brain and accurately localized to specific cortical and subcortical structures—a goal we hope to achieve in the new millennium. A glimpse of this dream has emerged in the closing years of the 20th century with the development of positron emission tomography (PET), which is based on tomographic mapping of radioactive tracers during their transit through the brain.

PET techniques first offered the alluring opportunity to see the human brain at work. This new perspective on human brain function has the advantage of allowing simultaneous investigation of activation within the full brain volume. Radiotracer methods thus became a valuable complement to the prevailing electroencephalographic (EEG) methods, which can only detect changes in electrical activity from the scalp surface. Another traditional way to investigate the brain's function is to study lesions in brain-damaged patients. However, the variability in the location and extent of lesions occurring naturally in humans is a major limitation of such studies. The functional reorganization that may result from lesions or pathological processes also limits generalization of the clinical findings to normal brain function. The new radiotracer methods avoid those problems by allowing the examination of normal brain function and thus providing a baseline to which abnormal brain function can be contrasted.

THE CAVEATS

Methodological limitations. Notwithstanding those promises, PET techniques have fallen short of meeting objectives for ideal brain imaging (see Chapter 4). The risks associated with radioisotope injection limit the number of investigations that can be performed on volunteer subjects or patients. The advantage of examining simultaneously the activity in multiple brain regions is achieved at the cost of limited spatial resolution (on a scale of millimeters). Poor temporal resolution further limits PET investigations to processes covering tens of seconds, in contrast to faster methods such as EEG, magnetoencephalography (MEG), and functional magnetic resonance imaging (fMRI). Furthermore, cerebral responses observed using PET only approximate neuronal activity by measuring changes in glucose consumption or blood flow. Finally, the relatively low sensitivity of PET techniques frequently requires the averaging of data from numerous subjects to detect reliable levels of pain-evoked activity.

Interpretative guidelines. The notion of *functional specialization* is inherent to the experimental design and interpretative framework of most or all brain-mapping studies. PET studies usually directly compare an "activation" condition and a neutral control condition (see Plate 1). In pain studies, comparison between the activation observed in painful and nonpainful conditions is designed to isolate the brain activity associated with pain. However, variations in the control condition have a profound impact on the results and may lead to misinterpretation. The "subtraction paradigm," first implemented in cognitive studies, assumes that the control condition includes all processes involved in the experimental condition except for the target process under study. The control condition should not include additional processes absent from the activation condition. As we will see, most investigators have administered innocuous sensation in their control condition, using the same physical source of stimulation (e.g., heat), applied at a lower intensity (e.g., nonpainful warmth), to the same body part, and following the same spatiotemporal pattern as the pain stimulation (e.g., painful heat). This choice is intended to control for factors associated with stimulus recognition, nonspecific orientation and attention, and evaluative processes that are independent of pain but inherent to any stimulation paradigm. However, this approach is not free of caveats because the activation and control conditions are not equivalent with respect to all processes other than pain. For example, some neurophysiological processes may be uniquely activated by the application of innocuous stimulation in the control condition; results from the subtraction of this control could then be interpreted as pain-related decreases. In turn, decreases in activity specifically evoked by the nonpainful stimulation may be falsely interpreted, after subtraction, as pain-related increases. Furthermore, areas involved in both painful and nonpainful sensations may be subtracted out, although their contribution to each type of sensation may be functionally and physiologically separable using methods with higher spatiotemporal resolution.

Second, activation studies only indirectly support the participation of a given area in the target process. Even in the ideal case where the control condition is well designed, and the process under study well isolated, the activation of a specific brain area does not ensure a significant or necessary contribution to the target process. In contrast, the persistence of a specific deficit resulting from a brain lesion provides more compelling evidence that the damaged area is necessary for normal function (although lesion studies have other limitations, as mentioned above).

Third, inherent problems confound the interpretation of negative findings in functional brain-imaging studies (also see Chapter 7). These problems result from (1) uncertainty about the specific mechanisms involved in the coupling between cerebral blood flow and neuronal activity, (2) the relatively poor spatiotemporal resolution and other technical limitations of the method, and (3) the limited power of the method in detecting small changes in activity (see Chapter 4). This last point is critical, as the power to detect a given response is statistically dependent upon the number of observations and the magnitude of the effect expected. The number of subjects and the experimental design currently used in PET studies are sensitive to differences of about 3–5% in regional cerebral blood flow (rCBF) between the activation and control conditions. Recent findings using fMRI indicate that in many experiments a significant response may occur below this level (see Chapters 6 and 7). Therefore, the absence of significant activation within a given brain area cannot be interpreted as a lack of involvement of this area in the process studied.

In spite of these limitations, human brain-imaging techniques using PET have provided a spectacular tool for exploring cerebral processes associated with pain perception. This chapter follows the emergence of these studies, describes their general theoretical implications, documents their major contributions to our understanding of human pain perception, and explores the possible implications for the understanding and treatment of clinical pain conditions.

THE SEARCH FOR THE "PAIN CENTER"

In retrospect, the concept of a "pain center" seems intuitively implausible, but this once-common expectation underscores how little was known, even in 1990, about possible cerebral processes underlying human pain perception. The most probable candidate for such a fundamental role in pain perception was the thalamus. Head and Holmes (1911) observed that lesions to the lateral thalamus could cause extensive sensory loss accompanied by spontaneous painful burning sensations, termed the *central pain syndrome.* They suggested that the negative symptoms were consequent to the interruption of somatosensory pathways, while positive symptoms arose from a disinhibition of activity in the medial thalamus. The medial thalamus was presumably involved in emotional aspects, and the increase in activity in this area led to the abnormal experience of pain. Observations of the neurosurgeon Wilder E. Penfield generally supported the idea that the cerebral cortex had little, if any, involvement in pain. Electrical stimulation of the somatosensory cortex of awake patients, undergoing surgery for the resection of epileptogenic brain tissue, only rarely led to the experience of pain (Penfield and Boldrey 1937). Moreover, the observation that localized cortical lesions seldom abolished pain (Head and Holmes 1911; White and Sweet 1969) was consistent with the notion that pain depends on subcortical processes. Thus, the first pain studies to use modern brain-imaging techniques faced a large unknown and asked only a simple question: Is the cerebral cortex involved in the perception of pain?

THE SIGNATURE OF PAIN IN THE BRAIN

The initial PET studies of brain activity associated with pain provided the first clear indication that the cerebral cortex is indeed activated during the application of noxious stimuli. Talbot et al. (1991) compared brain activity in response to painful versus nonpainful stimulation in eight normal individuals. Twelve short (5-second) phasic heat stimuli from a contact thermode were applied alternately to six spots on each subject's right volar forearm while cerebral blood flow was measured. Stimuli consisted of either painful (47°–49°C) or nonpainful (41°–42°C) temperatures applied during each of four 60-second scans. The direct comparison of the two conditions revealed greater rCBF during pain in the anterior cingulate cortex (ACC), over the postcentral gyrus in the primary somatosensory cortex (S1), and in the parietal operculum in the region of the secondary somatosensory cortex (S2). These sites were activated in the left hemisphere, contralateral to the stimulation. In this initial study, the thalamus was outside the scanner's field of view, but subsequent studies (see especially Jones et al. 1991a) documented thalamic activation during pain and confirmed the importance of pain-related activation in the ACC. Subsequent reports have added the insula to the sites consistently activated during pain (e.g., Coghill et al. 1994). These results have been replicated abundantly using phasic heat stimulation (recently reviewed by Treede et al. 1999). Four cortical areas (S1, S2, the ACC, and the insula) have been the major focus of our studies because animal studies have shown that these areas receive nociceptive input from spino-thalamocortical pathways (see below). Although the thalamus is not a simple transmission relay, the evidence for direct spinothalamocortical nociceptive input provided one of the basic criteria for identifying cortical areas likely to be involved in pain processes.

The S1 cortex receives its main thalamic afferent projections from the ventroposterior lateral (VPL) and ventroposterior medial (VPM) nuclei (Jones and Friedman 1982; Rausell and Jones 1991; Rausell et al. 1992). S1 receives additional input from the ventroposterior inferior nucleus (VPI) and from the central lateral (CL) nucleus of the intralaminar group (Gingold et al. 1991). The ventral thalamic nuclei receive nociceptive inputs from the dorsal horn of the spinal cord and contain neurons that respond to nociceptive stimulation of the skin and viscera (Casey and Morrow 1983; Albé-Fessard et al. 1985; Bushnell and Duncan 1987; Bushnell et al. 1993; Apkarian and Shi 1994; Brüggemann et al. 1994; Al-Chaer et al. 1996). Neurons responsive to nociceptive stimuli, while scarce in S1, are consistently found there in the monkey (Kenshalo and Isensee 1983; Kenshalo et al. 1988; Gingold et al. 1991). The receptive fields of these neurons are generally larger than those of non-nociceptive neurons, often covering more than one part of the body. Nociceptive neurons respond with higher discharge frequency to increasingly intense noxious mechanical or thermal stimulation. In addition, these neurons generally have a small, contralateral, *non*-nociceptive receptive field. This functional organization suggests that although few nociceptive neurons exist in S1, localized nociceptive stimuli may recruit a large population of S1 neurons distributed more widely across the cortical surface. The activation of these neurons probably underlies the pain-related increase in rCBF observed in S1 in functional brain-imaging studies in humans. However, in some studies, neuronal activity specifically associated with innocuous sensation in S1 during the control condition may have masked a distinct activation specifically associated with pain, due to the close spatial proximity of nociceptive and non-nociceptive S1 neurons and because of the dual role of some S1 nociceptors in signaling nociceptive and non-nociceptive stimuli.

The S2 cortex is located on the dorsal bank of the Sylvian fissure at the level of the ventral parietal operculum. This area receives thalamocortical afferent projections from VPI, VPL, CL, and the posterior nuclei (Friedman and Murray 1986), some of which have been shown to convey nociceptive information from spinothalamic afferents in the monkey (Stevens et al. 1993). Furthermore, corticocortical projections from S1 may contribute to nociceptive activity observed in S2 (Pons and Kaas 1986; Pons et al. 1992). Electrophysiological evidence from unit recordings in monkeys confirms the existence of nociresponsive neurons in S2. Most of these cells respond to somatic stimulation, but only a few display nociceptive properties (Robinson and Burton 1980a,b,c; Dong et al. 1989); their receptive fields are bilateral or contralateral and are of variable sizes. Adjacent regions, including the posterior insula and the lateral aspect of the parietal operculum (Broadmann area 7b), also contain a small proportion of nociceptive neurons (Robinson and Burton 1980a,b,c; Dong et al. 1994). Dong et al. (1989) suggested that the unit recording method may underestimate the nociceptive activity in S2 and in the parietal operculum because nociceptive neurons are grouped in clusters and may be missed by the electrode penetrations, and because nociceptive activity may not reach the threshold for the generation of action potentials. In contrast, the pain-related electrical potentials (Chudler et al. 1986), magnetic fields (Kitamura et al. 1995), and increases in rCBF that are consistently observed in this area imply the presence of currents or synaptic activity but do not require the production of action potentials. Thus, the activity observed in human functional brain-imaging studies may reflect the pain-related synaptic activity of neurons scattered within S2 and adjacent cytoarchitectonic areas.

Evidence for nociceptive activity in the insular region has been more elusive. The recent search for pain-related pathways to this area was partly motivated by the initial observations of pain-related activation in functional brain-imaging studies (see especially Coghill et al. 1994; Treede et al. 1999). The insula is a heterogeneous cortical area that receives afferent projections from thalamic, amygdaloid, and brainstem nuclei. In monkeys, the anterior insula receives projections from the posterior ventromedial posterior nucleus (VMpo) of the thalamus, which receives thermal and nociceptive inputs from the superficial lamina of the spinal cord (Craig et al. 1994; Craig 1996). An homologous region in the human thalamus, containing neurons with similar properties, has been localized in the posterior-inferior part of the principal sensory nucleus and is named the ventrocaudal nucleus (Vc) (Lenz et al. 1993). The anterior insula may also receive afferent signals directly and indirectly from the parabrachial and solitary nuclei of the brainstem and amygdala (Augustine 1996; Bernard et al. 1996; Craig 1996), and exhibits abundant connections with S2, the posterior insula, and the ACC. Electrophysiological recordings in the monkey further document the existence of thermoreceptive and nociceptive neurons in the insula (Dostrovsky and Craig 1996). These findings support the notion that insular activation in functional brain-imaging studies of pain reflects this nociceptive (Craig 1996) and thermoreceptive input (Craig et al. 1996, 2000). These observations also suggest that studies using substantial warm (e.g., Talbot et al. 1991) or cool stimuli in their control condition may be less sensitive to activation from heat pain or cold pain due to the masking effect of temperature-related activation. Thus, notwithstanding the complex interactions of thermoreceptive, nociceptive, and autonomic processing within the insular cortex (IC), numerous clinical studies support the role of this region in the perception of pain (Biemond 1956; Greenspan and Winfield 1992; Bassetti et al. 1993), in emotional responses to potentially painful stimuli (Berthier et al. 1988), and in autonomic functions probably related to pain perception (Oppenheimer et al. 1996).

The ACC is also a likely recipient of nociceptive spinothalamocortical input. This area receives thalamic projections from medial (e.g., mediodorsal) and intralaminar thalamic nuclei (e.g., parafascicularis), regions that exhibit nociceptive activity in the monkey (Vogt et al. 1979; Baleydier and Mauguiere 1980; Vogt et al. 1987; Bushnell and Duncan 1989; Zhang et al. 1996). Within area 24 of the ACC, nociceptive neurons have been recorded in anesthetized rabbits (Sikes and Vogt 1992), and unpublished observations from our laboratory suggest that these responses may also be found in the awake monkey. Recent data suggest a role for these nociceptive ACC neurons in anticipation or avoidance of painful stimuli (Koyama et al. 1998).

In human ACC, electrical potentials were demonstrated during the application of heat pain stimuli (Lenz et al. 1998a,b), and more recently, nociceptive neurons have been reported in this area (Hutchison et al. 1999). These
neurons might play a critical role in the pain-related activation of the ACC
observed in functional brain-imaging studies.

The consistent activation observed in the S1, S2, insula, and ACC in
response to various experimental painful stimuli in functional brain-imaging studies supports the existence of anatomical pathways conveying nociceptive signals to those areas in humans. Activation in these areas has been
observed in response to thermal and chemical stimulation of the skin, electrical stimulation of the muscle, and mechanical stimulation of the viscera
(also see Chapter 7). However, different studies have had inconsistent results, most notably for S1, with some reporting increases (Talbot et al. 1991),
some reporting decreases (Apkarian et al. 1992), and others finding no change
in rCBF in response to noxious stimuli (Jones et al. 1991a). These differences may be partly explained by methodological variations across studies
(see Bushnell et al. 1999a). For example, studies that maximize the sensitivity of the PET method (see Volkow et al. 1991) by acquiring data at the
onset of pain or by presenting phasic stimulation repeatedly throughout the
scans have generally found activation in S1 (e.g., Coghill et al. 1994). In
contrast, studies using a tonic stimulus in which the onset of data acquisition is not synchronized with the onset of pain may miss the initial peak
increase in rCBF. This possibility is consistent with electrophysiological
studies showing a peak response within 10–30 seconds after the onset of a
painful stimulus (Kenshalo and Isensee 1983). The late decrease in rCBF
observed in one study also suggests a further decrease in S1 activity in
response to prolonged stimulation (Apkarian et al. 1992). These effects may
also contribute to the failure to observe S1 activation in paradigms using
tonic stimuli and scan durations exceeding 60 seconds (Derbyshire and Jones
1998). Individual differences in sulcal anatomy may further reduce the capacity to detect changes in S1 because of the required between-subject averaging of pain-evoked activity (Bushnell et al. 1999a). Likewise, limited statistical power related to the small samples used in many studies may be
responsible for some negative findings (e.g., Jones et al. 1991a). Finally,
recent data further show that S1 activity is highly modulated by cognitive
factors (discussed below) that also may increase the variability in results
reported by different studies. Although many of these factors may contribute to the occasional absence of pain-related activation reported for S1, S2,
and the insula, activation of the ACC is observed in virtually all pain studies.

Other cortical and subcortical sites are activated less consistently across
PET studies (Treede et al. 1999). Additional sites of activation are often

observed in the premotor and supplementary motor areas (Coghill et al. 1994), and occasionally in the prefrontal and lateral posterior parietal cortices. Pain-related decreases in rCBF have been reported sporadically in the occipital, temporal, medial parietal, and prefrontal cortices. Subcortical activation is often observed in the thalamus (Jones et al. 1991a), either contralateral to the stimulation or bilaterally, and most likely reflects the activity of nociceptive neurons in many thalamic nuclei, as discussed above. Activation has also been found in the cerebellum and the basal ganglia, but different studies have reported peak locations in various subcompartments, in the putamen, the globus pallidus, or the claustrum, making the functional interpretation of these effects difficult. Other sites include the hypothalamus and the brainstem, whose nuclei contain nociresponsive neurons; these sites include the parabrachial nuclei and the periaqueductal gray (PAG). Activation found in the thalamus, the hypothalamus, and the brainstem cannot be localized precisely in specific nuclei because of the limited spatial resolution of the PET method. In some studies, these subcortical structures may be outside the field of view of the scanner.

Evidence provided by PET studies indicates that a variety of noxious stimuli activate the thalamus and multiple cortical areas, including S1, S2, the insula, and the ACC. The convergence of findings is remarkable, given the diversity of experimental noxious stimulation and experimental conditions used in these studies. This combined evidence suggests that the concurrent activation of this network of brain structures constitutes the signature of pain in the brain. This pattern of activation may reflect the complexity of the subjective experience of pain.

THE MULTIDIMENSIONAL NATURE OF PAIN

The concept of pain, as distinguished from nociception, has multiple facets. Defined as a subjective experience, pain includes sensory and affective dimensions (see Chapter 1; see also Melzack and Casey 1968). Sensory dimensions refer to the quality, intensity, and spatiotemporal dynamics of the experience. The affective dimension has been subdivided into two successive components (Wade et al. 1996). *Primary affect* refers to the immediate feeling of unpleasantness associated with the experience of a threat (see Price 2000); *secondary affect* refers to the emotion associated with the more elaborate evaluation of the significance and future consequences of this felt threat (Wade et al. 1996; Price 2000). The affective dimensions can be reliably dissociated from the sensory dimension of pain; this distinction has proven useful for describing both experimental (Rainville et al. 1992) and clinical pain (Price et al. 1987). Each of these separate dimensions is also a constituent of other types of subjective experiences. The experience of nonpainful body sensation is defined along the same sensory dimensions, while basic negative emotions, such as fear, are felt as unpleasant and may be accompanied by the experience of a threat. The uniqueness of pain resides in the particular combination of those dimensions.

   Given the multiple areas that are consistently activated when pain is felt, how are we to conceive the brain's representation of the sensory and affective dimensions of pain? This question raises further questions about the specificity of pain-related activity. Are components of this pattern specifically observed during pain? Are pain sensation and pain unpleasantness represented in specific areas or within multiple areas? The cortical regions activated by painful stimuli are also involved in diverse sensory, cognitive, autonomic, and motor functions that may point toward their specific or preponderant functional contributions to the experience of pain. One of the most influential models posited parallel lateral and medial spinothalamic pathways terminating in lateral thalamic and medial/intralaminar nuclei, and projecting in turn to somatosensory and "fronto-limbic" cortical areas (Melzack and Casey 1968; Albé-Fessard et al. 1985; Fields 1987). These two parallel pathways are generally thought to subserve sensory-discriminative and affective-motivational functions, respectively. Two approaches have provided partial answers to these questions. The first approach investigates the extent to which the structural network displays properties compatible with the representation of a given dimension of pain. The second approach hypothesizes that the different dimensions of the pain experience are not equally represented in each of the structures activated during the experience of pain; i.e., that there is some degree of anatomical-functional specialization. However, these two possibilities—distributed representation and anatomical-functional specialization—are not necessarily incompatible and may be viewed as complementary.

DISTRIBUTED REPRESENTATION OF PAIN INTENSITY

   The hypothesis that activity within cortical regions activated during the presentation of noxious stimuli is correlated to the experience of pain was first tested in a PET study in which tonic innocuous and noxious temperatures (35°–49°C) were applied to the index finger (Duncan et al. 1994). The standard subtraction analysis (49°–35°C) of pain-related rCBF changes was compared with regression analyses based on stimulus temperature and on subjective ratings of thermal intensity and pain (see Plate 1). The regression of rCBF on pain ratings was the most powerful model, resulting in the highest number of sites displaying rCBF levels that were correlated to the pain reported. This provocative result clearly indicates that cerebral activity is more proximal to the subjective experience of pain, indexed by subjective ratings, than to the physical intensity (temperature) of the noxious stimulus, or to the subjective perception of temperature. The correlation between pain ratings and changes in the contralateral S1, S2, insula, and ACC showed that the magnitude of pain-evoked increases in rCBF in these regions was related to the subjective experience of pain. These findings were largely confirmed and extended in a recent study (Coghill et al. 1999) in which rCBF levels in the contralateral S1 and bilateral S2, IC, and ACC correlated with the perceived intensity of pain. These observations suggest that the sensory intensity of pain could be represented in many areas of the brain, and not only in the somatosensory cortices. This redundancy in the representation of information related to pain intensity had been observed previously in electrophysiological recordings in the medial and lateral thalamus of the monkey, and had been argued to reflect a potential contribution of both medial and lateral pain pathways to the sensory discrimination of pain (Bushnell and Duncan 1989). This redundancy in cortical pain processing may further explain the persistence of basic pain perception abilities despite extensive cortical damage (Bernier et al. 1997), and sheds light on the relative ineffectiveness of neurosurgical approaches to alleviate chronic pain (White and Sweet 1969). A corollary of this concept of distributed processing implies that each area displaying activity correlated to pain intensity can, at least potentially, subserve the appreciation of the intensity of pain, and that a complete loss of pain sensation is unlikely even after extensive cortical damage. This distributed organization may further underlie the determinant influence of pain intensity on pain unpleasantness (e.g., Wade et al. 1996; Price 2000) by directly providing information about intensity to affect-related structures. However, despite this ubiquitous coding of pain intensity, some evidence suggests a privileged representation of sensory aspects of pain in the somatosensory cortex.

S1 AND THE SENSORY ASPECTS OF PAIN

An initial controversy surrounded pain studies regarding the prevalence and functional significance of activation within S1 (reviewed in Bushnell et al. 1999a). As discussed above, many technical and methodological factors may have contributed to this uncertainty. However, the debate first took place on interpretative grounds. The observation of S1 activation by Talbot and coworkers (1991) was not replicated by Jones and colleagues (1991a), who argued that S1 activity in Talbot's study was independent of pain and related only to spatiotemporal aspects of the contact heat stimuli that were applied to multiple spots on the subject's forearm. However, this argument neglected to take into account the control condition in which warm contact stimuli had been applied using the same methods and following the same spatiotemporal sequence; these incidental aspects of the stimulation were therefore controlled and could not account for the pain-related activation observed in S1 (Duncan et al. 1992). The results indicated that S1 activity was greater during heat pain than during similar warm stimulation and suggested a participation of S1 cortex in the process of pain perception. Although it is plausible that multiple applications of a painful stimulus during the scans may have contributed to the increased activation of S1 activation in Talbot's study, it is unlikely that this effect could be attributed to processes independent of pain. Studies reporting positive results during the ensuing decade of PET imaging (see Bushnell et al. 1999a) indicate that S1 is activated during various types of pain and experimental paradigms and that this activation often exceeds that found during the control innocuous stimulation.

Consistent with the notion of functional specificity, some studies also suggest a critical involvement of S1 in processes responsible for the spatial localization of pain and the discrimination of pain intensity. Somatotopic organization of pain-related activity has been most clearly observed in S1 (Andersson et al. 1997) and most likely contributes to the ability to localize pain. A role in the appreciation of the spatiotemporal dynamic of pain sensations may further depend on an interaction of somatosensory cortices with dorsolateral prefrontal and posterior parietal cortices that are involved in spatial and temporal aspects of attention (Coghill et al. 1999). However, this interaction remains to be demonstrated and its mechanism identified.

A critical involvement of S1 in the sensation of pain is also suggested by the more robust activation observed in experiments that focus on this aspect of the experience (see Bushnell et al. 1999a). For example, in the baseline conditions of an experiment on the hypnotic modulation of pain sensation that compared noxious versus innocuous stimulation, without cognitive manipulations (Hofbauer et al. 1998), and in a study on the discrimination of pain sensation intensity (Carrier et al. 1998), S1 activation was unequivocal, and stronger than the activation found in other areas. These results contrast with those usually found in studies that do not explicitly emphasize the sensory aspects of the pain experience, in which S1 pain-related activity is weakly significant or absent. Furthermore, during the application of heat pain stimuli of equal intensity, S1 activity is reliably modulated by hypnotic (Hofbauer et al. 1998) or attentional (Carrier et al. 1998) interventions directed primarily at the sensory aspect of pain. In these studies, subjective ratings of pain intensity were directly proportional to the activity measured in S1. Also consistent with these findings is the observation of deficits in pain discrimination immediately following lesions of S1 in monkeys (Kenshalo et al. 1991). The marked loss of discriminative functions and elevated pain threshold following damage to S1/S2 in stroke patients (Ploner et al. 1999) also suggest that S1 is a primary contributor to the sensory dimension of pain. However, the subsequent recuperation of the ability to discriminate the intensity of noxious stimuli that frequently follows such lesions could reflect the secondary representation of pain intensity in other areas, as suggested by Coghill et al. (1999).

THE DISSOCIATION OF PAIN AFFECT FROM PAIN SENSATION

Representation of the affective dimension of pain was initially hypothesized to depend on limbic prefrontal cortices (e.g., Melzack and Casey 1968; Fields 1987), but the precise area involved was left unspecified. The ACC now emerges as a likely candidate from the wealth of data yielded by PET imaging studies. This structure is activated in virtually all pain studies using a variety of stimulation, and activation of this site could constitute a necessary condition for the normal experience of pain. The specificity of pain-related activity was documented in a PET study using an illusion of pain (Craig 1996). The thermal grill illusion is produced by simultaneous innocuous warm and innocuous cool stimuli applied to the skin in spatial alternation. This complex stimulus is rated as painful and unpleasant although each of its constituents, applied alone uniformly, is perceived only as warm or cool. The application of the thermal grill replicated the pattern of pain-evoked cortical activation observed with heat or cold pain in the S1, S2, insula, and ACC. In contrast, uniform warm or cool stimuli activated only S1, S2, and the insula. The specific activation observed during heat pain, cold pain, and especially during the illusion of pain suggests a determinant role of ACC in pain perception. Most interestingly, the regression analysis of rCBF changes based on subjective pain ratings was highly significant in the ACC (A.D. Craig and M.C. Bushnell, unpublished observation). These results, combined with the activation of the ACC in all pain studies, strongly suggest that this area is critical for the normal experience of pain. Other regions are likely to participate in aspects of pain that are partly shared with innocuous somatosensory perception. As the experience of pain may be most clearly contrasted to other somatosensory experiences by its intrinsic affective dimension, we hypothesized that the activation of the ACC reflects this aspect of the experience.

This hypothesis was directly tested using hypnotic suggestions to modulate pain unpleasantness or pain intensity. Pain affect was dissociated from pain sensation by using hypnotic suggestions to alter the experience produced by immersion of the hand in painfully hot water (Rainville et al. 1999). In one experiment, suggestions were designed to decrease or increase pain affect by associating the pain sensation with either an increased or decreased feeling of comfort and well-being. These hypnotic suggestions produced the targeted modulation in pain unpleasantness without producing changes in the perception of pain intensity. A second set of suggestions was designed to modulate pain sensation; in this condition, both pain intensity and pain unpleasantness were modulated in a highly correlated fashion. These hypnotic suggestions for modulating pain affect or pain sensation produced strikingly different effects on rCBF responses to noxious thermal stimuli (Rainville et al. 1997; Hofbauer et al. 1998). Modulation of pain affect produced changes in pain-evoked activity in the ACC, but not in S1 (Plate 2A). Moreover, rCBF in the ACC, but not in S1, was positively correlated with pain unpleasantness. In contrast, the modulation of pain intensity produced the strongest change of pain-evoked activity in the S1 cortex (Plate 2B), which was positively correlated with the subjects' perception of pain intensity. These results are consistent with the proposed role of these regions in pain sensation and affect. However, when the modulation of pain

---

Plate 1. Basic methods of analysis used in PET studies. (A) The subtraction method relies on the direct comparison of one condition where pain is experienced (Pain) to another "control" condition in which no pain is felt (No Pain). Single scans in horizontal view show the normalized value (%rCBF) obtained for each voxel and represented by different colors. The percentages reported below each image refer to the value at the voxel indicated by a cross. Volumes are directly subtracted on a voxel-by-voxel basis to obtain pain-related changes in %rCBF (Pain − No Pain). This operation is repeated in each subject and a *t* test is performed at each voxel to assess the statistical significance of this difference across the group (*T*-volume). The statistical volume is overlaid in registry to an anatomical image to localize the sites of significant pain-related changes in rCBF (here S1). (B) The regression method relies on an analysis of the relationship between rCBF and a "regressor," which can be a variable related to the stimulus or experimental conditions (e.g., stimulus intensity), to another physiological measure (e.g., heart rate), or to a psychological variable such as the subjective ratings of pain. In the example, scans 1–4 are taken in a nonpainful condition and scans 5–8 in a painful condition. The normalized rCBF value at the voxel indicated by the cross is indicated with the pain ratings obtained after each scan. The regression analysis evaluates the significance of the relationship between pain ratings and rCBF for each voxel. A *T*-volume and a Pearson *r* volume are calculated to assess the significance of this relationship across the group. Each value is overlaid on the anatomical image to localize sites were rCBF is significantly correlated to the subjective ratings of pain (here S1). →

affect was secondary to the modulation of pain sensation intensity, the corresponding modulation of ACC did not reach significance. Although the interpretation of negative findings should be considered cautiously (see above), this observation is intriguing when contrasted with the changes observed in the ACC when pain unpleasantness was specifically, rather than secondarily, modulated by the hypnotic suggestions.

Consistent with this hypothesized dissociation of sensory and affective processing of pain perception, Ploner et al. (1999) have recently reported that subsequent to an infarction of the S1 and S2 cortex, the unpleasant "feeling" integral to pain was preserved, even in the absence of sensory discriminative capacity and first pain sensation. Taken together with the PET studies of hypnotic and attentional modulation of pain, these findings complement those of Coghill et al. (1999) discussed above, by suggesting a

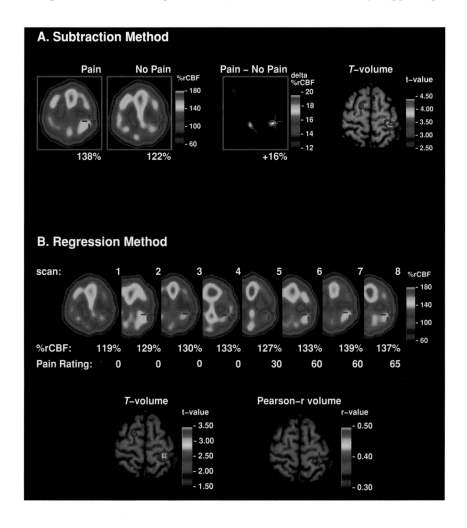

preponderant participation of the S1 cortex in pain sensation and of the ACC in pain affect (also see Tölle et al. 1999). It should be clear that this participation need not be exclusive and that these results are not incompatible with Coghill's suggestion that multiple areas may contribute to the representation of pain intensity.

Structures other than the ACC may very well contribute to various aspects of pain affect. For example, involvement of the IC in autonomic function, as a part of homeostatic regulation, is consistent with its participation in pain affect (Craig et al. 2000). The ACC and the IC are classical components of the limbic system and consist of multiple histologically defined subregions that most likely participate in different processes. In addition to pain, the ACC has been associated with arousal, attention, motor control, response selection, and autonomic activity (see Chapter 7; review by Devinsky et al. 1995; see also Vogt et al. 1992; Turken and Swick 1999). Similarly, the insula has been associated with pain, thermal, taste, and visceral sensation, as well as with autonomic control (Augustine 1996; Craig et al. 2000). The subjective experience of pain affect is probably influenced by the strength and efficacy of autonomic, cognitive, motor, and behavioral responses triggered by nociceptive processes. In turn, pain affect influences the voluntary behavioral responses and strategies adopted when facing a noxious stimulus (Wade et al. 1996; Price 2000). These cortical areas, therefore, may contribute to perception of affect through their regulation of autonomic and voluntary responses employed to interrupt or cope with pain.

PAIN AND EMOTIONS

In many circumstances the affective aspect of pain goes beyond its immediate unpleasantness. Secondary negative emotions can be triggered and experienced in response to the meanings and the perceived future consequences of pain (Price 1999). The interaction between pain and emotions may also take other forms. For example, the anticipation of pain may induce negative emotions, and emotional states may, in turn, influence the perception of pain (Rhudy and Meagher 2000).

Few brain-imaging studies have been performed on the experience of emotions. However, the results suggest that emotion- and pain-related brain activity may largely overlap. A recent PET study of emotions shows activation in the S2, insular, and cingulate cortices, in addition to the brainstem, the hypothalamus, and the orbitofrontal cortex, during the experience of emotions elicited by the recall of personal episodes marked with sadness, happiness, anger, or fear (Damasio et al. 2000). Likewise, a PET study of tactile phobia, without somatomotor stimulation, revealed activation of the somatomotor cortex, ACC, insula, and thalamus (Rauch et al. 1995). The unpleasant feeling of thirst also involves many structures activated during pain such as the thalamus, insula, and cingulate cortex (Denton et al. 1999). All these conditions—pain, emotion, and thirst—constitute affective states and recruit classical limbic cortices. These structures constitute potential candidates for the interaction between pain and emotions. However, the experience of pain produced in experimental studies generally lacks a strong emotional dimension because the subjects know that the experience will be brief and will not be accompanied by tissue damage or long-term adverse effects. Consequently, pain-related areas S1, S2, IC, and ACC may be more closely concerned with the immediate experience of pain. The orbitofrontal cortices activated during emotions may be recruited when pain is accompanied by strong feelings associated with the future consequences of pain. This possibility is consistent with clinical reports of prefrontal lobotomy, leucotomy, and orbitofrontal damage leading to a flattening of affect and insensitivity to consequences (Bechara et al. 1994). This convergence of activation associated with the experience of pain, emotional feelings, and motivational states, is consistent with a recent theoretical proposal that the subjective feelings of emotions and, more generally, conscious experience, are critically dependent upon the activity in brain structures involved in the representation of the body (Damasio 1999). The potential implications of this proposition for the understanding of pain and the interaction between pain and emotions will require further experimental exploration.

IMAGING CLINICAL PAIN

Functional brain-imaging studies of experimental pain provide the necessary basic knowledge to understand the brain's representation of pain and to start to investigate clinical pain states. A few studies have imaged brain activity in the course of an episode of acute clinical pain or during abnormal pain sensations such as hyperalgesia and allodynia, conditions characteristic of many clinical pain states. Furthermore, researchers are only beginning to investigate the cerebral correlates of persistent pain states. A major limitation of such studies is their inability to specify the causal mechanisms involved in the observed central changes. Abnormal brain activity observed in pathological pain states may passively reflect plastic changes occurring at lower levels of the neuraxis, or may reflect active plastic changes involving cerebral mechanisms, or, most likely, both. In any case, brain-imaging studies can reveal the specific areas most likely to contribute to abnormal

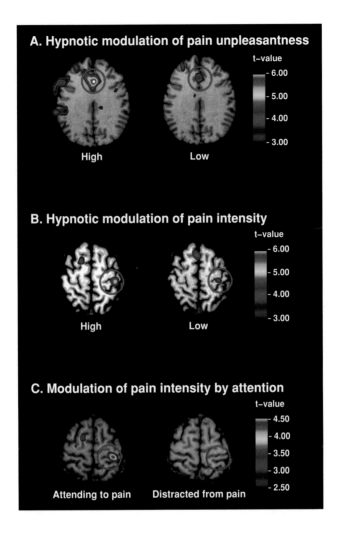

Plate 2. Modulation of pain-related activity by cognitive intervention. The modulation of pain by hypnosis or attention/distraction changes brain activity in pain-related areas. (A) The specific increase (high) or decrease (low) of pain unpleasantness by hypnotic suggestion directed at the affective dimension of pain modulated pain-related activity in the ACC (red circle). (B) In contrast, hypnotic suggestions that primarily affected pain sensation intensity produced changes mainly in S1 (red circle). (C) Similarly, pain ratings are higher and pain-related activity in S1 (red circle) is stronger when subjects pay attention to the painful stimulus than when they are distracted from pain.

pain states in humans. The evaluation of neurophysiological hypotheses about the mechanisms involved in the generation of abnormal pain states requires a combination of physiological studies in animals and brain-imaging studies in humans.

IMAGING VISCERAL PAIN

Most clinical pain arises from deep structures, such as joints, muscles, and viscera, yet little is known about how the brain processes visceral pain. Brain imaging, including PET, is now being used to examine the forebrain representation of visceral pain in humans. As indicated above, several cortical and subcortical forebrain structures are involved in processing cutaneous pain, which probably reflects the multidimensional nature of pain, involving sensory, affective, and motivational components. However, the experience described as "visceral pain" differs substantially from that associated with cutaneous pain in all of these dimensions. Whereas cutaneous pain is localizable and has distinct sensory qualities consistent with the type of tissue damage (e.g., burning, pricking, or pinching), visceral pain is difficult to localize, is often referred to a distant region (e.g., cardiac ischemia is felt as pain in the arm), and is frequently described as variable and difficult to define, but with a strong affective component (Schott 1994; McMahon et al. 1995). Most strikingly, visceral and cutaneous pain elicit highly divergent behavioral and autonomic responses. Whereas cutaneous pain evokes quick protective reflexes, tachycardia, hypertension, and increased alertness, visceral pain produces quiescence, bradycardia, hypotension, and loss of interest in the environment (Lewis 1942).

Little is known about the role of various cortical regions in visceral pain processing. As described above, the cortical regions most consistently activated by cutaneous pain are S1, S2, the ACC, and the IC (Jones et al. 1991a; Coghill et al. 1994; Hsieh et al. 1995; Casey et al. 1996). In two PET studies examining visceral pain, both found activation in the ACC, and one also showed activation in the IC (Aziz et al. 1997; Silverman et al. 1997). Silverman et al. (1997) observed that ACC activation was in a region that may be rostral to that most commonly activated by cutaneous pain, suggesting the possibility of a segregation between visceral and cutaneous representation in the ACC. A similar segregation of visceral and cutaneous nociceptive processing has been demonstrated in some animal studies of the brainstem. Keay et al. (1994) demonstrated in rats that noxious stimulation of the skin increases *c-fos* labeling in the lateral PAG, whereas stimulation of the viscera increases *c-fos* labeling in the ventrolateral PAG. Correspondingly, behavioral reactions evoked by microstimulation in the lateral PAG are similar to those produced by cutaneous pain, while behavioral reactions evoked by microstimulation in the ventrolateral PAG are similar to those produced by visceral pain. A fine-grain spatial comparison of ACC or other cortical representation of visceral and cutaneous pain will probably be achieved in future fMRI studies.

Evidence from Silverman et al. (1997) suggests that the specific brain regions engaged by noxious visceral stimulation in chronic pain patients may be different from those activated in normal healthy subjects under the same experimental conditions. Whereas painful colorectal distension activated the ACC in normal subjects, in patients with irritable bowel syndrome, the ACC failed to respond to the same stimuli. In contrast, these stimuli activated the left prefrontal cortex, mainly in Brodmann's area 10. Other studies of persistent aberrant pain have found that these pain states may sometimes engage cortical regions not activated by "normal" pain (see below).

IMAGING PERSISTENT PAIN STATES

Several investigators have used PET in patients with neuropathic pain of central or peripheral origin to determine changes in pain processing that could account for such symptoms as ongoing pain, hyperalgesia, and allodynia. Given the difficulties of applying PET to small, heterogeneous populations of patients and the differing pathological conditions studied, no consistent effects have emerged. In patients with peripheral neuropathic pain, one study described a unilateral decrease in thalamic activity (Iadarola et al. 1995), while another found both decreased activity in the resting thalamus and increased activity within a number of pain-related cortical regions, including the ACC and IC (Hsieh et al. 1995). In patients with central pain, one PET imaging study associated the pain with hyperexcitability in the thalamus (Cesaro et al. 1991) and another with hyperexcitability in the cerebral cortex (Canavero et al. 1993). Some data suggest that allodynia, whether related to clinical neuropathic pain or to experimental capsaicin application, is processed differently in the cerebral cortex than is nociceptive pain. Whereas the ACC is almost always activated in PET or fMRI studies of nociceptive pain, Peyron and colleagues (1998, 2000) failed to find ACC activation during allodynia in central pain patients. Similarly, Baron et al. (1999) observed no ACC activation when examining dynamic tactile allodynia during a capsaicin model in normal subjects and suggested that A-fiber-mediated pain has a unique cortical presentation. Other data do not support this interpretation, but rather suggest that pain arising from either aberrant or normal processes ultimately activates the same cortical structures. For example, ACC activation has been reported during dynamic tactile allodynia, both after capsaicin injection in normal subjects (Iadarola et al. 1998), and in patients with peripheral neuropathic pain (Petrovic et al. 1999). Additionally, Craig et al (1996) found ACC activation during the thermal grill pain illusion, an experimental model of central pain. These varying and seemingly contradictory results among PET imaging studies of chronic neuropathic pain suggest that multiple pathological mechanisms may contribute to similar clinical signs and symptoms.

USE OF PET TO EXAMINE CEREBRAL BASIS OF ANALGESIC TREATMENTS

FOREBRAIN MECHANISMS OF OPIOID ANALGESIA

The μ-opioid receptor has been identified at many levels of the neuraxis, including primary afferent fibers, spinal cord, thalamus, and cerebral cortex (Arvidsson et al. 1995). Although much research has been directed at the role of peripheral and spinal opioid receptors, little is known about opioid pain modulation in the forebrain. Casey et al. (2000) used PET to examine regional changes in CBF related to cold water pain, fentanyl administration, and the fentanyl-related modulation of cold water pain. After fentanyl, but not placebo, pain perception was reduced, as were all cortical and thalamic responses to painful cold (Plate 3). Fentanyl alone increased rCBF in the ACC, particularly in the perigenual region. On the other hand, fentanyl had no effect on either the perception or the cortical activation evoked by vibratory stimuli (Plate 4). These results suggest a selective fentanyl-mediated suppression of nociceptive spinothalamic transmission to the forebrain, indicating that the ACC may be a site of opioid analgesia.

NEURAL MECHANISMS OF STIMULATION-PRODUCED ANALGESIA

For more than 25 years, neurosurgeons have used electrical thalamic stimulation to treat intractable central and peripheral neuropathic pain, with varying success (Hosobuchi et al. 1973; Mazars et al. 1973). More recently, Tsubokawa et al. (1991, 1993) introduced electrical motor cortex stimulation for treatment of central pain. About half of the patients in which such stimulation has been tried show substantial pain relief of more than 60% (Katayama et al. 1998); however, the mechanisms underlying this stimulation-produced analgesia are unclear and may be multifaceted.

Several laboratories have used PET to investigate the mechanisms underlying therapeutic electrical brain stimulation for the treatment of neuropathic pain. The original theoretical basis for thalamic stimulation presumed that chronic pain could be relieved by activating tactile thalamocortical pathways that had been deafferented by nerve damage or neuronal lesions (Mazars et al. 1960, 1974). To examine possible neural pathways that could be activated using this therapeutic approach, Duncan et al (1998) measured

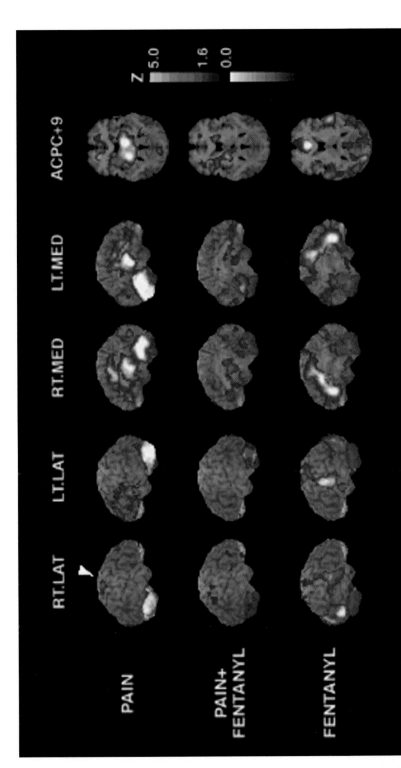

RT.LAT   LT.LAT   RT.MED   LT.MED   ACPC+9

PAIN

PAIN+
FENTANYL

FENTANYL

Z
5.0
1.6
0.0

rCBF in five patients who had received successful long-term pain relief with thalamic stimulation. Consistent with Mazar's original idea of activating tactile thalamocortical pathways, increased rCBF was observed to some extent in the S1 cortex during the thalamic stimulation. However, a much more robust activation was noted in the anterior insular cortex, a region known to be activated in humans by thermal stimulation, whether painful or innocuous (Casey et al. 1996; Craig et al. 1996). The increased activity in the anterior insula during therapeutic thalamic stimulation suggests that activation of temperature pathways may be an important component of the analgesia for these patients. This hypothesis is supported by patients' reports of stimulation-related thermal sensations (in addition to the tingling tactile paresthesiae) and by physiological and clinical data showing that pain perception is modulated by cutaneous temperature (Bini et al. 1984; Schoenfeld et al. 1985; Wahren et al. 1989; Osgood et al. 1990; Yarnitsky and Ochoa 1990; Strigo et al. 1999). Using similar methods, Davis et al. (2000) examined five other patients during thalamic stimulation. In these patients, the most robust activation was observed in the ACC, suggesting that other mechanisms may also be involved in producing successful analgesia with thalamic stimulation.

Mechanisms underlying the therapeutic effect of motor cortex stimulation are, likewise, unclear and may be multifaceted. Motor cortex stimulation achieves pain control at intensities below the threshold for muscle contraction (Tsubokawa et al. 1993), indicating that peripheral feedback generated by muscle contraction and activation of corticospinal tract neurons do not play a necessary role. PET studies performed during motor cortex stimulation indicate a robust activation of the motor thalamus (ventralis lateralis, VL), with additional activation of medial thalamic nuclei and limbic cortical structures that could be involved in pain modulation (Peyron et al. 1995; Garcia-Larrea et al. 1997, 1999). Many patients experience tingling paresthesiae, suggesting that motor cortex stimulation produces activation of non-nociceptive third- or fourth-order somatosensory neurons within the VL or somatosensory cortex, respectively, which in turn could inhibit hyperactive nociceptive neurons.

← **Plate 3.** Fentanyl-related modulation of noxious cold water pain. Sagittal and horizontal brain slices of PET activation are shown for each of three conditions, cold-water PAIN, PAIN + FENTANYL, and FENTANYL alone. After fentanyl, all cortical and thalamic responses to painful cold were reduced. Fentanyl alone increased rCBF in the ACC, particularly in the perigenual region. (Reprinted with permission from Casey et al. 2000).

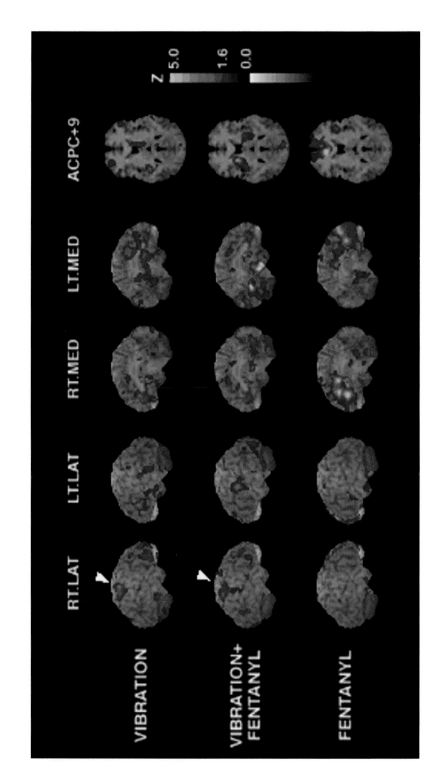

PSYCHOLOGICAL INTERVENTIONS

Human brain imaging has also revealed possible mechanisms related to analgesic psychological interventions, including attentional modulation of pain (Peyron et al. 1999; Bushnell et al. 1999b; Petrovic et al. 2000) and hypnotic analgesia (Rainville et al. 1997; Wik et al. 1998). Studies of attentional modulation of pain show that when subjects are required to perform tasks that direct their attention toward either auditory or visual stimuli, their estimates of both the intensity and the unpleasantness of concurrently presented noxious stimulation decrease significantly (Miron et al. 1989; Carrier et al. 1998). Likewise, Bushnell et al. (1999a) found that while the subject's attention is directed away from painful stimuli, there is a significant reduction in pain-evoked rCBF within the S1 cortex, as shown in Plate 2C. Similarly, Petrovic et al. (2000) recently described a significant reduction in pain-evoked activity in S2 when human subjects were distracted from cold pain by performing a maze task. Thus, these studies are consistent with the notion that cognitive manipulations that alter a subject's perception of pain intensity may operate through modulation of pain-related activity within sensory processing regions of the cerebral cortex, such as S1 and S2 (for an opposing view, see Peyron et al. 1999).

Hypnotic suggestions allow another form of psychological or cognitive intervention, in which subjects can be instructed to reinterpret the sensations produced by noxious stimuli, rather than direct their attention away from the noxious stimulation. As was discussed earlier, hypnotic suggestions that alter perceived pain intensity (Hofbauer et al. 1998; Bushnell et al. 1999a) are associated with a modulation of pain-evoked activity in S1, similar to that observed during attentional distraction within a sensory discrimination paradigm (Plate 2). In contrast, hypnotic suggestions that alter the perceived unpleasantness of a painful stimulus, without changing the perceived intensity, result in a preferential modulation of pain-evoked activity in the ACC (Rainville et al. 1997). These PET studies reveal a possible specialization in the cerebral processing that may underlie the multidimensional nature of analgesia, and further document the neurophysiological consequences of psychological interventions used as analgesic treatments.

← **Plate 4.** Fentanyl-related modulation of innocuous vibrotactile stimulation. Sagittal and horizontal brain slices of PET activation are shown for each of three conditions, VIBRATION, VIBRATION + FENTANYL, and FENTANYL alone. Fentanyl produces no significant change in the cortical activation evoked by vibratory stimuli. (Reprinted with permission from Casey et al. 2000).

THE USE OF PET TO EXAMINE PAIN-RELATED CHANGES IN NEUROTRANSMITTER SYSTEMS

Whereas most of the PET studies that address pain mechanisms use radiolabeled water to image pain-related changes in rCBF, PET can also be used to radiolabel neurotransmitter systems. Little work has been done using radioligand binding in relation to pain, but opioid systems have been most extensively studied. Various neuropharmacological studies have revealed multiple sites of antinociceptive actions for morphine, including the PAG (Basbaum et al. 1976; Jensen and Yaksh 1989; Alvarez-Royo et al. 1991), the spinal cord dorsal horn (Jones et al. 1990; Morgan et al. 1991), and the medial thalamus (Reyes-Vazquez et al. 1986; Carr and Bak 1988; Reyes-Vazquez et al. 1989; Dafny et al. 1990). Autoradiographic studies have confirmed that all these areas have high concentrations of opioid receptors (Simon and Hiller 1978; Pfeiffer et al. 1982; Warmsley et al. 1982; Atweh and Kuhar 1983; Sadzot et al. 1991; Jones et al. 1991b). The cortical site with the highest concentration of opioid receptors in humans is the ACC (Sadzot et al. 1991), which as described above is activated during pain and following the administration of fentanyl.

Using ^{11}C-diprenorphine (a nonspecific opioid antagonist) and PET, Jones and colleagues (1994, 1999) investigated the possible role of cortical opioid receptors in chronic pain states by measuring changes in opioid receptor binding during pain resulting from rheumatoid arthritis or trigeminal neuralgia. Jones et al. (1994) tested the hypothesis that inflammatory pain is associated with a change in cerebral endogenous opioid systems. Four patients were studied both when they were in pain and when their pain was relieved by local administration of steroids or by spontaneous remission. A significant increase in ^{11}C-diprenorphine binding was correlated with a reduction in pain. In addition to a generalized increase in binding throughout the brain, significant region-specific increases occurred in the frontal, cingulate, and temporal cortices. These findings suggest that opioid receptors in these regions may contribute to analgesia. When an individual is experiencing pain, endogenous opioid mechanisms may be activated, so that fewer receptor sites are available to exogenously administered opioids. When the pain is reduced, these sites become available. Similar results were observed when ^{11}C-diprenorphine binding was examined during trigeminal neuralgic pain and after relief by thermocoagulation (Jones et al. 1999). The ^{11}C-diprenorphine binding was increased in the prefrontal, insular, cingulate, and inferior parietal cortices, as well as in the thalamus and basal ganglia, suggesting a widespread circuit of opioid pain modulation in the forebrain.

CONCLUSIONS

Human brain imaging provides an exquisite bridge between classical neurophysiological studies of nociception and psychophysiological studies of human pain perception. Nevertheless, studies using these brain-imaging techniques need not be given mystical status (nor marginalized). At its base, brain imaging is simply classical neurophysiology, or more precisely, functional neuroanatomy. Numerous imaging studies have now confirmed the relationship between sensory stimulation and the activation of visual (Watson 1999), auditory (Millen et al. 1995; Tzourio et al. 1997), and somatosensory (Burton et al. 1993) pathways. Human pain research has especially benefitted from recent brain-imaging techniques, which allow us to go beyond the simple study of nociception and ask broader questions involving the neural basis of the subjective experience of pain. In addition to the obvious contribution to pain relief that the increased understanding of cerebral pain processes may bring to suffering patients, this endeavor may further advance our understanding of the neurophysiological basis of consciousness itself (Bushnell et al. 1999b; Damasio 1999; Price 1999).

The functional imaging of hemodynamic parameters such as blood flow has been the focus of most PET studies to date. The emerging technique of fMRI provides a number of advantages over PET for functional imaging, including better temporal and spatial resolution, reduced cost, increased availability, and the absence of radioactivity. However, fMRI is currently stimulus-dependent, while PET offers the advantage of assessing abnormalities of rCBF distribution in the resting condition. This feature is critical for studying chronic pathological conditions in which baseline activity may be abnormal in selected structures. A major contribution of PET to the future study of pain mechanisms may well lie in its application to the study of neurotransmitter systems. Using the competitive receptor-binding approach described above, we are now able to examine the role of different neurotransmitter systems and specific receptors in pain transmission and analgesia produced by a variety of techniques.

ACKNOWLEDGMENT

Dr. Rainville is supported by the Human Frontier Science Program.

REFERENCES

Al-Chaer ED, Lawand NB, Westlund KN, Willis WD. Visceral nociceptive input into the ventral posterolateral nucleus of the thalamus: a new function of the dorsal column pathway. *J Neurophysiol* 1996; 76:2661–2674.

Albé-Fessard D, Berkley KJ, Kruger L, Ralston HJ, Willis WD. Diencephalic mechanisms of pain sensation. *Brain Res Rev* 1985; 9:217–296.

Alvarez-Royo P, Clower RP, Zola-Morgan S, Squire LR. Stereotaxic lesions of the hippocampus in monkeys: determination of surgical coordinates analysis of lesions using magnetic resonance imaging. *J Neurosci Methods* 1991; 38:223–232.

Andersson J, Lilja A, Hartvig PH. Somatotopic organization along the central sulcus, for pain localization in humans, as revealed by positron emission tomography. *Exp Brain Res* 1997; 117:192–199.

Apkarian AV, Shi T. Squirrel monkey lateral thalamus. I. Somatic nociresponsive neurons and their relation to spinothalamic terminals. *J Neurosci* 1994; 14: 6779–6795.

Apkarian AV, Stea RA, Manglos SH, et al. Persistent pain inhibits contralateral somatosensory cortical activity in humans. *Neurosci Lett* 1992; 140:141–147.

Arvidsson U, Riedl M, Chakrabarti S, et al. Distribution and targeting of a mu-opioid receptor (MOR1) in brain and spinal cord. *J Neurosci* 1995; 15:3328–3341.

Atweh SF, Kuhar MJ. Distribution and physiological significance of opioid receptors in the brain. *Br Med Bull* 1983; 39:47–52.

Augustine JR. The insular lobe in primates including humans. *Neurol Res* 1996; 7:2–10.

Aziz Q, Andersson JLR, Valind S. Identification of human brain loci processing esophageal sensation using positron emission tomography. *Gastroenterology* 1997; 113:50–59.

Baleydier C, Mauguiere F. The duality of the cingulate gyrus in monkey. Neuroanatomical study and functional hypothesis. *Brain* 1980; 103:525–554.

Baron R, Baron Y, Disbrow EA, Roberts TPL. Brain processing of capsaicin-induced secondary hyperalgesia: a functional MRI study. *Neurology* 1999; 53:548–557.

Basbaum AI, Clanton CH, Fields HL. Opiate and stimulus-produced analgesia: functional anatomy of a medullospinal pathway. *Proc Natl Acad Sci USA* 1976; 73:4685–4688.

Bassetti C, Bogousslavsky J, Regli F. Sensory syndromes in parietal stroke. *Neurology* 1993; 43:1942–1949.

Bechara A, Damasio AR, Damasio H, Anderson SW. Insensitivity to future consequences following damage to human prefrontal cortex. *Cognition* 1994; 50:7–15.

Bernard JF, Bester H, Besson JM. Involvement of the spino-parabrachio amygdaloid and hypothalamic pathways in the autonomic and affective emotional aspects of pain. *Prog Brain Res* 1996; 107:243–255.

Bernier J, Bushnell MC, Ptito M, Ptito A, Marchand S. Touch, pain and temperature perception in hemispherectomized patients. *Soc Neurosci Abstr* 1997; 23.

Berthier M, Starkstein S, Leiguarda R. Asymbolia for pain: a sensory-limbic disconnection syndrome. *Ann Neurol* 1988; 24:41–49.

Biemond A. The conduction of pain above the level of the thalamus opticus. *Arch Neurol Psychiat* 1956; 75:231–244.

Bini G, Cruccu G, Hagbarth K-E, Schady W, Torebjork E. Analgesic effect of vibration and cooling on pain induced by intraneural electrical stimulation. *Pain* 1984; 18:239–248.

Brüggemann J, Shi T, Apkarian AV. Squirrel monkey lateral thalamus. II. Viscerosomatic convergent representation of urinary bladder, colon, and esophagus. *J Neurosci* 1994; 14:6796–6814.

Burton H, Videen TO, Raichle ME. Tactile-vibration-activated foci in insular and parietal-opercular cortex studied with positron emission tomography: mapping the second somatosensory area in humans. *Somatosens Mot Res* 1993; 10:297–308.

Bushnell MC, Duncan GH. Mechanical response properties of ventroposterior medial thalamic neurons in the alert monkey. *Exp Brain Res* 1987; 67:603–614.

Bushnell MC, Duncan GH. Sensory and affective aspects of pain perception: is medial thalamus restricted to emotional issues? *Exp Brain Res* 1989; 78:415–418.

Bushnell MC, Duncan GH, Tremblay N. Thalamic VPM nucleus in the behaving monkey. I. Multimodal and discriminative properties of thermosensitive neurons. *J Neurophysiol* 1993; 69:739–752.

Bushnell MC, Duncan GH, Hofbauer RK. Pain perception: is there a role for primary somatosensory cortex? *Proc Natl Acad Sci USA* 1999a; 96:7705–7709.

Bushnell MC, Duncan GH, Hofbauer RK. Human functional brain imaging: the bridge from neurophysiology to the mind. *Pain Forum* 1999b; 8:133–135.

Canavero S, Pagni CA, Castellano G, et al. The role of cortex in central pain syndromes: preliminary results of a long-term technetium-99 hexamethylpropyleneamineoxime single photon emission computed tomography study. *Neurosurgery* 1993; 32:185–191.

Carr KD, Bak TH. Medial thalamic injection of opioid agonists: mu-agonist increases while kappa-agonist decreases stimulus thresholds for pain and reward. *Brain Res* 1988; 441:173–184.

Carrier B, Rainville P, Paus T, Duncan GH, Bushnell MC. Attentional modulation of pain-related activity in human cerebral cortex. *Soc Neurosci Abstr* 1998; 24(1):1135.

Casey KL, Morrow TJ. Ventral posterior thalamic neurons differentially responsive to noxious stimulation of the awake monkey. *Science* 1983; 221:675–677.

Casey KL, Minoshima S, Morrow TJ, Koeppe RA. Comparison of human cerebral activation patterns during cutaneous warmth, heat pain, and deep cold pain. *J Neurophysiol* 1996; 76:571–581.

Casey KL, Svensson P, Morrow TJ, et al. Selective opiate modulation of nociceptive processing in the human brain. *J Neurophysiol* 2000; 84:525–533.

Cesaro P, Mann MW, Moretti, JL, et al. Central pain and thalamic hyperactivity: a single photon emission computerized tomographic study. *Pain* 1991; 47:329–336.

Chudler E H, Dong WK, Kawakami Y. Cortical nociceptive responses and behavorial correlates in the monkey. *Brain Res* 1986; 397:46–60.

Coghill RC, Talbot JD, Evans AC, et al. Distributed processing of pain and vibration by the human brain. *J Neurosci* 1994; 14:4095–4108.

Coghill RC, Sang CN, Maisog JM, Iadarola MJ. Pain intensity processing within the human brain: a bilateral, distributed mechanism. *J Neurophysiol* 1999; 82:1934–1943.

Craig AD. Pain, temperature, and the sense of the body. In: Franzen O, Johansson R, Terenius L (Eds). *Somesthesis and the Neurobiology of the Somatosensory Cortex*. Basel: Birkhauser, 1996, pp 27–39.

Craig AD, Bushnell MC, Zhang E-T, Blomqvist A. A thalamic nucleus specific for pain and temperature sensation. *Nature* 1994; 372:770–773.

Craig AD, Reiman EM, Evans AC, Bushnell MC. Functional imaging of an illusion of pain. *Nature* 1996; 384:258–260.

Craig AD, Chen L, Brandy D, Reiman EM. Thermosensory activation of insular cortex. *Nat Neurosci* 2000; 3:184–190.

Dafny N, Reyes-Vazquez, C, Qiao JT. Modification of nociceptively identified neurons in thalamic parafascicularis by chemical stimulation of dorsal raphe with glutamate, morphine, serotonin and focal dorsal raphe electrical stimulation. *Brain Res Bull* 1990; 24:717–723.

Damasio AR. *The Feeling of What Happens: Body and Emotion and the Making of Consciousness*. New York: Harcourt Brace, 1999.

Damasio AR, Grabowski TJ, Bechera A, et al. Subcortical and cortical brain activity during the feeling of self-generated emotions. *Nat Neurosci* 2000; in press.

Davis KD, Taub E, Duffner F, et al. Activation of the anterior cingulate cortex by thalamic stimulation in patients with chronic pain: a positron emission tomography study. *J Neurosurg* 2000; 92:64–69.

Denton D, Shade R, Zamarippa F, et al. Neuroimaging of genesis and satiation of thirst and an interoceptor-driven theory of origins of primary consciousness. *Proc Natl Acad Sci USA* 1999; 96:5304–5309.

Derbyshire SWG, Jones AKP. Cerebral responses to a continual tonic pain stimulus measured using positron emission tomography. *Pain* 1998; 76:127–135.

Devinsky O, Morrell MJ, Vogt BA. Contributions of anterior cingulate cortex to behaviour. *Brain* 1995; 118:279–306.

Dong WK, Salonen LD, Kawakami Y, et al. Nociceptive responses of trigeminal neurons in SII-7b cortex of awake monkeys. *Brain Res* 1989; 484:314–324.

Dong WK, Chudler EH, Sugiyama K, Roberts VJ, Hayashi T. Somatosensory, multisensory, and task-related neurons in cortical area 7b (PF) of unanesthetized monkeys. *J Neurophysiol* 1994; 72:542–564.

Dostrovsky JO, Craig AD. Nociceptive neurons in primate insular cortex. *Soc Neurosci Abstr* 1996; 22:111.

Duncan GH, Bushnell MC, Talbot JD, et al. Localization of responses to pain in human cerebral cortex. *Science* 1992; 255:215–216.

Duncan GH, Morin C, Coghill RC, et al. Using psychophysical ratings to map the human brain: regression of regional cerebral blood flow (rCBF) to tonic pain perception. *Soc Neurosci Abstr* 1994; 20:1572.

Duncan GH, Kupers RC, Marchand S, et al. Stimulation of human thalamus for pain relief: possible modulatory circuits revealed by positron emission tomography. *J Neurophysiol* 1998; 80:3326–3330.

Fields HL. *Pain*. New York: McGraw-Hill, 1987.

Friedman DP, Murray EA. Thalamic connectivity of the second somatosensory area and neighboring somatosensory fields of the lateral sulcus of the macaque. *Comp Neurol* 1986; 252:348–374.

Garcia-Larrea L, Peyron R, Mertens P, et al. Positron emission tomography during motor cortex stimulation for pain control. *Stereotact Funct Neurosurg* 1997; 68:141–148.

Garcia-Larrea L, Peyron R, Mertens P, et al. Electrical stimulation of motor cortex for pain control: a combined PET-scan and electrophysiological study. *Pain* 1999; 83:259–273.

Gingold SI, Greenspan JD, Apkarian AV. Anatomic evidence of nociceptive inputs to primary somatosensory cortex: relationship between spinothalamic terminals and thalamocortical cells in squirrel monkeys. *J Comp Neurol* 1991; 308:467–490.

Greenspan JD, Winfield JA. Reversible pain and tactile deficits associated with a cerebral tumor compressing the posterior insula and parietal operculum. *Pain* 1992; 50:29–39.

Head H, Holmes G. Sensory disturbances from cerebral lesions. *Brain* 1911; 34:102–254.

Hofbauer RK, Rainville P, Duncan GH, Bushnell MC. Cognitive modulation of pain sensation alters activity in human cerebral cortex. *Soc Neurosci Abstr* 1998; 24:1135.

Hosobuchi Y, Adams JE, Rutkin B. Chronic thalamic stimulation for the control of facial anesthesia dolorosa. *Arch Neurol* 1973; 29:158–161.

Hsieh JC, Belfrage M, Stone-Elander S, Hansson P, Ingvar M. Central representation of chronic ongoing neuropathic pain studied positron emission tomography. *Pain* 1995; 63:225–236.

Hutchison WD, Davis KD, Lozano AM, Tasker RR, Dostrovsky JO. Pain-related neurons in the human cingulate cortex. *Nat Neurosci* 1999; 2:403–405.

Iadarola MJ, Max MB, Berman KF, et al. Unilateral decrease in thalamic activity observed with positron emission tomography in patients with chronic neuropathic pain. *Pain* 1995; 63:55–64.

Iadarola MJ, Berman KF, Zeffiro TA, et al. Neural activation during acute capsaicin-evoked pain and allodynia assessed with PET. *Brain* 1998; 121(Pt 5):931–947.

Jensen TS, Yaksh TL. Comparison of the antinociceptive effect of morphine and glutamate at coincidental sites in the periaqueductal gray and medial medulla in rats. *Brain Res* 1989; 476:1–9.

Jones AKP, Brown WD, Friston KJ, Qi LY, Frackowiak RSJ. Cortical and subcortical localization of response to pain in man using positron emission tomography. *Proc R Soc Lond B Biol Sci* 1991a; 244:39–44.

Jones AK, Qi LY, Fujirawa T, Luthra SK, et al. In vivo distribution of opioid receptors in man in relation to the cortical projections of the medial and lateral pain systems measured with positron emission tomography. *Neurosci Lett* 1991b; 126:25–28.

Jones AKP, Cunningham VJ, Ha-Kawa S, et al. Changes in central opioid receptor binding in relation to inflammation and pain in patients with rheumatoid arthritis. *Br J Rheumatol* 1994; 33:909–916.

Jones AK, Kitchen ND, Watabe H, et al. Measurement of changes in opioid receptor binding in vivo during trigeminal neuralgic pain using [^{11}C]diprenorphine and positron emission tomography. *J Cereb Blood Flow Metab* 1999; 19:803–808.

Jones EG, Friedman DP. Projection pattern of functional components of thalamic ventrobasal complex on monkey somatosensory cortex. *J Neurophysiol* 1982; 48:521–544.

Jones SL, Sedivec MJ, Light AR. Effects of iontophoresed opioids on physiologically characterized laminae I and II dorsal horn neurons in the cat spinal cord. *Brain Res* 1990; 532:160–174.

Katayama Y, Fukaya C, Yamamato T. Poststroke pain control by chronic motor cortex stimulation: neurological characteristics predicting a favorable response. *J Neurosurg* 1998; 89:585–591.

Keay KA, Clement CI, Owler B. Convergence of deep somatic and visceral nociceptive information onto a discrete ventrolateral midbrain periaqueductal gray region. *Neuroscience* 1994; 61:727–732.

Kenshalo DR Jr, Isensee O. Responses of primate SI cortical neurons to noxious stimuli. *J Neurophysiol* 1983; 50:1479–1496.

Kenshalo DR Jr, Chudler EH, Anton F, Dubner R. SI nociceptive neurons participate in the encoding process by which monkeys perceive the intensity of noxious thermal stimulation. *Brain Res* 1988; 454:378–382.

Kenshalo DR Jr, Thomas DA, Dubner R. Primary somatosensory cortical lesions reduce the monkey's ability to discriminate and detect noxious thermal stimulation. *Soc Neurosci Abstr* 1991; 17:1206–1206.

Kitamura Y, Kakigi R, Hoshiyama M, et al. Pain-related somatosensory evoked magnetic fields. *Electroencephalogr Clin Neurophysiol* 1995; 95:463–474.

Koyama T, Ikami A, Ikami A. Nociceptive neurons in the macaque anterior cingulate activate during anticipation of pain. *Neuroreport* 1998; 2663–2667.

Lenz FA, Rios M, Zirh A, et al. Painful stimuli evoke potentials recorded over the human anterior cingulate gyrus. *J Neurophysiol* 1998a; 79:2231–2234.

Lenz FA, Gracely RH, Baker FH, et al. Reorganization of sensory modalities evoked by microstimulation in region of the thalamic principal sensory nucleus in patients with pain due to nervous system injury. *J Comp Neurol* 1998b; 399:125–138.

Lenz FA, Seike M, Richardson RT. Thermal and pain sensations evoked by microstimulation in the area of human ventrocaudal nucleus. *J Neurophysiol* 1993; 70:200–212.

Lewis T. *Pain.* New York: MacMillan, 1942.

Mazars G, Roge R, Mazars Y. Resultats de la stimulation du faisceau spino-thalamique et leur incidence sur la physiopathologie de la douleur. *Rev Neurol (Paris)* 1960; 103:136–138.

Mazars GJ, Merienne L, Ciolocca C. Stimulations thalamiques intermittentes antalgiques. *Rev Neurol (Paris)* 1973; 128:273–279.

Mazars G, Merienne L, Cioloca C. Traitement de certains types de douleurs par des stimulateurs thalamiques implantables. *Neuro-Chirurgie* 1974; 2:117–124.

McMahon SB, Dmitrieva N, Koltzenburg M. Visceral pain. *Br J Anaesth* 1995; 75:132–144.

Melzack R, Casey KL. Sensory, motivational and central control determinants of pain: a new conceptual model. In: Kenshalo DR (Ed). *The Skin Senses.* Springfield, IL: Thomas, 1968, pp 423–443.

Millen SJ, Haughton VM, Yetkin Z. Functional magnetic resonance imaging of the central auditory pathway following speech and pure-tone stimuli. *Laryngoscope* 1995; 105:1305–1310.

Miron D, Duncan GH, Bushnell MC. Effects of attention on the intensity and unpleasantness of thermal pain. *Am Pain Soc Abstr* 1989; 27:53.

Morgan MM, Gold MS, Liebeskind JC, Stein C. Periaqueductal gray stimulation produces a spinally mediated, opioid antinociception for the inflamed hindpaw of the rat. *Brain Res* 1991; 545:17–23.

Oppenheimer SM, Kedem G, Martin WM. Left-insular cortex lesions perturb cardiac autonomic tone in humans. *Clin Auton Res* 1996; 6:131–140.

Osgood PF, Carr DB, Kazianis A, et al. Antinociception in the rat induced by a cold environment. *Brain Res* 1990; 507:11–16.

Penfield W, Boldrey E. Somatic motor and sensory representation in the cerebral cortex of man as studied by electrical stimulation. *Brain* 1937; 60:389–443.

Petrovic P, Ingvar M, Stone-Elander S, Petersson KM, Hansson P. A PET activation study of dynamic mechanical allodynia in patients with mononeuropathy. *Pain* 1999; 83:459–470.

Petrovic P, Petersson KM, Ghatan PH, Stone-Elander S, Ingvar M. Pain-related cerebral activation is altered by a distracting cognitive task. *Pain* 2000; 85:19–30.

Peyron R, Garcia-Larrea L, Deiber MP, et al. Electrical stimulation of precentral cortical area in the treatment of central pain: electrophysiological and PET study. *Pain* 1995; 62:275–286.

Peyron R, Garcia-Larrea L, Gregoire MC, et al. Allodynia after lateral-medullary (Wallenberg) infarct. A PET study. *Brain* 1998; 121(Pt 2):345–356.

Peyron R, Larrea L, Goire MC, et al. Haemodynamic brain responses to acute pain in humans: sensory and attentional networks. *Brain* 1999; 122:1765–1780.

Peyron R, Larrea L, Goire MC, et al. Parietal and cingulate processes in central pain. A combined positron emission tomography (PET) and functional magnetic resonance imaging (fMRI) study of an unusual case. *Pain* 2000; 84:77–87.

Pfeiffer A, Pasi A, Mehraein P, Herz A. Opiate receptor binding sites in human brain. *Brain Res* 1982; 248:87–96.

Ploner M, Freund HJ, Schnitzler A. Pain affect without pain sensation in a patient with a postcentral lesion. *Pain* 1999; 81:211–214.

Pons TP, Kaas JH. Corticocortical connections of area 2 of somatosensory cortex in macaque monkeys: a correlative anatomical and electrophysiological study. *J Comp Neurol* 1986; 248:313–335.

Pons TP, Garraghty PE, Mishkin M. Serial and parallel processing of tactual information in somatosensory cortex of rhesus monkeys. *J Neurophysiol* 1992; 68:518–527.

Price DD. *Psychological Mechanisms of Pain and Analgesia,* Progress in Pain Research and Management, Vol. 15. Seattle: IASP Press, 1999.

Price DD. Psychological and neural mechanisms of the affective dimension of pain. *Science* 2000; 288:1769–1772.

Price DD, Harkins SW, Baker C. Sensory-affective relationships among different types of clinical and experimental pain. *Pain* 1987; 28:297–308.

Rainville P, Feine JS, Bushnell MC, Duncan GH. A psychophysical comparison of sensory and affective responses to four modalities of experimental pain. *Somatosens Mot Res* 1992; 9:265–277.

Rainville P, Duncan GH, Price DD, Carrier B, Bushnell MC. Pain affect encoded in human anterior cingulate but not somatosensory cortex. *Science* 1997; 277:968–971.

Rainville P, Carrier B, Hofbauer RK, Bushnell MC, Duncan GH. Dissociation of sensory and affective dimensions of pain using hypnotic modulation. *Pain* 1999; 82:159–171.

Rauch SL, Savage CR, Alpert NM, et al. A positron emission tomographic study of simple phobic symptom provocation. *Arch Gen Psychiatry* 1995; 52:20–28.

Rausell E, Jones EG. Chemically distinct compartments of the thalamic VPM nucleus in monkeys relay principal and spinal trigeminal pathways to different layers of the somatosensory cortex. *J Neurosci* 1991; 11:226–237.

Rausell E, Bae CS, Viñuela A, Huntley GW, Jones EG. Calbindin and parvalbumin cells in monkey VPL thalamic nucleus: distribution, laminar cortical projections, and relations to spinothalamic terminations. *J Neurosci* 1992; 12:4088–4111.

Reyes-Vazquez C, Enna SJ, Dafny N. The parafasciculus thalami as a site for mediating the antinociceptive response to GABAergic drugs. *Brain Res* 1986; 383:177–184.

Reyes-Vazquez C, Qiao J-T, Dafny N. Nociceptive responses in nucleus parafascicularis thalami are modulated by dorsal raphe stimulation and microiontophoretic application of morphine and serotonin. *Brain Res Bull* 1989; 23:405–411.

Rhudy JL, Meagher MW. Fear and anxiety: divergent effects on human pain thresholds. *Pain* 2000; 84:65–75.

Robinson CJ, Burton H. Organization of somatosensory receptive fields in cortical areas 7b, retroinsula, postauditory and granular insula of M. fascicularis. *J Comp Neurol* 1980a; 192:69–92.

Robinson CJ, Burton H. Somatic submodality distribution within the second somatosensory (SII), 7b, retroinsular, postauditory, and granular insular cortical areas of M. fascicularis. *J Comp Neurol* 1980b; 192:93–108.

Robinson CJ, Burton H. Somatotopographic organization in the second somatosensory area of M. fascicularis. *J Comp Neurol* 1980c; 192:43–67.

Sadzot B, Price JC, Mayberg HS, et al. Quantification of human opiate receptor concentration and affinity using high and low specific activity [^{11}C]diprenorphine and positron emission tomography. *J Cereb Blood Flow Metab* 1991; 11:204–219.

Schoenfeld AD, Lox CD, Chen CH, Lutherer LO. Pain threshold changes induced by acute exposure to altered ambient temperatures. *Peptides* 1985; 6:19–22.

Schott GD. Visceral afferents: their contribution to 'sympathetic dependent' pain. *Brain* 1994; 117:397–413.

Sikes RW, Vogt BA. Nociceptive neurons in area 24 of rabbit cingulate cortex. *J Neurophysiol* 1992; 68:1720–1732.

Silverman DHS, Munakata JA, Ennes H, et al. Regional cerebral activity in normal and pathological perception of visceral pain. *Gastroenterology* 1997; 112:64–72.

Simon EJ, Hiller JM. The opiate receptors. *Annu Rev Pharmacol Toxicol* 1978; 18:371–394.

Stevens RT, London SM, Apkarian AV. Spinothalamocortical projections to the secondary somatosensory cortex (SII) in squirrel monkey. *Brain Res* 1993; 631:241–246.

Strigo I, Carli F, Bushnell MC. The effect of ambient temperature on human pain perception. *Anesthesiology* 1999; 92:699–707.

Talbot JD, Marrett S, Evans AC. Multiple representations of pain in human cerebral cortex. *Science* 1991; 251:1355–1358.

Tölle TR, Kaufmann T, Siessmeier T, et al. Region-specific encoding of sensory and affective components of pain in the human brain: a positron emission tomography correlation analysis. *Ann Neurol* 1999; 45:40–47.

Treede RD, Kenshalo DR, Gracely RH, Jones AK. The cortical representation of pain. *Pain* 1999; 79:105–111.

Tsubokawa T, Katayama Y, Yamamoto T, Hirayama T, Koyama S. Chronic motor cortex stimulation for the treatment of central pain. *Acta Neurochir* 1991; 52:137–139.

Tsubokawa T, Katayama Y, Yamamoto T, Hirayama T, Koyama S. Chronic motor cortex stimulation in patients with thalamic pain. *J Neurosurg* 1993; 78:393–401.

Turken AU, Swick D. Response selection in the human anterior cingulate cortex. *Nat Neurosci* 1999; 2(10):920–924.

Tzourio N, Massioui FE, Crivello F, et al. Functional anatomy of human auditory attention studied with PET. *Neuroimage* 1997; 5:63–77.

Vogt BA, Rosene DL, Pandya DN. Thalamic and cortical afferents differentiate anterior from posterior cingulate cortex in the monkey. *Science* 1979; 204:205–207.

Vogt BA, Pandya DN, Rosene DL. Cingulate cortex of the rhesus monkey: I. Cytoarchitecture and thalamic afferents. *J Comp Neurol* 1987; 262:256–270.

Vogt BA, Finch DM, Olson CR. Functional heterogeneity in cingulate cortex: the anterior executive and posterior evaluative regions. *Cereb Cortex* 1992; 2:435–443.

Volkow ND, Mullani N, Gould LK, Adler SS, Gatley SJ. Sensitivity of measurements of regional brain activation with oxygen-15-water and PET to time of stimulation and period of image reconstruction. *J Nucl Med* 1991; 32:58–61.

Wade JB, Dougherty LM, Archer CR, Price DD. Assessing the stages of pain processing: a multivariate analytical approach. *Pain* 1996; 68:157–167.

Wahren LK, Torebjörk E, Jorum E. Central suppression of cold-induced C fibre pain by myelinated fiber input. *Pain* 1989; 38:313–319.

Warmsley JK, Zarbin MA, Young WS, Kuhar MJ. Distribution of opiate receptors in the monkey brain: an autoradiography study. *Neuroscience* 1982; 7:595–613.

Watson JD. Functional imaging of human visual cortex. *Clin Exp Pharmacol Physiol* 1999; 23:926–930.

White JC, Sweet WH. *Pain and the Neurosurgeon: A Forty-Year Experience.* Springfield, IL: Thomas, 1969.

Wik G, Fischer H, Bragee B, Finer B, Fredrikson M. Functional anatomy of hypnotic analgesia: a PET study of patients with fibromyalgia. *Eur J Pain* 1998; 3:7–12.

Yarnitsky D, Ochoa JL. Release of cold-induced burning pain by block of cold-specific afferent input. *Brain* 1990; 113:893–902.

Zhang ET, Han ZS, Craig AD. Morphological classes of spinothalamic lamina I neurons in the cat. *J Comp Neurol* 1996; 367:537–549.

Correspondence to: Pierre Rainville, PhD, Department of Neurology, University of Iowa Hospitals and Clinics, Iowa City, IA 52242, USA. Fax: 319-356-4505; email: pierre-rainville@uiowa.edu.

Pain Imaging, Progress in Pain Research and
Management, Vol. 18, edited by Kenneth L.
Casey and M. Catherine Bushnell, IASP Press,
Seattle, © 2000.

6

Functional Magnetic Resonance Imaging: Technical Aspects

G. Bruce Pike[a] and Richard D. Hoge[b,c]

[a]McConnell Brain Imaging Center, Montreal Neurological Institute, McGill University, Montreal, Quebec, Canada; [b]Nuclear Magnetic Resonance Center, Massachusetts General Hospital, Charlestown, Massachusetts, USA; [c]Department of Radiology, Harvard University Medical School, Charlestown, Massachusetts, USA

Since its inception in the early 1970s (Lauterbur 1973), magnetic resonance imaging (MRI) has evolved to be the neuroradiology modality of choice because of its superb soft tissue contrast and exquisite anatomical detail. However, while dominant in the anatomical arena, MRI has only recently been exploited to image brain function. Information on brain function has traditionally been obtained using radioactive tracer techniques, such as positron emission tomography (PET), to measure changes in cerebral blood flow (CBF) in response to functional activations. However, the past 5–7 years have witnessed the birth of functional MRI (fMRI), which now holds the promise of advancing functional imaging in the same way that MRI enhanced anatomical imaging.

Functional MRI does not image brain activity directly but is based on the detection of changes in various physiological correlates of neuronal activation. These include cerebral blood volume, blood flow, and blood oxygenation. The most common approach is based on blood oxygenation changes, and the signal contrast thus generated has been termed BOLD, for blood oxygenation level dependent. BOLD fMRI is now widely used in brain-mapping studies due to the availability of MRI facilities and the lack of health risk associated with MRI.

This chapter reviews the fundamental concepts surrounding fMRI. We will begin with a brief introduction to the essential physics of MRI, which is necessary to understand the fMRI signal being recorded, how the signal is affected by acquisition parameters, and the limitations imposed by fundamental principles and practical hardware. We will consider the primary fMRI contrast mechanisms and acquisition methodologies and present the use of these techniques in various experimental designs. The analysis of fMRI data involves the detection of small signals in the presence of significant noise and therefore requires statistical methods. We will review these techniques and the compensation for effects such as motion.

MAGNETIC RESONANCE IMAGING

NUCLEAR MAGNETIC RESONANCE

MRI was originally, and more accurately, described by the term *nuclear magnetic resonance imaging* (NMRI) as it is based on the same physical phenomenon as used in NMR spectroscopy. (Loss of the "N" to form MRI may have been motivated by the perceived negative connotations of the word *nuclear* by the general public.) The discovery of NMR in 1946 is attributed to two groups working independently: one at Stanford under the direction of Bloch (Bloch et al. 1946) and the other at Harvard under Purcell (Purcell et al. 1946).

The essence of the NMR phenomenon is that when certain atomic nuclei (those with an odd number of protons, neutrons, or both) are placed in a magnetic field and irradiated with a radio frequency (RF) excitation field at their resonant frequency, they absorb and re-emit energy at the same frequency. While a complete and accurate description of NMR is beyond the scope of this book, the phenomenon originates from the interaction of the nuclei's magnetic moment and angular momentum with the external magnetic field. The relationship between the resonance frequency, ω, and the applied magnetic field, B_0, is given by the Larmor equation:

$$\omega = \gamma B_0$$

where the constant of proportionality, γ, is unique for a given nuclear species. For hydrogen nuclei, which are observed in conventional MRI, γ is 42.58 MHz/T. Therefore, for a 1.5-T MRI scanner, hydrogen nuclei have a resonant frequency of approximately 64 MHz (at the bottom of your FM radio dial). This simple linear relationship between resonant frequency and magnetic field strength is central to both spectroscopy and imaging. In spectroscopy, magnetic field variations due to chemical environment are exploited to differentiate nuclei in different chemical milieus. In imaging, magnetic field variations are intentionally introduced to allow spatial localization of the signal based on resonant frequency.

RELAXATION—T_1, T_2, AND T_2^*

When a population of hydrogen nuclei is placed in a magnetic field, the rules of quantum mechanics dictate that they will assume one of two orientations: parallel or anti-parallel to the applied field. At thermal equilibrium a small net excess of nuclei (approximately 1–10 nuclei per million at MRI field strengths) will assume the lower energy state (aligned with B_0). The net effect of all these nuclei is the formation of a small bulk magnetization, M_0, oriented in the direction of B_0. It is this quantity that we manipulate and measure in MRI.

Upon initial placement of a sample in a magnetic field, M_0 does not form instantaneously but instead approaches its equilibrium value via a first-order process known as spin-lattice relaxation. The time constant of the exponential growth of M along the direction of B_0 (conventionally referred to as the z direction or the longitudinal direction) is T_1. This process of spin-lattice relaxation occurs whenever M is changed from its equilibrium state, M_0. Spin-lattice relaxation is illustrated in Fig. 1a for three samples with different T_1's. The equilibrium amplitude of M_0 reflects the number of nuclei present in the sample and is called the proton density, or simply ρ, and is often referenced to water. For example, for CSF $\rho \approx 1$, while for white matter $\rho \approx 0.65$.

While the equilibrium magnetization points along the longitudinal direction (i.e., $M = M_z = M_0$), this magnetization cannot be directly detected. MRI can only measure the component of magnetization perpendicular to B_0 (i.e., in the transverse plane) that precesses at its resonant frequency. Transverse magnetization is generated using an RF excitation pulse that rotates M away from the longitudinal direction. An RF excitation pulse producing a 90° rotation of M (sometimes called a *flip angle*) would rotate all longitudinal magnetization into the transverse plane and thereby maximize the detected signal. The component of M that is in the transverse plane, M_{xy}, will precess at its Larmor frequency but will also decay via a process called spin-spin relaxation, with a time constant T_2. Spin-spin relaxation comes about due to the loss of coherence between precessing transverse magnetization because the frequency of precession will fluctuate slightly over space and time as the nuclei experience the fluctuating magnetic fields of their environment. In addition to the naturally occurring random field variations, static field inhomogeneities often enhance the loss of coherence (also called dephasing) and hence increase the rate of decay of M_{xy}. The M_{xy} therefore decays exponentially, with a total observed time constant of T_2^* ($1/T_2^* = 1/T_2 + 1/T'_2$), where T'_2 is the decay time constant due just to field inhomogeneities. T_2 and T_2^* decay curves are illustrated in Fig. 1.

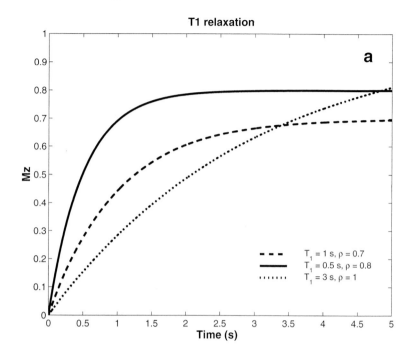

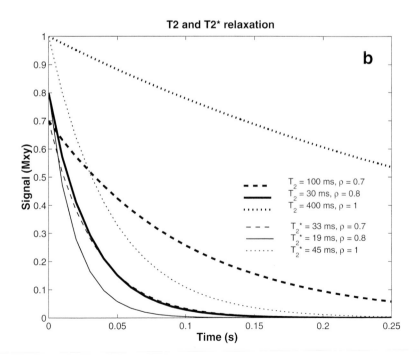

While static field inhomogeneity and the resulting accelerated signal decay are often considered undesirable effects, they can also be of explicit interest, as in BOLD fMRI. There are two basic types of MRI acquisitions, which enable either T_2^* or T_2 signal dependence. Excitation followed, after a time delay of TE (echo time), by signal measurement is referred to as *gradient-echo* (GE) imaging, and the received signal will have decayed according to T_2^* (i.e., $M_{xy} \propto \exp[-TE/T_2^*]$). If, at a time of TE/2, a 180° pulse is added, the M_{xy} dephasing due to static field inhomogeneities can be reversed, and an echo will form at TE that will have an amplitude dependent only upon T_2 (i.e., $M_{xy} \propto \exp[-TE/T_2^*]$). This technique is called *spin-echo* (SE) imaging, and the 180° pulse used to correct for static inhomogeneities is called a *spin-echo pulse*.

Clearly, TE can be adjusted to give variable sensitivity to T_2 (SE) or T_2^* (GE). To achieve sensitivity to T_1, the time between excitations, also called the *repetition time* (TR), can be varied: the shorter the TR, the greater is the T_1 weighting that is introduced. Another method of introducing T_1 weighting is known as *inversion recovery* (IR) imaging. In IR imaging the experiment begins with a 180° pulse that inverts M_z. After an inversion time delay (TI), during which M_z recovers according to T_1, an excitation pulse is used to measure the partially recovered longitudinal magnetization by converting it into observable transverse magnetization (M_{xy}). IR sequences are extensively used in perfusion-based fMRI techniques.

IMAGING

To produce images, linear magnetic field gradients (i.e., magnetic fields whose amplitude varies linearly with position) are used to establish a direct relationship between resonant frequency and location along the gradient. These gradient fields are much smaller than the main field and cause a dispersion of frequencies about the main resonant frequency (e.g., a 1.5-T magnet with a gradient of 10-mT per meter would produce frequencies of approximately 64 ± 0.04 MHz for a 20-cm field of view). Since position is encoded as frequency, a Fourier transform (which calculates the frequency spectrum of a signal) is used to reconstruct images in MRI. (A more complete

---

← **Fig. 1.** (a) Spin-lattice and (b) spin-spin relaxation curves for three fictitious materials. Spin-lattice relaxation is the process by which the magnetization (M_z) forms along the direction of the external magnetic field (B_0) and is characterized by the time constant T_1. Spin-spin relaxation describes the decay of transverse magnetization (signal) following an excitation and is characterized by the time constants T_2 (thick lines) and T_2^* (thin lines), which exclude and include magnetic field inhomogeneities, respectively.

description of Fourier transforms and MRI, written for biological scientists, can be found in Pike 1988.)

In conventional MRI acquisitions (Fig. 2, left), the raw data required to reconstruct an image are measured on a Cartesian grid. One line is measured per TR (repetition time). Therefore, for example, the acquisition of all the data for a 256×256 matrix image with an imaging pulse sequence (the term pulse sequence refers to the sequence of RF pulses, magnetic field gradients, and data sampling that make up the entire imaging experiment) having a 100-ms TR would require 25.6 s. While this type of acquisition is sufficient for most routine anatomical imaging, it is relatively slow for imaging dynamic physiological processes and can suffer from artifacts created by changes in the subject (e.g., motion) during data acquisition.

ECHO PLANAR IMAGING

Many fast imaging methods have been developed to reduce motion artifacts and increase temporal resolution for sequential measurements. The fastest of these techniques are referred to as *single-shot* methods because all the data required to reconstruct an image are acquired after a single excitation. The most common single-shot technique is *echo-planar imaging* (EPI), which derives its name from the fact that a plane (two-dimensional grid) of data is collected from a single echo (Fig. 2b, right). A typical 64×64 matrix EPI acquisition takes less than 50 ms and therefore avoids the problem of intrascan movement artifacts by effectively "freezing" most motion. How-

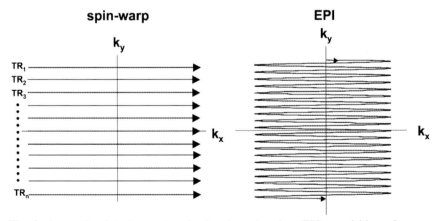

Fig. 2. Conventional (spin-warp) and echo-planar imaging (EPI) acquisitions. In conventional MRI, raw data are acquired one line per repetition (TR) on a Cartesian grid. In EPI, a single excitation is followed by an extremely rapid measurement (usually <100 ms) of all the necessary raw data for image reconstruction using an oscillating data-sampling trajectory.

ever, interscan movement remains a problem for fMRI using single-shot EPI and is usually addressed via careful head restraint and post-processing techniques (as discussed below).

The most common approach to imaging a volume of tissue with EPI is to acquire a series of slices sequentially. Considering the data sampling time, echo time, and other small pulse sequence delays, the minimum interslice interval is typically on the order of 100 ms. Thus, for the 20–30 slices required to image the entire brain, the minimum total scan time per volume is approximately 2–3 s. On some scanners, the time delay between slices is always minimized, and any extra time before the next prescribed volume acquisition is collected together at the end of the sequence. On other systems, the default is to evenly space the slice acquisitions over the prescribed repeat time for volume acquisition. The order of slice acquisition is usually under user control and may be linear, reverse linear, or interleaved, for example. Whichever approach is used, it is important to account for the time difference between slices when analyzing the functional data, since the analysis is usually based on the relationship between the time course of the stimulus or task and that of the observed MRI signal. This issue is particularly important in event-related fMRI experiments because the imaging time per volume is significant compared to the time constants of the hemodynamic response.

HARDWARE

An MRI scanner consists of the following basic components: a large static magnet, a set of linear gradient coils, radiofrequency (RF) excitation and reception coils, amplifiers to drive the gradient and RF coils, data sampling electronics, and computers to control the various components, reconstruct images, and handle all image viewing and archiving. While a discussion of all these components is beyond the scope of this chapter, we will briefly consider those features most relevant to fMRI from the point of view of both performance and safety.

Main magnetic field strength. Functional MRI experiments are performed almost exclusively at field strengths of 1 T and above (1 Tesla is approximately 20,000 times the strength of the earth's magnetic field). To achieve such high fields, superconducting magnets are employed. These magnets consist of very long windings (many kilometers) wrapped around a hollow cylinder and immersed in liquid helium. At this temperature (4.2° Kelvin), the windings become superconducting (i.e., have no resistance), and a large injected current continues to flow without a power source. These magnets are thus always "on." The force with which they can attract ferromagnetic objects represents perhaps the most significant safety hazard for subjects and operators. The presence of the static magnetic field has no known negative biological consequences.

The primary limitations on magnetic field strength are related to engineering aspects of their manufacture. For MRI in general, the advantage of increasing the magnetic field strength is to increase the received signal due to an increase in the induced magnetization amplitude (i.e., M_0) and resonance frequency. The exact relationship between magnetic field strength and the signal-to-noise ratio (SNR) in a specific imaging context is complicated by the fact that the relaxation rates also have a field dependence. However, for fMRI the BOLD signal for cortical gray matter increases in proportion to the field strength to the power of 1.6 (i.e., BOLD fMRI signal $\propto B_0^{1.6}$) (Gati et al. 1997). Thus, a 2% BOLD signal at 1.5 T would be expected to be approximately 10% at 4 T. This substantial signal advantage has motivated the development and purchase of very high field systems for fMRI. However, there are some advantages to operating at 1.5 T, such as shorter T_1's and easier fine-tuning of field homogeneity. The most common magnetic field strength for clinical imaging is 1.5 T, while approximately 20–30 systems worldwide are in the 3–4 T range and a few systems are under development in the range of 5–8 T. While 1.5 T may not be the final optimal field strength for (BOLD) fMRI, it has proven sufficient, and a large volume of functional neuroscience research continues to be conducted on these instruments. The potential advantages of stronger magnets lie mainly in the requirement for less signal averaging for a given experiment, in the possibility for true single-subject, single-event trials, and in the potential for greater spatial resolution.

Magnetic field gradients. Magnetic field gradients are produced by an additional set of (nonsuperconducting) coils that are driven by large amplifiers under the control of the scanner's computer. The knocking or banging sound produced during MRI scanning originates from the mechanical forces between the gradients and the main magnetic field. Single-shot imaging is very demanding on the gradient system as it dictates both large amplitudes and fast switching. The technical challenges of gradient system design and production relate to the problems of switching very large currents very quickly without overheating the amplifiers or coils. For this reason many scanners use water-cooled coils and amplifiers. Gradient systems that permitted single-shot EPI were not widely available on commercial scanners until the late 1990s and were often purchased as third-party add-on systems by larger research centers prior to that time. Today gradient systems capable of EPI are available from most scanner manufactures as a "high-end" option. In addition to strength and speed, the ability to scan frequently without pausing (i.e., with a high-duty cycle) is an important gradient (and computer) system feature for fMRI.

While technical developments continue to enable stronger and faster gradients, the final limitations will not be technical but biological. Basic electromagnetics tells us that a changing magnetic field (*dB/dt*) will induce current in a conductor (by the same principle as in an electrical generator). Tissue constitutes a conducting medium, so a rapidly changing magnetic field, such as that produced by an MRI gradient coil, can induce a current; if strong enough (large *dB/dt*), this current can produce nerve stimulation. This is exactly the principle of transcranial magnetic stimulation (TMS), in which a small coil is placed directly on the head, and a large magnetic pulse is used to stimulate the underlying cortex (Gates 1995). While carefully controlled focal stimulation is the goal of TMS, the potential for less predictable and controlled stimulation from body-sized MRI gradient coils represents a safety concern, particularly if *dB/dt* reaches a level sufficient to cause cardiac stimulation. Current body-sized MRI gradient coils used in EPI can generate *dB/dt*'s capable of peripheral nerve stimulation, which is an order of magnitude lower than that required for cardiac stimulation, but the coils are usually operated below this level. Since *dB/dt* increases with distance along the gradient, one solution to extending the range of safe *dB/dt* is to use shorter gradients that are specifically designed for neurological applications. These systems are often designed with a smaller diameter, thereby requiring less current for a given gradient amplitude, and are integrated with an RF head coil.

Radiofrequency coils. As discussed above, an RF coil is necessary for excitation and reception. For excitation the goal is to achieve a uniform RF field (B_1), and hence pulse angle, across the volume to be imaged, and for fMRI this is almost always achieved with a head coil (designed to fit over the subject's head). For reception there are two competing goals: spatially uniform sensitivity and maximal signal-to-noise ratio (SNR). The greatest SNR is achieved by using a coil that just encompasses the volume of interest, while a larger coil will provide greater uniformity. If, for example, only the primary visual cortex is of interest, then a surface coil (which is placed on the surface of the body) just large enough to cover the occipital pole would produce the best SNR. However, the sensitivity of surface coils is spatially nonuniform and therefore results in images with large variations in intensity across the field of view. This lack of uniform sensitivity does not present a problem for fMRI per se, but it does restrict the study to a predetermined region of the brain. In our visual fMRI example, a surface coil over the occipital pole would provide excellent data for visual areas V1 and V2, but not for the lateral geniculate nucleus. A head coil, on the other hand, would provide lower SNR for the occipital lobes but a much more uniform sensitivity over the entire cortex. Since anatomical images are also usually acquired during an imaging session for registration with functional maps and transformation into stereotactic space, uniform image intensity can also simplify postscan processing. These conflicting goals can be somewhat ameliorated on scanners that allow the simultaneous use of both a head coil and surface coil.

The safety aspects of RF coils and excitation are related to power deposition and hence the possibility of heating. The maximal allowable power deposition in MRI is regulated by government agencies (e.g., the Food and Drug Administration in the United States); most commercial MRI scanners have both software and hardware safety mechanisms to avoid exceeding these conservative limits. One potential danger for fMRI is the possibility of electrical coupling if additional conductors are introduced into the magnet for stimulus delivery or subject monitoring. These problems can usually be avoided through careful wiring configurations, but great care should be exercised and technical expertise obtained.

fMRI CONTRAST MECHANISMS

fMRI ACTIVATION PHYSIOLOGY

The goal of fMRI is to identify regions of increased neuronal activity by detecting MRI-visible physiological effects. To understand how this is possible, we will now look at some of the biological events that occur when neural tissue is stimulated (see also Chapter 2 for details on the physiology of synaptic activity and regional blood flow).

The immediate effect of increasing the electrical activity of neurons is to raise the burden of adenosine triphosphate (ATP)-dependent ion pumps found on the neuronal cell membrane, thus increasing the demand for glucose and oxygen, the basic substrates of ATP production in the brain. This greater demand is met through accelerated tissue perfusion (Roy and Sherrington 1890; Fox et al. 1986; Frostig et al. 1990). The relationship between perfusion and brain electrical activity has formed the basis for activation studies using PET and single photon emission computed tomography (SPECT), in which a radioactive tracer is introduced into the blood stream, and imaging is performed to determine the tracer distribution in brain tissue during rest and activation. Increased blood flow during brain activation can also be detected using perfusion-sensitive fMRI methods, as discussed below.

Perfusion rates are accelerated by increasing the diameter of the arterioles feeding a tissue domain, thus decreasing their resistance to flow and causing an elevation of blood pressure on the venous side. This increase in arteriolar diameter, coupled with swelling of the highly extensible venous vessels due to increased pressure, increases the total blood content of the tissue (Grubb et al. 1974). This increase in cerebral blood volume (CBV) is another of the physiological events that can be detected using fMRI, as discussed below.

Under steady-state resting conditions, approximately 70% of the oxygen delivered by the blood is extracted by brain tissue (Schmidt and Thews 1983), leading to the presence of deoxyhemoglobin in the cortex. Deoxyhemoglobin, due to its paramagnetic properties, exerts a significant attenuating effect on the intensity of T_2*-weighted MR images acquired at rest (Thulborn et al. 1982; Brooks and Di Chiro 1987). Variations in blood flow and in the rate of oxygen consumption during brain activation cause shifts in the level of tissue deoxyhemoglobin, which can be detected using T_2*-weighted fMRI.

Although considerable evidence indicates that oxygen consumption increases during brain activation (Frostig et al. 1990; Marrett and Gjedde 1997; Davis et al. 1998; Hoge et al. 1999a,b; Mandeville et al. 1999), there is an overwhelming consensus that these metabolic changes are generally accompanied by proportionately larger increases in blood flow. The consequence, as discussed in more detail below, is that the BOLD fMRI signal increases during brain activation, instead of decreasing, as one might expect, given the known acceleration of oxidative metabolism (and hence increased deoxyhemoglobin production).

The most plausible theory regarding the observed imbalances between aerobic metabolism and blood flow is that the diffusibility of oxygen from blood to brain limits the rate at which it can be used at a given perfusion level. Several quantitative models of oxygen delivery have been introduced (Buxton and Frank 1997; Gjedde 1997; Hyder et al. 1998; Hudetz 1999), all predicting that disproportionately large flow increases are required to produce a given increase in oxygen delivery by increasing blood–brain gradients. In the sections that follow, we will discuss the physical mechanisms by which these processes are transduced into MRI-visible signals.

fMRI BASED ON CEREBRAL BLOOD VOLUME

The first human fMRI brain maps were obtained by Belliveau et al. (1991) using a CBV technique. Their approach consisted of rapidly imaging the passage through the brain of a bolus of paramagnetic contrast agent (gadolinium diethylenetriamine penta-acetic acid) using T_2 or T_2^*-weighted acquisitions (Rosen et al. 1990; Belliveau et al. 1991). The effect of the paramagnetic agent is to produce magnetic field inhomogeneities at the microvascular scale and thus to enhance the rate of decay of the transverse magnetization. Therefore, as the intravascular contrast agent passes through the brain, a signal attenuation is observed that is linearly proportional to the concentration of the contrast agent. Integrating the area under such a concentration time curve provides a measure of CBV. By repeating this experiment in baseline and activation conditions and subtracting the calculated CBV images, one can produce a functional activation map. The major shortcomings of this fMRI technique are the poor temporal resolution and the requirement for an exogenous contrast agent, which limits the number of functional measurements that can be performed.

New intravascular contrast agents can remain at stable concentrations in the blood for several hours, alleviating the requirement for bolus injection methods. One example is monocrystalline iron oxide nanocolloid (MION), which has been used in rats to provide a fivefold increase in SNR over BOLD contrast at 2 T (Mandeville et al. 1998). While the MION concentrations used in these experiments are considerably higher than those approved for humans, initial testing of stable blood-pool contrast agents in humans has begun (Scheffler et al. 1999).

The advantages of this approach are the potentially high SNR, good temporal resolution, and physiologically quantitative nature of the measured signal (which is directly proportional to CBV). As with gadolinium-DTPA bolus methods, toxicity issues may limit the number and frequency of studies that can be performed on an individual.

PERFUSION-BASED fMRI

MRI methods for imaging flow are well developed (e.g., MR angiography is now widely used clinically), but to be useful for fMRI, blood flow must be measured at the microvascular scale (perfusion) because macrovascular flow changes can be quite remote from the activated region. The use of such perfusion-sensitive methods for fMRI represents the closest parallel to PET CBF-based functional imaging. Various approaches to perfusion imaging have been developed over the past 10–15 years, each with its own advantages and shortcomings. For fMRI, the most promising class of techniques is *arterial spin labeling* (ASL), which is conceptually very similar to radiotracer techniques such as PET. In ASL (Plate 1), arterial water is magnetically labeled (e.g., inverted by a 180° pulse) upstream and is allowed to flow into the region of interest and exchange with tissue water

(Detre et al. 1992; Williams et al. 1992). When the measurement is repeated with and without the upstream tagging (to form tag and control images) and the control image is subtracted from the tag image, an image with an intensity-dependent perfusion is formed. The typical use of ASL in fMRI therefore consists of the repeated acquisition of tag and control images during some modulation of the activation condition. These images are then pairwise subtracted to form a time series of perfusion-weighted images.

The first application of ASL to detect activation-induced flow changes was by Kwong et al. (1992), who used an inversion pulse in the imaging plane to effectively tag inflowing blood as fully relaxed magnetization. Notable variations of this method include EPI-STAR (echo planar imaging with signal targeting and alternating radiofrequency) (Edelman et al. 1994) and FAIR (flow alternating inversion recovery) (Kim 1995). More recent developments have focused on multiple slice imaging and quantification. An example of a slice from a multiple-slice FAIR data set is shown in Fig. 3.

The primary shortcomings of ASL-based fMRI are poor SNR, difficulty in acquiring volumetric data, and limited temporal resolution. The main potential advantage is that it provides a more direct view (compared to BOLD-based fMRI) of CBF change, which is a well-established correlate of neuronal activity.

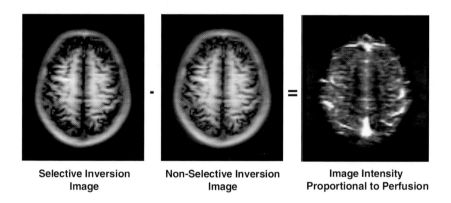

| Selective Inversion Image | Non-Selective Inversion Image | Image Intensity Proportional to Perfusion |

Fig. 3. One image from a multiple-slice FAIR perfusion imaging sequence. The image on the left was acquired after selectively inverting the magnetization within the imaging region only (selective IR image). Blood flowing into this region will have a different magnetization state (tag) than blood within the region, and the image intensity will be flow dependent. The middle image (nonselective IR image) was acquired after inverting the magnetization over the entire head. All blood within the brain has the same magnetization state, so the image intensity is flow independent (control). A difference image is shown on the right (scaled to show the small signal difference) that isolates the flow-dependent signal. A time series of such images is collected in perfusion-based fMRI.

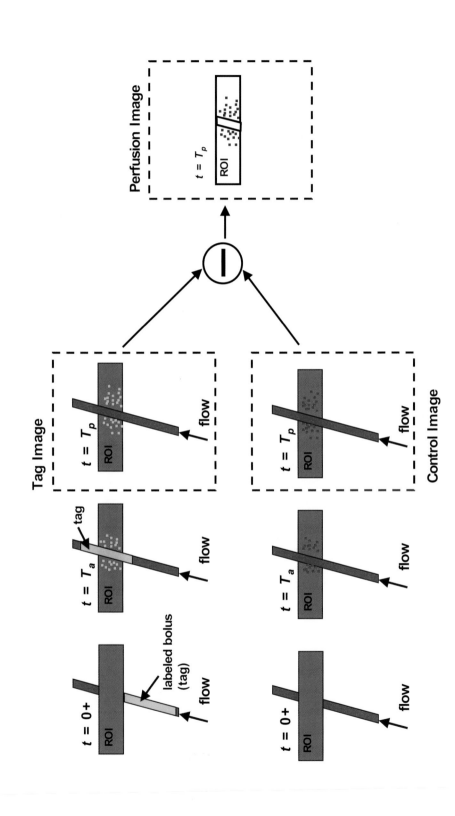

BOLD-BASED fMRI

It has long been known that the magnetic susceptibility of hemoglobin depends upon its oxygenation state (Pauling and Coryell 1936) and that the transverse relaxation rate of whole blood depends in part on oxygen saturation (Thulborn et al. 1982; Wright et al. 1991). Deoxyhemoglobin is paramagnetic and thus acts as an endogenous contrast agent that creates microscopic magnetic field inhomogeneities that enhance the rate of decay of transverse magnetization (i.e., it shortens T_2 and T_2^*). A BOLD signal arises in T_2^*-weighted MR images of the brain because the local image intensity is attenuated by deoxyhemoglobin, which is introduced into venous blood as tissues extract oxygen for aerobic metabolism (Plate 2). Increasing the perfusion rate in tissues generally leads to dilution of venous deoxyhemoglobin. The resultant increase in signal intensity is the BOLD response, which forms the basis for fMRI brain mapping (Kwong et al. 1992; Ogawa et al. 1992). In fact, the BOLD technique is so predominant in functional brain imaging that its use is generally implicit when referring to fMRI.

As discussed earlier, increases in blood flow rate also distend the highly compliant venous vessels. The resultant increase in the fraction of tissue volume occupied by deoxygenated blood partially counteracts the diluting effect of the perfusion increase. If the rise in perfusion is due to heightened neuronal activity, then metabolic oxygen extraction also increases, accelerating the production of deoxyhemoglobin and further counteracting the dilution effect. While both these effects attenuate the BOLD signal, the disproportionately large increase in blood flow dilutes deoxyhemoglobin in a net steady-state response to activation. Hence a positive signal change is observed in areas of focal activation in T_2^*-weighted images. The differing time courses of these counteracting effects, however, is likely to contribute to the signal over- and undershoots commonly seen in BOLD fMRI.

CBV is highly correlated with steady-state perfusion over a broad range of flow rates (Grubb et al. 1974). Perfusion, in turn, is regulated by the diameter of arterioles feeding a region of tissue. This mechanism generally sustains tissue metabolism at different levels of activity, but pharmacological perturbations, such as CO_2 inhalation and infusion of L-arginine or

---

← **Plate 1.** Illustration of arterial spin labeling (ASL) perfusion imaging. The top row represents the acquisition of a tag image. Blood flowing into the region of interest is magnetically labeled (e.g., inverted with a 180° pulse) upstream and is allowed to flow through the region and exchange with tissue water before an image is acquired (dotted box). The bottom row shows the acquisition of a control image in a manner identical to the tag image but without the labeling. The difference between the tag and control image depends only on the tissue perfusion.

acetazolamide, can induce arteriolar dilation independent of tissue metabolism (Bruhn et al. 1994; Zaharchuk 1997).

Although neurally mediated arteriolar dilation regulates CBF, the influence of arterial blood on the BOLD signal is probably insignificant because it comprises a relatively small fraction (~25%) of total CBV and contains negligible amounts of deoxyhemoglobin. MRI-relevant changes in total CBV are therefore primarily due to the passive inflation of venules caused by the elevation of venous blood pressure that occurs when arteriolar resistance is lowered (Mandeville et al. 1998). Because of their passive, mechanical nature, steady-state venous CBV changes are believed to be simple correlates of CBF, independent of the cause of the perfusion increase.

Similar to the correlation of CBV with blood flow, recent fMRI research indicates that a fixed relationship between CBF and cerebral metabolic rate of oxygen consumption, analogous to Grubb's formula, may apply during brain activation if systemic physiological parameters are stabilized (Davis et al. 1998; Hoge et al. 1999b). The emerging consensus that blood flow and oxygen consumption are coupled, but with disproportionately large CBF increases, represents a significant endorsement of BOLD as a measure of neuronal activity. However, investigation of brain activation physiology and of the exact meaning of the BOLD signal remains an area of active research.

fMRI EXPERIMENT DESIGN

Most fMRI experiments involve controlled variations in experimental conditions while serial images of the brain are acquired. The objective is generally to identify regions of the brain exhibiting condition-correlated signal changes. The rapid imaging rates possible with current MRI technology allow great flexibility in the design of experiments. However, biological and statistical considerations impose constraints on what is practical and effective. In this section, we will review the main classes of fMRI experiment design and discuss their suitability for various scientific or clinical objectives.

NOISE SOURCES IN fMRI

In designing optimally sensitive fMRI experiments, it is important to consider the two primary sources of noise (i.e., interfering signals). The first is purely thermal noise generated by thermodynamic processes in the subject and added by the scanner's RF receiver electronics (it is called "thermal" noise because it would vanish at absolute zero temperature). Thermal noise would occur during imaging of an inanimate object, and its severity varies according to relatively simple physical rules. The second source of noise consists of ongoing physiological processes in living subjects that are capable of affecting the fMRI signal. These include pulsatile blood flow through the tissue, respiratory modulation of tissue blood oxygenation and regional static field values, and tissue motion. The thermal component of the noise is additive to the "true" signal, while the physiological component is generally multiplicative.

Depending on the exact parameters used for data acquisition, either the thermal or physiological noise component may dominate. Thermal noise is likely to be dominant at high spatial resolution, especially at lower field strengths and when whole-head receiver coils are used. The relative importance of thermal noise drops very rapidly as voxel (image volume element) dimensions increase, however, and may be further reduced at high magnetic field strengths and through the use of localized surface receiver coils. Because task-induced BOLD responses and the physiological noise component are both multiplicative effects (possibly acting via the same physical mechanisms), the ratio of functional contrast to physiological noise is likely to be relatively independent of imaging parameters. It is therefore very difficult to completely eliminate physiological noise (although some strategies for dealing with cardiac and respiratory noise have been proposed; e.g., Biswal et al. 1996).

The physiological noise component also differs from the thermal noise in that it has a strong content of slow fluctuation and drift. Thus, when it comes to averaging out physiological noise, images that are closely spaced in time are not really independent measurements. The improvement in statistical power with increasingly rapid imaging is thus less than would be expected based on the assumption of purely "white" (uncorrelated) noise. It is important to avoid stimulus presentation timing that is likely to cause responses resembling the slow signal drift that is often prominent in physiological noise.

OPTIMIZATION OF SIGNAL-TO-NOISE RATIO

Because the task-induced contrast in fMRI experiments is small (often only marginally above noise), it is important to acquire as many independent measurements as possible in order to improve sensitivity by increasing statistical power. It is, of course, also desirable to design the experimental task or stimulus so that it maximizes the response amplitude, to the extent possible without compromising selectivity for the brain function of interest.

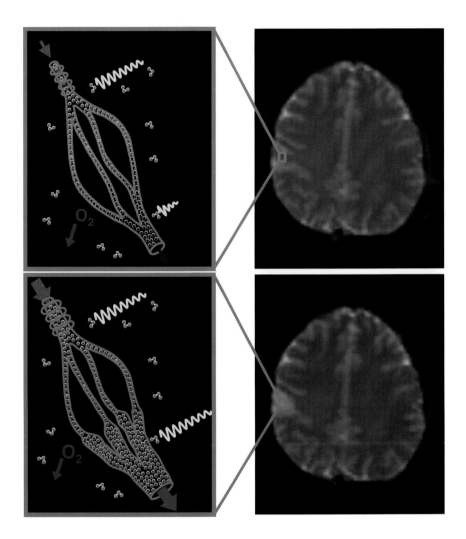

Plate 2. Physical basis of the BOLD fMRI signal. In the baseline condition (top row), oxygenated arterial blood (red) enters the capillary network. Oxyhemoglobin has a magnetic susceptibility similar to that of the surrounding tissue, so it does not significantly affect the MRI signal (yellow) from the surrounding tissue water (light blue). As oxygen is extracted for aerobic metabolism, deoxyhemoglobin is produced (dark blue), and its paramagnetism enhances the rate of decay of the water signal in and around the venous compartment. During activation (bottom row), blood flow is increased in excess of the increase in oxygen consumption, causing dilution of the deoxyhemoglobin (reddening of the venous blood) and distension of the venous vessels. The net effect is still a reduction in the absolute concentration of deoxyhemoglobin and thus an increase in the water signal in and around the venous vessels in the area of activation (region shown as brighter on the bottom-right T_2^*-weighted image; the signal increase is exaggerated here for the purpose of illustration).

The statistical requirement for many independent measurements can be met by imaging either fast and/or for a long time. There are, however, practical limits to the gains that can be made using either strategy. Rapid imaging generates large numbers of measurements but, as stated above, the most severe physiological noise may be at low frequencies. Rapid imaging also causes signal attenuation due to incomplete T_1 recovery (see "Relaxation—T_1, T_2, and T_2*" above). Fig. 4a shows the relative signal-to-noise ratio (SNR) attainable in brain tissue plotted as a function of imaging rate (accounting for incomplete T_1 recovery and assuming continuous optimization of flip angle). The SNR increases dramatically up to one image per second but

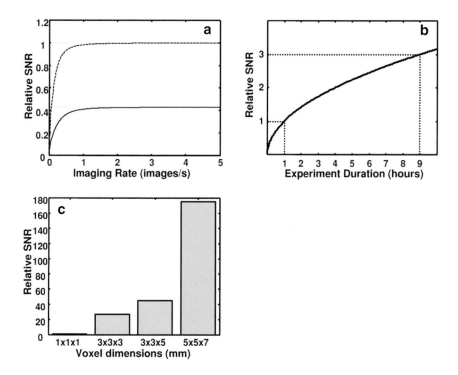

Fig. 4. Signal-to-noise behavior in fMRI; effects of varying acquisition parameters are shown. All plots show idealized signal-to-noise ratio (SNR), ignoring special characteristics of physiological noise. (a) Relative SNR as a function of imaging rate at 1.5 T (solid line) and 3.0 T (dashed line), taking into account T_1 attenuation, statistical enhancement, and field strength (see text). T_1 values of 900 ms and 1300 ms for 1.5 T and 3.0 T, respectively, are assumed. RF excitation flip angle is continuously adjusted to maximize SNR at a given imaging rate. SNR improvement plateaus at about 1 image per second. (b) Relative SNR as a function of experiment duration, showing statistical enhancement as square root of imaging time. Increases in sensitivity are costly in terms of scan time. (c) Relative SNR as a function of voxel dimensions. Increasing spatial resolution leads to rapid degradation of SNR (with SNR normalized to that of a 1-mm^3 voxel).

shows little improvement at higher rates. For multi-slice imaging of the entire brain, most MRI systems can acquire data at the same rate of about one image per second.

As noted above, another means of increasing statistical power is to perform longer experiments. There is no physical limit on the duration of imaging sessions, but the SNR of an experiment increases only as the square root of the number of measurements performed. This means that significant increases in statistical power come at a huge cost in terms of scan time. For example, increasing the SNR of a 1-hour experiment by a factor of three would require 9 hours of scanning time (Fig. 4b). This lengthy ordeal is clearly intolerable for an individual subject, so when this level of sensitivity is required a multi-subject experiment would generally be performed. When a high SNR is required in a single individual, as is usually the case in a clinical setting, gains in SNR may be achieved by lowering the spatial resolution (Fig. 4c).

MAIN CLASSES OF EXPERIMENTAL DESIGN

The distinction between "block design" and "event-based design" in this chapter is somewhat artificial. These terms are generally used to describe opposite extremes in the time scale on which experimental conditions are modulated, and the two designations tend to imply rather different approaches to experiment design and data analysis. A third experimental design, phase-encoded mapping, falls outside either definition and is discussed separately below. Traditional experimental design concepts, such as factorial design, may be applied to any of these fMRI experiment types by planning the study so that conventional statistical methods can be applied to task-evoked response magnitudes.

Block design. In block design experiments, intervals of fixed experimental condition are sustained for periods ranging from several seconds to a few minutes. Multiple blocks containing different conditions are appended together to produce scanning runs that typically last from 2 to 10 minutes. It is customary to represent the evolution of experimental state in fMRI experiments using plots that show the value of some experimental variables as a function of time during an imaging run. An example of such a plot, summarizing conditions in a simple block-design fMRI experiment, is shown in Fig. 5. In a pain study, the variable plotted might be the pulse amplitude of an electrical stimulator. Often, different experimental conditions cannot be described in terms of a concrete physical variable. In such cases the variable plotted can be thought of as an index identifying the condition.

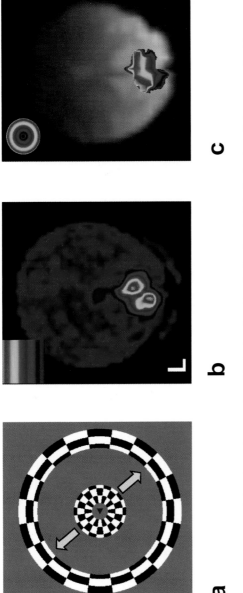

Plate 3. Phase-encoded retinotopic mapping. (a) A circular visual stimulus (radial checkerboard) is presented with an annular region masked out (middle gray ring with arrows). The radial boundaries of the masked region are gradually increased over time during imaging. Several cycles are repeated, and the BOLD signal at each spatial location in the image series is Fourier transformed. (b) Image showing Fourier transform magnitude at the repetition frequency of mask sweeping; retinotopically organized visual areas are selectively identified. (c) Fourier transform phase at the same frequency, showing progression of visual field projection radius (eccentricity) from posterior to anterior.

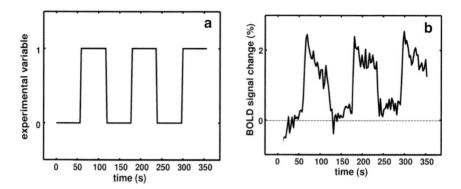

Fig. 5. Block-design approach to fMRI. (a) Plot of manipulated experimental variable as a function of time. (b) Plot of BOLD response over time in activated tissue. The signal consists of recorded fMRI data during modulation of visual input (on a 1.5-T MRI system).

Fig. 5 shows one possible stimulus modulation waveform, with six condition blocks, each of 60 seconds' duration. The main considerations in designing the stimulation schedule for a given study are the duration and number of blocks to use. Because physiological noise in the fMRI signal usually contains a strong content of slow fluctuation and drift, a relatively rapid modulation frequency is desirable so that the condition-induced responses are readily discernible from physiological background noise. The slowness of the perfusion response places an upper limit on the feasible modulation frequency, however, so block durations of at least 10 seconds are advisable. It is not mandatory for the stimulus modulation waveform to be periodic. It is possible to include blocks of different stimulus type in a single scanning run.

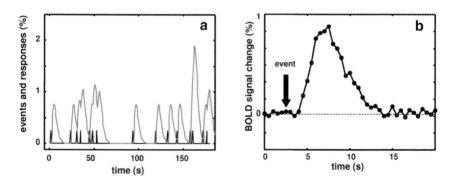

Fig. 6. Event-based design in fMRI. (a) A series of short events (black line) produces a corresponding series of responses (gray line), which overlap additively in time (simulated data). (b) Average event-related response (actual data), which can be computed through deconvolution.

Although the event-based approach described below is becoming increasingly important in fMRI, block design may still be preferred in certain cases. The main advantages of block over event-based design are that: (1) block-design experiments generally do not require the assumption of linear response combination, unlike event-based designs (see below); (2) experiment control is more straightforward; and (3) data analysis is generally simpler. However, the condition of interest must be meaningfully sustained over the desired block lengths. In some cases, psychophysical adaptation limits block duration.

Event-based design. When the condition of interest is transient or spontaneous, or when anticipatory responses are a potential confounding factor, an event-based design is required. In the most general sense, an event-based experiment involves one or more types of events at arbitrary (possibly random) time points while serial images of the brain are acquired. Typical events include short stimulus bursts, instructions to the subject to perform a task, self-generated actions performed by the subject, and spontaneous events such as bursts of epileptic spiking activity or the onset of some painful clinical episode.

Fig. 6 shows a series of events and associated responses (it is assumed we are looking at activated tissue), as would be observed in an event-based fMRI experiment with randomized event timing. Each event evokes a response waveform whose shape can be seen clearly by looking at the first event, which in this case is not affected by overlap from subsequent events. It is generally assumed that overlapping responses combine additively and that the contribution of individual events does not vary over time, properties known as *linearity* and *time invariance*. To the extent that these assumptions are true, a given series of events $x(t)$ is transformed into the observed fMRI signal $y(t)$ through the mathematical operation of convolution (designated by an asterisk) with the event-related hemodynamic response function $h(t)$:

$$y(t) = x(t) * h(t) + \text{noise}.$$

For discretely sampled functions like fMRI time series, convolution can be expressed as a matrix multiplication. The convolution operation is invertible via matrix arithmetic so, given a recorded fMRI signal $y(t)$ and a function $x(t)$ representing the event series, the average event-related response function $h(t)$ at a particular voxel can be computed through deconvolution:

$$h(t) = y(t) *^{-1} x(t).$$

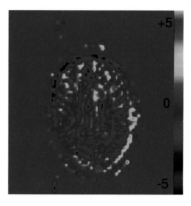

Plate 4. Image showing misregistration artifacts at brain boundaries. Colors denote *t*-statistic values. Imaging was performed while the subject was at rest but poorly immobilized. Note the complementary nature of edge enhancement on opposite sides of the brain.

Noise present in the observed signal is carried over into noise in the estimated event-related response function $h(t)$.

Studies suggest that fMRI responses are sufficiently linear for the above approach to work well (Dale and Buckner 1997; Burock et al. 1998). However, this indication has not been exhaustively tested. Permitting response overlap with randomly timed events (as shown in Fig. 6) can significantly boost statistical sensitivity by allowing large numbers of events to occur. If there are concerns about linearity, however, events can be timed to eliminate overlap between responses. In this case, the deconvolution operation is equivalent to simply averaging the responses seen following each event.

Because the convolution operations described above must be performed on discretely sampled (as opposed to continuous) signals, they are simplified if randomized event times are also discrete so that events coincide with scanning time points. The temporal resolution of the estimated event-related response will then be limited to the scan repetition rate, however. If higher temporal resolution is desired, the event times may be set to be fractions of an interscan interval. The event-related response function can then be computed on this finer time grid by resampling the fMRI time series onto the same grid, filling the time points between scans with zeros, and deconvolving with the input event series as described above. This technique is equivalent to a re-resorting of the originally sampled time points, depending on the temporal offset of the preceding stimulus, prior to computation of the average event-related signal.

The event-based view of experiment design described here is quite general, and there is no reason why the deconvolution methods described above

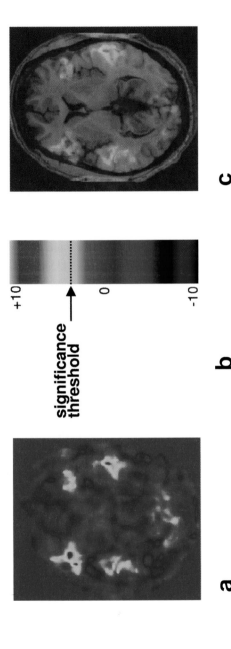

Plate 5. fMRI statistical map and threshold. (a) Map of *t*-statistic values computed from data acquired during performance of a language task. (b) Color legend indicating threshold of statistical significance (4.1). (c) Statistical map superimposed on an anatomical MR image.

could not also be used to compute responses to sustained, block-type conditions (except that overlapping stimulus blocks are not likely to produce
linear responses). Treating block onsets (e.g., the rising edges in Fig. 5a) as
"events" and deconvolving these from the observed signal would yield the
average block response. Note that the deconvolution approach to computing
event-related responses alleviates the need for counterbalancing that exists
with some statistical approaches. It must be stressed that linear combination
of overlapping responses is an important requirement for deconvolution.

Phase-encoding design.   If topographic organization of brain function
is orderly and specific within a cortical area, phase-encoding methods may
be useful. Examples of such organization include the retinotopic arrange-
ment of the visual cortex, tonotopic organization in the auditory cortex, and
somatotopic representation in the sensorimotor cortex.

At typical fMRI resolution, adjacent voxels within such cortical areas
all respond to the same type of input, differing only in their preferred value
of some variable stimulus parameter. Such areas can be identified and mapped
with great selectivity by performing fMRI experiments in which the input
required to activate the cortical area of interest is continuously presented
while the topographically encoded parameter is repeatedly varied through
some range of values.

Because the stimulus of interest is constantly presented, brain regions
that respond to the input but are not topographically organized will not
exhibit any response modulation during this type of experiment. In regions
that react selectively to specific values of the variable stimulus parameter,
however, the fMRI signal will fluctuate with the same periodicity as the
stimulus parameter modulation. Fourier transform methods may then be used
to identify and map regions whose signal fluctuates strongly at the parameter modulation frequency. Phase-encoded retinotopic mapping (Plate 3), in
which the eccentricity or polar angle of a visual stimulus is continually
varied, is an example of this type of procedure (Sereno et al. 1995).

fMRI DATA ANALYSIS

Above we discussed different ways of varying experimental conditions
during fMRI scanning to produce condition-related signal changes in the
images. In this section we cover the basic issues involved in detecting those
changes, including techniques used to remove artifacts and enhance the
noise characteristics of data prior to statistical analysis.

MOTION CORRECTION

During serial acquisition of functional MR images, investigators repeatedly sample a fixed spatial grid of voxels and try to ensure that the subject's brain never moves relative to this grid. Nonetheless, subject motion is difficult to completely eradicate, with the consequence that large fluctuations in intensity over time are often observed at tissue boundaries in functional image series. Sensitivity to this effect, often called a misregistration artifact, increases with spatial resolution. The large signal fluctuations associated with misregistration artifact can obliterate the small responses caused by neuronal stimulation, and can also mimic brain activation if subject motion is correlated with the deliberate variations in experimental condition. Plate 4 shows a misregistration artifact in an fMRI statistical map that was acquired with no change in experimental condition (all apparent responses are therefore artifactual).

Another source of spurious signal fluctuation associated with subject motion is disruption of the RF excitation history at a given spatial sampling location. If the tissue sampled at a given location is replaced with tissue that has more fully relaxed longitudinal magnetization, large intensity modulations can occur. This effect is small at long TRs (>3 s at 1.5 T) but can be severe at short ones (<1 s).

The first type of motion-associated signal corruption, misregistration artifact, can be corrected to some extent through retrospective alignment of all images in a series with the first image of the series (or some other reasonable target). This involves two steps: (1) computation of the geometric shift and rotation that has occurred between a particular (possibly shifted) source image and the target and (2) interpolation of voxel intensities in the shifted image onto the "correct" spatial sampling grid, which is derived from the target image.

The alignment process can be complicated by several factors. The first is that, as discussed above in "Echo Planar Imaging," the slices of volumetric fMRI scans are acquired not simultaneously but over a period up to several seconds long. Thus, if significant motion occurs during acquisition of the stack of slices, then the apparent shape of the brain will be distorted in a complex fashion. Aligning two objects with different shapes is a more difficult problem than that of aligning identical objects, and the solution may not be well defined. Another factor that can compromise realignment of brain images is related to the fact that, rather than a full three-dimensional (3-D) volumetric image of the brain, often only a limited cross-sectional portion of the brain is sampled. Although it should theoretically be possible to perform the required alignment based on image details within the sampled

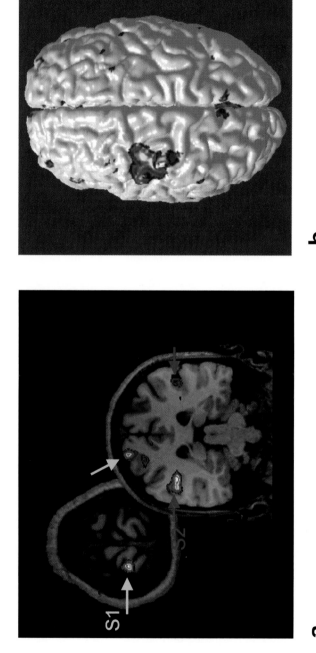

Plate 6. Superposition of functional and anatomical MR images. (a) Thresholded activation map from a simple block-design heat pain study superimposed on axial and coronal cross-sectional anatomical images. (b) Thresholded statistical map from a hand movement experiment overlaid on a 3-D surface rendering of the subject's brain.

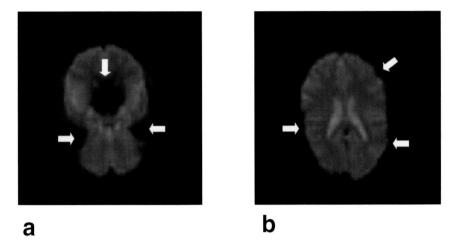

a   **b**

Fig. 7. Signal dropout and distortion in T_2^*-weighted echo-planar images. (a) Image showing signal dropout near air-filled sinus spaces (arrows). (b) Image slightly superior to (a) showing subtle image distortions (arrows).

volume, correction of large displacements perpendicular to the slice plane may be less robust due to the loss of information on the position of the brain boundaries. Development of algorithms for accurate and robust alignment of functional MR images is an active area of research, and several software packages are available to facilitate this task (Collins et al. 1994; Friston et al. 1995; Woods et al. 1998).

The second step of realignment, that of interpolation, must be done carefully to minimize the possibility of image degradation. The important factor here is use of the proper weighting function for interpolating intensity values of the shifted images onto the target sampling grid. Types of interpolation available include nearest-neighbor, tri-linear, tri-cubic, and 3-D sinc. Nearest-neighbor and tri-linear interpolation causes image degradation that is generally considered unacceptable for fMRI (Hajnal et al. 1995; Ostuni et al. 1997). Tri-cubic and sinc interpolation lead to superior image quality but are more computationally intensive, although sinc interpolation can be efficiently implemented using fast Fourier transforms.

Another form of misregistration that can occur involves spatial distortions that arise in echo-planar images due to inhomogeneities in the static magnetic field (see "Imaging"). Distortion does not necessarily impede detection of activated regions, but it can prevent accurate superposition of activation maps on undistorted anatomical images. The level of distortion present in echo-planar images varies greatly over different brain regions; if

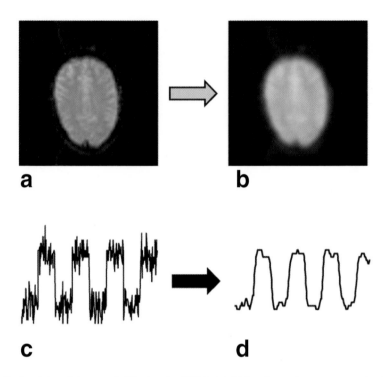

Fig. 8. Spatial and temporal filtering in fMRI. (a) Echo-planar image as acquired on scanner (left) and filtered version (right). (b) fMRI signal containing high-frequency noise (left) and filtered version (right).

severe, it may be removed using field-mapping techniques (Reber et al. 1998; Chen and Wyrwicz 1999). In much of the brain the distortion is negligible, given the relatively low spatial resolution of functional MR images. In inferior and frontal brain regions that are close to air-filled sinuses, however, distortion can be severe and is usually accompanied by signal dropout (dark regions caused by extreme T_2^* shortening). Fig. 7 shows examples of signal dropout and distortion. Shortening the echo time (with no other change) reduces dropout but does not change distortion.

Certain parts of the brain, such as the brainstem, undergo considerable displacement during the cardiac cycle due to strong pulsatile pressures in nearby blood vessels. An effective strategy in such cases is to perform cardiac-gated imaging, whereby image acquisition is initiated by the subject's heart beat. Because a given slice is always imaged during the same phase of the cardiac cycle, pulsating brain structures will be minimally displaced between images. Variations in heart rate can cause intensity fluctuations due to differences in T_1 recovery, but these highly deterministic shifts can easily be corrected (Guimaraes et al. 1998).

SPATIAL AND TEMPORAL FILTERING

Functional MRI detects brain activation through perfusion responses, which occur on a relatively slow time scale and are spatially diffuse. Nonetheless, typical fMRI signals include noise which, although heavily weighted towards low frequencies, contains significant high-frequency components that could not possibly reflect an activation-induced perfusion response. There are also strong components of noise at cardiac and respiratory frequencies, which can be detected by appropriate monitoring. Thermal noise exhibits minimal spatial autocorrelation in fMRI, so activation maps may show considerable high-frequency thermal noise. Spatial and temporal filtering procedures can be used to remove such components, enhancing the detectability of the response of interest at the expense of detail (Fig. 8).

Spatial filtering, performed prior to statistical detection operations, can also reduce the impact of misregistration artifacts by lowering the effective resolution of the images. Due to the natures of thermal noise and MRI data acquisition, images filtered to a given resolution will not achieve the (higher) SNR of images originally acquired at the lower resolution. Images acquired at lower resolution are more subject to severe intensity dropout in regions of static field inhomogeneity. If the brain region of interest is close to an air-filled sinus, it may be desirable to image at a higher spatial resolution than normal and then recover some of the lost SNR by aggressive filtering. Spatial filtering operations have an impact on the statistical interpretation of fMRI data, which will be discussed below. It is generally preferable to perform spatial filtering prior to statistical analysis, since many statistical operations used in fMRI are nonlinear with respect to combination of input signals.

Temporal filtering can also improve the detectability of activation-evoked responses by removing high-frequency noise from the fMRI signal (Biswal et al. 1996). Low-frequency components can be removed by fitting a low-order polynomial to the time-series data and removing linear and, if desired, higher order terms (Press et al. 1992). Components related to cardiac and respiratory signals that were recorded can be removed from the fMRI signal. As with spatial blurring, the statistical implications must be considered whenever temporal filtering is performed. In many cases the categorization of time periods that is implicit in statistical analysis is equivalent to a filtering operation, so temporal filtering may not contribute greatly to sensitivity; this measure is generally more useful for signal plotting and display.

STATISTICAL ANALYSIS

Once any preprocessing operations such as motion correction and temporal or spatial filtering have been performed, the final step in an fMRI experiment is usually to generate and interpret some form of statistical map. Virtually all of the statistical operations used take the time-series data for each voxel as an input and transform it into a single number that represents the response magnitude at that location. This number is then assigned to the corresponding voxel in the output statistical map.

The mathematical operations used to transform time series into scalar statistics are generally designed in such a way that repeated application to a large set of pure noise signals, containing no evoked responses, will produce a well-defined distribution of output values. For such transformations to be useful as statistical tests, it must be possible to compute this probability distribution based on the properties of the transformation and on readily available knowledge about the experiment such as the number of independent measurements in the signal (such knowledge is used to determine the number of degrees of freedom of the distribution). Application of the transformation to a signal containing (sufficiently) large task-induced effects should produce output scalar values that are highly unlikely to occur by chance, as dictated by the computed probability distribution. For a given output scalar statistic, it must be possible to compute the probability of observing that value given a pure noise input (note that the "noise" here is assumed to have the same characteristics as that present in the measured signal). It is common practice to set an arbitrary probability threshold below which the null hypothesis of no response is declared false. The response is thereby deemed to be statistically significant.

The statistical operations used in fMRI can be broadly grouped into parametric and nonparametric methods. Parametric methods assume that the set of measurements comprising the fMRI time series follow a particular probability distribution and attempt to estimate the parameters needed to describe that distribution. Student's t test, in which the mean and standard deviation of the measurement values at baseline and during activation are estimated and compared, is an example of a parametric test. Mean and standard deviation are statistics describing a normal distribution, with an implicit assumption that the measurement errors follow this distribution. If they do not, then hypothesis testing based on the t-statistic may be misleading. Another example of a parametric test used in fMRI is linear correlation. This test yields the correlation coefficient r, which is a measure of the degree of correlation between the fMRI signal level and the value of an experimental variable (see Fig. 5). Here too, the probability of a particular r value can only be computed accurately if the fMRI signal and the experimental variable function jointly form a binormal distribution (Press et al. 1992). Examples of other parametric test statistics that are important in fMRI include the Z score and F ratio (Friston et al. 1994a; Worsley 1997).

Under conditions where thermal RF noise dominates in the fMRI signal, the assumption of normality is likely to apply, and parametric statistical procedures are preferred. Non-normal noise distributions can arise when physiological noise dominates, however. Also, artifactual effects such as subject motion can produce huge spikes in the fMRI signal that would be highly improbable under the normal distribution. Under these conditions, nonparametric statistics may be useful.

Nonparametric methods do not depend on a particular distribution of measurement errors. The main advantage of this type of test is greatly enhanced robustness in the presence of outlier values in the fMRI signal. The disadvantage is generally some loss of sensitivity; that is, some responses that would be statistically significant in a parametric test would not appear so with a nonparametric test. An example of a nonparametric test that can be applied to fMRI data is the Spearman rank-order correlation (SROC) test (Press et al. 1992). This test is identical to linear correlation, except that the correlation operation is performed on the ranks of the fMRI signal and condition waveform (each measurement is assigned an integer indicating the order in which its magnitude ranks among those of all the other measured values; ties are handled in a special way). This procedure can be used to produce a statistic whose distribution can be computed, regardless of the noise distributions of the input data. Another nonparametric test used in fMRI is the Kolmogorov-Smirnov (KS) test. Here the cumulative distributions of measurement values during the baseline and activated states are computed and the maximum difference between them is determined. This difference is the KS statistic, whose distribution can also be computed without knowledge of the distributions of the fMRI signal and experimental waveform.

Regardless of the type of statistical test used, some form of correction for multiple comparisons is usually performed in fMRI. This correction is carried out to ensure that the false-positive rate predicted by the chosen probability threshold is accurate over the imaged volume as opposed to each voxel. Because fMRI activation maps may contain huge numbers of voxels, a small voxelwise false-positive rate can nonetheless ensure a significant number of false-positive voxels in the entire volume. Multiple comparisons are usually corrected for by first determining the effective number of resolution elements within the imaged volume. This number may be different from the number of voxels because of spatial smoothing and intrinsic spatial autocorrelation in the images. Next, this number plus a model of the noise characteristics is used to adjust the voxelwise probability threshold so that it can be applied across the entire volume with the desired false-positive rate (Friston et al. 1994b).

The computation of significance levels is also influenced by temporal autocorrelation in the data. The exact distribution shapes of all of the test statistics described above depend on the number of independent measurements used to compute the statistic. Physiological noise in fMRI, which has a strong low-frequency content, exhibits significant autocorrelation. This means that consecutively acquired functional MR images do not really constitute completely independent measurements, since they are likely to be sampling the same low-frequency noise fluctuations. Computing the test statistic distribution based on the total number of images is therefore likely to overestimate the significance of a given response, resulting in excessive false-positive rates. Fortunately, the autocorrelation characteristics of the fMRI signal can be determined and this information used to correctly calculate the required probability distribution (Friston et al. 1994a).

VISUALIZATION

The next step in data analysis (assuming a mapping experiment) is to display the statistical map (Plate 5). It is important to indicate the threshold of statistical significance, and it has become customary to do this by excluding parts of the statistical map that fall below this value prior to superposition on an anatomical MR image (Plate 6a). This process really serves more to provide anatomical context than to aid in assessment of the activation map. An alternate means of expressing threshold values, which leads to considerably less information loss, is to display the entire statistical map and indicate the threshold on a color legend, as shown in Plate 5b. Maps can be superimposed either on cross-sectional anatomical images (Plates 5c, 6a) or on 3-D renderings of the brain surface (Plate 6b).

Surface-based 3-D visualization (Dale et al. 1999; Fischl et al. 1999) is extremely useful for determining the position of activated regions in terms of sulcal anatomy, but does not show subcortical structures. Sophisticated computer-processing methods are required for generation and manipulation of surface renderings, and existing technology may require the manual intervention of a skilled user. Surface generation in the presence of abnormal anatomy (congenital defect, surgical resection, or tumor) may be impossible.

Planar 2-D visualization, which is the default mode of viewing MR images, gives little information about sulcal anatomy, but provides cross-sectional views showing subcortical structures and permitting simultaneous depiction of brain regions that would not be possible on a 3-D surface. Planar visualization is considerably more robust in the presence of abnormal anatomy than are surface-based methods, and relies on simpler anatomical data processing procedures with minimal manual intervention. Ideally, both surface and cross-sectional views should be consulted for optimal interpretation of fMRI results.

CONCLUSIONS

MRI developments over the past decade have revolutionized the area of functional brain imaging by providing a widely available and safe tool for neuroscientists to study neuronal activation. The spatial and temporal resolution of fMRI are far superior to PET and provide tremendous potential for the investigation of the steady-state and transient neuronal response associated with pain. Furthermore, the lack of ionizing radiation enables the repeated and detailed investigation of single subjects and patients. Unfortunately, in its current form, fMRI does not provide the absolute quantitation available with PET, nor does it have the sensitivity to detect picomolar concentrations of labeled compounds. However, basic research continues to clarify the exact physical and physiological origin of fMRI signals and should lead to a more rigorous and quantitative interpretation in the coming years. Advances in MRI technology (e.g., higher magnetic field strengths), experiment design, and statistical analysis will also enable the pursuit of more sophisticated hypotheses about the brain's functional organization. The contribution of fMRI in future pain research will come from the ability to perform repeated detailed studies of normal subjects and patients. This will enhance the exploration of cognitive processes, drugs, hypnosis, and the placebo effect.

REFERENCES

Belliveau JW, Kennedy DN Jr, McKinstry RC, et al. Functional mapping of the human visual cortex by magnetic resonance imaging. *Science* 1991; 254:716–719.

Biswal B, DeYoe A, Hyde J. Reduction of physiological fluctuations in fMRI using digital filters. *Magn Reson Med* 1996; 35:107–113.

Bloch F, Hansen WW, Packard M. The nuclear induction experiment. *Phys Rev* 1946; 70:474–485.

Brooks R, Di Chiro G. Magnetic resonance imaging of stationary blood: a review. *Med Phys* 1987; 14(6):903–913.

Bruhn H, Kleinschmidt A, Boecker H, et al. The effect of acetazolamide on regional cerebral blood oxygenation at rest and under stimulation as assessed by MRI. *J Cereb Blood Flow Metab* 1994; 14:742–748.

Burock M, Buckner R, Woldorff M, Rosen B, Dale A. Randomized event-related experimental designs allow for extremely rapid presentation rates using functional MRI. *Neuroreport* 1998; 19:3735–3739.

Buxton RB, Frank LR. A model for the coupling between cerebral blood flow and oxygen metabolism during neural stimulation. *J Cereb Blood Flow Metab* 1997; 1:64–72.

Chen N, Wyrwicz A. Correction for EPI distortions using multi-echo gradient-echo imaging. *Magn Reson Med* 1999; 41(6):1206–1213.

Collins DL, Neelin P, Peters TM, Evans AC. Automatic 3D registration of MR volumetric data in standardized Talairach space. *J Comput Assist Tomogr* 1994; 18(2):192–205.

Dale A, Buckner R. Selective averaging of rapidly presented individual trials using fMRI. *Hum Brain Mapp* 1997; 5:329–340.

Dale A, Fischl B, Sereno M. Cortical surface-based analysis. I: Segmentation and surface reconstruction. *Neuroimage* 1999; 9(2):179–194.

Davis T, Kwong K, Weisskoff R, Rosen B. Calibrated functional MRI: mapping the dynamics of oxidative metabolism. *Proc Natl Acad Sci USA* 1998; 95:1834–1839.

Detre JA, Leigh JS, Williams DS, Koretsky AP. Perfusion imaging. *Magn Reson Med* 1992; 23:37–45.

Edelman RR, Siewert B, Darby DG, et al. Qualitative mapping of cerebral blood flow and functional localization with echo-planar MR imaging and signal targeting with alternating radio frequency. *Radiology* 1994; 192:513–520.

Fischl B, Sereno M, Dale A. Cortical surface-based analysis. II: Inflation, flattening, and a surface-based coordinate system. *Neuroimage* 1999; 9(2):195–207.

Fox P, Mintun M, Raichle M, et al. Mapping human visual cortex with positron emission tomography. *Science* 1986; 323(6091):806–809.

Friston K, Jezzard P, Turner R. Analysis of functional MRI time-series. *Hum Brain Mapp* 1994a; 1:153–171.

Friston K, Worsley K, Frackowiak R, Maziotta J, Evans A. Assessing the significance of focal activations using their spatial extent. *Hum Brain Mapp* 1994b; 1:210–220.

Friston K, Ashburner J, Frith C, et al. Spatial registration and normalization of images. *Hum Brain Mapp* 1995; 2:165–189.

Frostig R, Lieke E, Tso D, Grinvald A. Cortical functional architecture and local coupling between neuronal activity and the microcirculation revealed by in vivo high-resolution optical imaging. *Proc Natl Acad Sci USA* 1990; 87(16):6082–6086.

Gates JR. Transcranial magnetic stimulation. *Neuroimaging Clin N Am* 1995; 5:711–720.

Gati JS, Menon RS, Ugurbil K, Rutt BK. Experimental determination of the BOLD field strength dependence in vessels and tissue. *Magn Reson Med* 1997; 38:296–302.

Gjedde A. The relation between brain function and cerebral blood flow and metabolism. In: Bajter H, Caplan L (Eds). *Cerebrovascular Disease*. Philadelphia: Lippincott-Raven, 1997, pp 23–40.

Grubb R, Phelps M, Eichling J. The effects of vascular changes in $PaCO_2$ on cerebral blood volume, blood flow and vascular mean transit time. *Stroke* 1974; 5:630–639.

Guimaraes A, Melcher J, Talavage T, et al. Imaging subcortical auditory activity in humans. *Hum Brain Mapp* 1998; 6(1):33–41.

Hajnal J, Saeed N, Soar E, et al. A registration and interpolation procedure for subvoxel matching of serially acquired MR images. *J Comput Assist Tomogr* 1995; 19(2):289–296.

Hoge R, Atkinson J, Gill B, et al. Investigation of BOLD signal dependence on CBF and $CMRO_2$: the deoxyhemoglobin dilution model. *Magn Reson Med* 1999a; 42(5):849–863.

Hoge RD, Atkinson J, Gill B, et al. Linear coupling between perfusion and oxygen consumption in activated human cortex. *Proc Natl Acad Sci USA* 1999b; 96:9403–9408.

Hudetz A. Mathematical model of oxygen transport in the cerebral cortex. *Brain Res* 1999; 817:75–83.

Hyder F, Shulman R, Rothman D. A model for the regulation of cerebral oxygen delivery. *J Appl Physiol* 1998; 85:554–564.

Kim SG. Quantification of relative cerebral blood flow change by flow-sensitive alternating inversion recovery (fair) technique: application to functional mapping. *Magn Reson Med* 1995; 34:293–301.

Kwong KK, Belliveau JW, Chesler DA, et al. Dynamic magnetic resonance imaging of human brain activity during primary sensory stimulation. *Proc Natl Acad Sci USA* 1992; 89:5675–5679.

Lauterbur PC. Image formation by induced local interactions: examples using nuclear magnetic resonance. *Nature* 1973; 242:190–191.

Mandeville J, Marota J, Kosofsky B, et al. Dynamic functional imaging of relative cerebral blood volume during rat forepaw stimulation. *Magn Reson Med* 1998; 39:615–624.

Mandeville J, Marota J, Ayata C, Moskowitz M, Weisskoff R. MRI measurement of the temporal evolution of relative $CMRO_2$ during rat forepaw stimulation. *Magn Reson Med* 1999; 42(5):944–951.

Marrett S, Gjedde A. Changes of blood flow and oxygen consumption in visual cortex of living humans. *Adv Exp Med Biol* 1997; 413:205–208.

Ogawa S, Tank DW, Menon R, et al. Intrinsic signal changes accompanying sensory stimulation: functional brain mapping with magnetic resonance imaging. *Proc Natl Acad Sci USA* 1992; 89:5951–5955.

Ostuni J, Santha A, Mattay V, et al. Analysis of interpolation effects in the reslicing of functional MR images. *J Comput Assist Tomogr* 1997; 21(5):803–810.

Pauling L, Coryell CD. The magnetic properties and structure of hemoglobin, oxyhemoglobin, and carbonmonoxyhemoglobin. *Proc Natl Acad Sci USA* 1936; 22:210–216.

Pike GB. *Multi-Dimensional Fourier Transforms in Magnetic Resonance Imaging.* Boston: Birkhauser, 1988, pp 89–128.

Press W, Teukolsky S, Verrerling W, Flannery B. *Numerical Recipes in C.* New York: Cambridge, 1992.

Purcell EM, Torrey HC, Pound RV. Resonance absorption by nuclear magnetic moments in solids. *Phys Rev* 1946; 69:127.

Reber P, Wong E, Buxton R, Frank L. Correction of off resonance-related distortion in echo-planar imaging using EPI-based field maps. *Magn Reson Med* 1998; 39(2):328–330.

Rosen BR, Belliveau JW, Vevea JM, Brady TJ. Perfusion imaging with NMR contrast agents. *Magn Reson Med* 1990; 14:249–265.

Roy C, Sherrington C. On the regulation of the blood supply of the brain. *J Physiol* 1890; 11:85–105.

Scheffler K, Seifritz E, Haselhorst R, Bilecen D. Titration of the bold effect: separation and quantitation of blood volume and oxygenation changes in the human cerebral cortex during neuronal activation and ferumoxide infusion. *Magn Reson Med* 1999; 42:829–836.

Schmidt R, Thews G. *Human Physiology.* Berlin: Springer-Verlag, 1983.

Sereno M, Dale A, Reppas J, et al. Borders of multiple visual areas in humans revealed by functional magnetic resonance imaging. *Science* 1995; 268:889–893.

Thulborn KR, Waterton JC, Matthews PM, Radda GK. Oxygenation dependence of the transverse relaxation time of water protons in whole blood at high field. *Biochim Biophys Acta* 1982; 714:265–270.

Williams DS, Detre JA, Leigh JS, Koretsky AP. Magnetic resonance imaging of perfusion using spin inversion of arterial water [published erratum appears in Proc Natl Acad Sci USA 1992; 89(9):4220]. *Proc Natl Acad Sci USA* 1992; 89:212–216.

Woods R, Grafton S, Watson J, Sicotte N, Maziotta J. Automated image registration: II. Intersubject validation of linear and nonlinear models. *J Comput Assist Tomogr* 1998; 22(1):153–165.

Worsley K. An overview and some new developments in the statistical analysis of PET and fMRI data. *Hum Brain Mapp* 1997; 5:254–258.

Wright GA, Hu BS, Macovski A. Estimating oxygen saturation of blood in vivo with MR imaging at 1.5 T. *Magn Reson Imaging* 1991; 1:275–283.

Zaharchuk G, Sasamata S, Mandeville J, Moskowitz M, Rosen B. Increased perfusion after acetazolamide challenge demonstrated in the ischemic rat brain using echo-planar arterial spin label perfusion imaging. In: *Proceedings of the 5th Annual Meeting of the ISMRM.* Berkeley: International Society of Magnetic Resonance in Medicine, 1997, p 604.

Correspondence to: G. Bruce Pike, PhD, Room WB-316, Montreal Neurological Institute, 3801 University Street, Montreal, Quebec, Canada H3A 2B4. Tel: 514-398-1929; Fax: 514-398-2975; email: bruce@bic.mni.mcgill.ca.

Pain Imaging, Progress in Pain Research and
Management, Vol. 18, edited by Kenneth L.
Casey and M. Catherine Bushnell, IASP Press,
Seattle, © 2000.

7

Studies of Pain Using Functional Magnetic Resonance Imaging

Karen D. Davis

Division of Neurosurgery, Toronto Western Research Institute; and Department of Surgery, University of Toronto, Toronto, Ontario, Canada

HISTORICAL BACKGROUND

Over 100 years ago, Roy and Sherrington (1890) noted that "the chemical products of cerebral metabolism ... cause variations of the caliber of the cerebral vessels. ... [The brain] is well fitted to provide for a local variation of the blood supply in accordance with local variations of the functional activity." The idea of a relationship between neuronal activity and its resultant metabolic demand provides a conceptual framework for modern imaging technologies (see Chapter 2). Positron emission tomography (PET) and functional magnetic resonance imaging (fMRI) technology is based on the ability of these techniques to provide an indirect measure of neuronal activity. In the early 1990s, fMRI was developed from magnetic resonance imaging (MRI) to image function rather than structure. This technology was advanced by the demonstration that MRI signals depend on blood oxygen levels (Ogawa et al. 1990a). This breakthrough was quickly followed by the first functional images of the human brain (Belliveau et al. 1991; Kwong et al. 1992).

HOW DOES fMRI WORK?

Functional MRI is a rapidly advancing technology that can be used for refined imaging of pain. The physiological basis of the fMRI signal is discussed in detail in Chapter 6. The basic concept derives from the sensitivity of fMRI to the oxygen saturation of blood and blood flow. This concept led to the development of technologies that exploited the blood-oxygenation-level-dependent (BOLD) effect (Ogawa et al. 1990a). The ability of the microvasculature to supply oxygen exceeds the ability of active neuronal tissue to extract oxygen. As a result of this increased perfusion, oxygen saturation of venous blood in active neuronal areas is higher than that of inactive areas. Since oxyhemoglobin and deoxyhemoglobin have different magnetic properties, the latter essentially acts as an endogenous contrast agent. Functional MRI is capable of measuring and localizing this difference, thus allowing generation of brain maps of "active" tissue (Ogawa et al. 1990a,b; DeYoe et al. 1994). The advantages of fMRI are its noninvasive nature (no radioactive substances are injected), its speed (hundreds of milliseconds), and its high spatial resolution (within several millimeters) (Prichard and Brass 1992; Crease 1993; Cohen and Bookheimer 1994). These features permit visualization of sites activated by brief stimuli in the human brain. A "functional" image is created when images obtained during a control state are compared to those obtained during a task. The term *activation* is commonly used to refer to statistically significant increases in magnetic resonance (MR) signal intensity in one or more given pixels related to a particular task. Activations reflect the hemodynamic response that occurs for several seconds after the onset of a stimulus or task (Kim and Ugurbil 1997). The precise relationship between action potential propagation and synaptic events are not fully understood, although synaptic activity most likely demands a large hemodynamic response (Akgören et al. 1996). Rees and colleagues (2000) recently presented evidence for a quantitative relationship between the average firing rate of a neuronal population and the magnitude of the fMRI BOLD signal.

TECHNICAL ISSUES

Despite the advantages of fMRI over other imaging techniques in terms of noninvasiveness and high resolution, several technical issues determine the extent to which fMRI can enhance pain studies.

Scanner. The strength, availability, and type of MRI system affect study design. Although standard 1.5-T clinical scanners can and have been used for fMRI studies of pain, a dedicated system with high field strength (e.g., 4 T) can provide superior imaging capability in human and animal studies requiring an enhanced signal-to-noise ratio. Some newer MRI "open" designs improve the accessibility of the body to stimulation devices. Memory capabilities of the MRI computer affect data collection and experiment duration and hence the overall study design. The typical capacity of many MRI systems allows for imaging up to 10,000 images in 10 minutes.

Experimental devices. All devices used in pain studies must be compatible with the MRI scanner. Devices made from wood, aluminum, brass, or other nonferromagnetic materials pose no difficulty. However, ferromagnetic components must be removed, replaced, or specially shielded to avoid interference with imaging, damage to equipment, or risk to the subject. This limitation of MRI restricts the selection of devices to deliver noxious stimuli, systems used to present tasks, and ways to monitor performance. MRI-compatible devices have been used successfully to deliver electrical stimuli to the median nerve (Davis et al. 1995, 1997) and to apply thermal stimuli to the skin (e.g., see (Davis et al. 1998a,b). An MRI-compatible pain-rating system recently has been developed to enable collection of continuous pain ratings online during imaging (Davis et al. 1998a) (Fig. 1).

Sources of noise. Several factors can contribute to "noisy" images such as interference from non-MRI-compatible equipment or overt head movement. Simple devices like a pillow can provide sufficient stabilization. Physiological noise can occur if overt movement of the body generates a signal (for example, MRI activation can occur if the subject moves a limb).

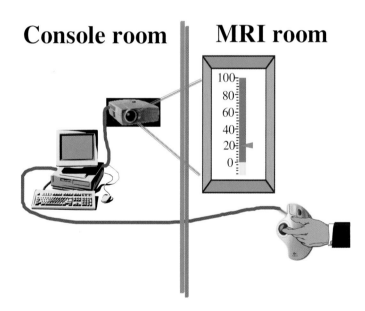

Fig. 1. Magnetic resonance-compatible continuous ratings system with a visual analogue scale (VAS). The subject uses a trackball device to adjust the arrow position within the VAS to indicate the level of pain throughout the fMRI experiment. The ratings are sampled at 2–5 Hz and are stored for offline analysis.

TYPE OF STUDIES

Several approaches can be used to image pain, depending on the question being asked. The question: "What brain areas become more or less active when pain is increased or decreased?" calls for activation or interference studies. These *task-related* studies rely on the investigators' ability to either induce pain or somehow reduce or interfere with evoked or chronic pain. A similar approach can be taken to probe connectivity questions such as: "What brain regions are affected by activity in another region?" However, if the question is: "Is there a chronic abnormality in the basal (resting) activity within certain brain areas?" then fMRI may not be the appropriate method of study because current techniques can only evaluate responses to stimulation.

EXPERIMENTAL DESIGNS

Many experimental designs are available to determine task-related activations related to pain, typically consisting of interleaved periods of painful and control (nonpain) stimulation. Most designs fall into one of two main categories based on the duration of the tasks: block and single-trial designs. Some examples of both design types are shown schematically in Fig. 2. In a block design, each period of painful or nonpainful stimulation is long, often 40–60 seconds or longer (see Fig. 2a). Within each block, the painful stimulus can be delivered in many ways. A single level of painful stimulus intensity can be delivered tonically. A tonic painful stimulus provides a consistent stimulus but may result in sensitization or habituation of the pain or signal within a stimulus cycle or after repetitive cycles (Becerra et al. 1999). To reduce complications associated with tissue damage, the noxious stimuli can be delivered in a sinusoidal fashion within each block (Davis et al. 1998b). Various levels of painful stimuli can be delivered within each block, as either a slow ramp or staircase. These designs permit correlation of the stimulus level with the resultant fMRI signal. In a single-trial (event-related) design, each stimulus is applied for a relatively short time. Whereas single-trial fMRI techniques in other sensory modalities, as when testing visual or auditory responses, can employ very short stimuli (≤ 1 second), the shortest duration of a single painful stimulus may be slightly longer, depending on the stimulation device (see below). Single-trial pain stimuli can be of constant or variable intensity.

Many factors deserve consideration in choosing a suitable design for a particular study. Ultimately, the design must be able to yield data with sufficient statistical power. The maximum amount of data obtained during any experiment is limited by the memory and storage capabilities of the MRI

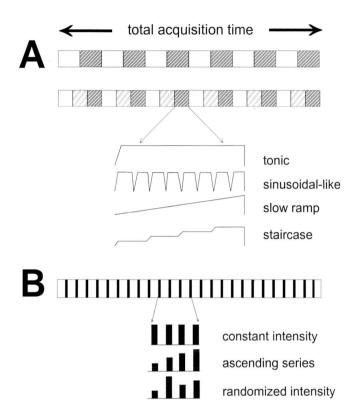

Fig. 2. (A) Blocked and (B) single-trial designs. (A) Blocked designs may consist of interleaved periods of pain (dark hatching) and one (upper bar) or two (second bar) types of control stimuli. The painful stimuli within each "pain" block can be maintained or delivered in a sinusoidal, slow ramp, or staircase fashion. (B) Single-trial designs consist of shorter painful stimuli (dark bars) of equal or differing intensity interleaved with a control (open bars). The control task is typically a lower intensity, nonpainful stimulus.

system. Therefore, a major consideration is the number of data points obtained during each pain task and its control. The duration of each scan (frame) and number of slices determine the number of images obtained for each slice during each stimulus. The hemodynamic response profile, which can be up to ~12 seconds, must also be considered for its impact on interstimulus durations. The type of stimulation device also presents some design limitations. Equipment such as Peltier-type thermal stimulators and certain mechanical devices require some "ramp-up" time and thus cannot deliver the desired stimulus intensity instantaneously. In this instance, a block design is often the best choice, although careful planning can allow for shorter single-trial designs. Laser and electrical devices have no such limitations.

DATA ANALYSIS APPROACHES

Imaging of pain with fMRI can be used to study general trends across the population and to look at specific individual subject responsivity. Both approaches have useful applications. Similarly, all data can be inspected for pain-related responses, or a directed search can be used to inspect activations within particular brain regions associated with pain, such as the primary and secondary somatosensory cortex (S1, S2), the insula, and the anterior cingulate cortex (ACC). The underlying assumptions in this approach are that we have already identified the boundaries of the structures of interest and that these brain regions are consistently activated across most subjects. Consistency across subjects of precise activation loci allows for transformation into standard space and averaging of data. Averaging of data, when appropriate, can improve the signal-to-noise ratio, reduce the complexity of the data, and facilitate comparison of data across laboratories via a standardized coordinate system (Talairach and Tournoux 1988). However, this process also produces spatial blurring. If a study is particularly concerned with pain-related activations that are small, spatially variable across subjects, or may only be present in a subset of subjects, then an individual subject analysis is necessary. Pain imaging in patients for diagnostic or presurgical mapping purposes or in experimental animals also precludes Talairach transformation and requires an individual subject analysis.

Data obtained during a pain and control task can be statistically compared by using a simple boxcar-type model whereby the stimulus levels are approximated by a square wave ("on-off"). For long blocks of stimuli this approach most likely suffices. Hemodynamic response characteristics have a greater influence in shorter blocks and in single-trial designs. A gamma variate function can be used to model the hemodynamic response (Cohen 1997) in these cases. This function can also be convolved with the time course of the stimuli to most appropriately model the expected signal change (Apkarian et al. 1999; Davis et al. 2000). If the psychophysical pain response varies within the experiment, the MRI signals can be correlated to the subjects' perception to obtain pain-related rather than stimulus-related activations (Porro et al. 1998; Apkarian et al. 1999; Davis et al. 2000). Time course analysis of pain-related activations provides another means of imaging pain. Although in its infancy, the study of temporal patterns of activation promises new approaches to the study of transient pain signals, aberrant signals, activity related to sensitization or habituation, and connectivity or networks.

NEGATIVE FINDINGS

An unresolved issue in pain imaging is the interpretation of negative findings. What can we say about a lack of activation within a particular brain region, particularly in an area known to be part of a nociceptive pathway? One possibility is that the area might not be involved in the process under study. An alternate possibility is that the area is involved in the process of interest, but that the technical constraints of imaging or the physiological characteristics of the response within or across subjects have precluded its detection. For instance, a response that habituates over time may not be detected if the data are probed for consistent task-related responses. Some new approaches to detecting fMRI activations, such as independent component analysis (Friston 1998; McKeown and Sejnowski 1998; McKeown et al. 1998), may be useful ways to probe data that may not have predictable responses. Pain-related cortical and thalamic responses may be particularly suitable to these new approaches because the central effects of maintained or repetitive noxious stimuli may habituate due to peripheral and descending modulatory influences. Also, the recruitment of some brain areas may depend on the magnitude of pain or may have a specific stimulus-response relationship for a particular aspect of the pain experience. Furthermore, little is known concerning the location of nociceptive neurons in the human brain. A few electrophysiological single-cell studies in the thalamus (Lenz et al. 1993, 1994) and ACC (Hutchison et al. 1999) found only a few nociceptive neurons concentrated in small areas of these regions. Therefore, pain-related responses might be confined to relatively small areas within particular brain regions. This possibility would hamper detection with fMRI, especially when using Gaussian filtering or averaging across subjects. Another possible confounding factor, noted by one group that found no heat-pain-related cortical activation (Disbrow et al. 1998), is that non-nociceptive and nociceptive neurons are intermingled within certain cortical regions. This anatomical complexity influences the identification of pain-related activations because the control task may activate spatially similar areas.

ACUTE SOMATIC PAIN

The designs and activations reported in fMRI studies of acute somatic pain are summarized in Table I. Most of these studies focused on only a portion of the brain to take advantage of fMRI's exceptional spatial and temporal resolution. Therefore, unlike PET, which allows for whole-brain

Table I
Functional magnetic resonance imaging studies of acute pain

Study	Pain Stimulus			Mean Pain (0–10 VAS)
	Modality	Site	Design	
Davis et al. 1995	electrical	median n.	block: 41 s	
Davis et al. 1997	electrical	median n.	block: 28 s	41
Bucher et al. 1998	electrical	neck	block: 96 s	mild to moderate
Berman et al. 1998	contact heat contact cold	hand/foot	block: 40 s	
Davis et al. 1998b	contact heat contact cold	palm	block: 40 s	6
Davis et al. 1998a	contact heat contact cold	palm	single trial: 1 s single trial: 3 s	~6–10
Disbrow et al. 1998	electrical contact heat mechanical	digit forearm hand	block: 32 s	
Oshiro et al. 1998	electrical	digit	block: 20 s	mild
Porro et al. 1998	chemical (ascorbic acid)	foot (s.c.)	one injection: 12 min pain	48
Becerra et al. 1999	contact heat	dorsal hand	block: 29 s	6.6–7.3
Bushnell et al. 1999	contact heat	calf	block: 9 s	
Gelnar et al. 1999	contact heat	digits 2–5	block: 35 s	3.4
Ploghaus et al. 1999	contact heat	hand	block: 11 s	moderate to strong
Davis et al. 2000	contact heat	hand	single trial ~4–20 s	~3–8

imaging, many fMRI studies have not attempted to identify all possible pain-related activations. However, technological advances now allow whole-brain fMRI scanning with better resolution than PET. The summary in Table I is confined to the thalamus, S1, S2, insula, ACC, and motor regions because most of the studies used a directed search to specifically examine pain-related effects in these areas. Various stimulus modalities have been used to study experimentally induced acute pain, including electrical stimuli (applied to a nerve or skin; Davis et al. 1995, 1997; Bucher et al. 1998; Oshiro et al. 1998), noxious thermal stimuli (heat or cold; Berman et al. 1998; Davis et al. 1998a,b; Apkarian et al. 1999; Becerra et al. 1999; Bushnell et al. 1999; Gelnar et al. 1999; Ploghaus et al. 1999), and noxious mechanical (e.g., pinch; Disbrow et al. 1998) or chemical stimuli (Porro et al. 1998). An example of pain-evoked activations in the thalamus and cortex is presented in Plate 1, which shows the fine resolution that can be achieved.

Table I
Continued

Study	Type of Analysis	N	Th	S1	S2	Insula	ACC	Motor
Davis et al. 1995	single subject	9		x		x		
Davis et al. 1997	single subject	10				x		
Bucher et al. 1998	single subject	6	x			x		x
Berman et al. 1998	single subject	8		x				
Davis et al. 1998b	single subject	12	x		x	x	x	x
Davis et al. 1998a	single subject	4	x		x	x	x	
Disbrow et al. 1998	single subject	12		x	x			x
								x
								x
Oshiro et al. 1998	single subject	6	x	x	x	x		
Porro et al. 1998	single subject, group*	24		x			x	x
Becerra et al. 1999	single subject, group	12	x	x	x	x	x	x
Bushnell et al. 1999	single subject	3		x				
Gelnar et al. 1999	single subject, group	9		x	x	x		x
Ploghaus et al. 1999	single subject, group	12	x	x	x	x	x	x
Davis et al. 2000	single subject*	10	x		x	x	x	

* Includes correlational analysis of evoked pain (during fMRI) to magnetic resonance signal.
Abbreviations: ACC = anterior cingulate cortex; Th = thalamus; S1 = primary somatosensory cortex; S2 = secondary somatosensory cortex; motor = motor areas including M1, premotor, SMA, or cerebellum.

Noncontact laser heat stimuli have not yet been used in fMRI because of the difficulty in using laser devices in an MR environment. The block paradigm is the approach typically used to study pain (Table I), although more recent studies have incorporated shorter stimuli for single-trial, event-related imaging. The overall pattern that emerges across all studies is that painful stimuli will activate the thalamus and the four cortical areas studied (S1, S2, insula, and ACC). Negative findings may be attributed to technical or physiological factors, as discussed above. Intersubject variability in the presence and precise location of pain-related activations has been reported in several studies (Davis et al. 1998b; Porro et al. 1998; Bushnell et al. 1999; Gelnar et al.

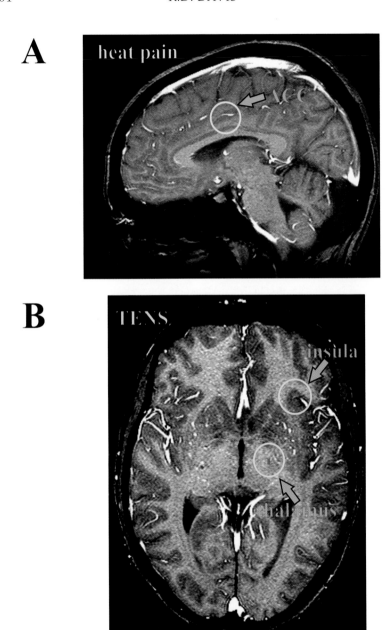

Plate 1. Examples of pain-evoked fMRI activations derived from block design experiments on a 1.5-T echospeed scanner. (A) The anterior cingulate cortex (ACC) activation shown was obtained during application of painful heat stimuli to the hand. (B) The thalamus and anterior insula activations were evoked during painful electrical stimulation of the median nerve with a transcutaneous electrical nerve stimulation (TENS) unit.

1999; Ploghaus et al. 1999) and may also be a factor in the results of group-averaged data. Variable psychophysical responses to painful stimuli are also important sources of variation in imaging results (see below).

VISCERAL PAIN

Few fMRI studies have been published on visceral pain. Binkofski et al. (1998) reported activations related to esophageal distension at nonpainful and painful intensities in normal volunteers. Their study revealed premotor and bilateral S1 and S2 activation during nonpainful distensions with additional bilateral anterior insular activations at higher intensities that were unpleasant but not painful. Painful distensions were associated with an additional activation in the caudal ACC. These findings are significant because they separate "pre-pain" unpleasantness from pain. The data suggest a participatory role for the insula in unpleasant internal sensations that may or may not be painful, in contrast to pain-specific activation of the caudal ACC.

Functional fMRI has also been used to examine central visceral pathways originating from the colon. Preliminary fMRI studies of rectal distension in the anesthetized monkey suggest that the dorsal columns play a role in visceral pain (Al-Chaer et al. 1999). Although pain imaging in the anesthetized monkey is in its infancy, it may provide a new opportunity to test hypotheses concerning visceral pain that are difficult to address in awake human volunteers.

SEPARATING THE STIMULUS FROM THE PERCEPTION

The challenge of imaging pain with fMRI begins with an appreciation of the complex cognitive, sensory, and motor events set in motion by a noxious stimulus. Careful consideration of confounding factors can improve experimental designs and help determine appropriate controls, but we have no way of controlling or even monitoring all psychophysical events associated with pain. However, we can begin to dissect these events by obtaining psychophysical information about the stimuli used during fMRI. This information can be analyzed in correlation with the evoked fMRI signal intensity data. Correlation analyses can help to separate the signal changes that are related merely to the presence of the stimulus from those that vary according to the temporal and intensity characteristics of a particular sensation. Nonspecific cognitive factors such as attention, arousal, and memory may contribute to stimulus-related activations. Information about cortical contributions to the experience of pain intensity have been inferred by correlation of the MR signal with the magnitude and temporal properties of pain intensity ratings obtained during imaging (Davis et al. 1998a, 2000; Porro et al. 1998) or in parallel psychophysical experiments (Apkarian et al. 1999). However, these findings should be interpreted carefully because of the similarity of the magnitude and time course of many components of the pain experience, such as intensity and affect (see Davis et al. 2000).

ATTENTION, ANTICIPATION, AND PAIN

Clearly, attention can alter noxiously evoked activity in central nociceptive pathways (Duncan et al. 1987; Bushnell and Duncan 1989) and can influence pain perception (Bushnell et al. 1985; Miron et al. 1989). The relationship between attention and pain has been studied to determine the overlap and the interaction between the two systems. An fMRI study of individual subject responses demonstrated that pain and attention tasks activated nonoverlapping regions of the posterior and anterior ACC, respectively (Davis et al. 1997). In this study, the attention task was not associated with the pain task in any way. However, the anticipation or expectation of pain, inherent to many pain-imaging studies, has recently been examined with high-field fMRI. Ploghaus et al. (1999) demonstrated that pain and its anticipation activate a common network including the thalamus, S1, S2, and basal ganglia. However, nearby but separate subregions within the ACC, insula, and cerebellum were identified for pain and anticipation. During the pain itself, activations were localized to the posterior ACC, mid-insula, and posterior cerebellum, whereas anticipation of the pain was associated with activations within the anterior ACC, anterior insula, and anterior cerebellum. The increasing magnitude of such "anticipation" activations over successive trials, unlike the consistent "pain" activations, suggests a learning effect. These data highlight the possible interactions between pain and related cognitive processes that may be altered during injury or chronic pain.

ALTERED STATES: CHRONIC PAIN, HYPERALGESIA, AND ANALGESIA

Functional fMRI was developed to detect signal changes that occur within the relatively short period of time in which a subject lies in the scanner. Chronic pain is thus a particularly difficult topic of study with fMRI. However, gross changes that accompany chronic pain across groups of subjects or within large brain regions of an individual may be detectable using signal averaging and multiple imaging sessions. Several laboratories are developing this approach for application to various patient populations. For example, fMRI has revealed less phantom limb pain associated with cortical reorganization in amputees who use a myoelectric prosthesis (Lotze et al. 1999). Clues about central mechanisms and plasticity in chronic pain can also be derived from studies that manipulate pain levels in patients with chronic pain. A recent preliminary report demonstrated that transient pain exacerbation evoked by leg raising can be used to study chronic back pain (Krauss et al. 1999).

Models of chronic pain and hyperalgesia can also be used to study central sensitization in normal volunteers. For example, injection of capsaicin into normal skin can produce mechanical, secondary hyperalgesia. A recent fMRI study of capsaicin-induced mechanical hyperalgesia reported that the most significant activations associated with static mechanical hyperalgesia (compared to nonpainful tactile stimulation) included the prefrontal and motor and inferior frontal areas (Baron et al. 1999). These activations were attributed to the various cognitive processes (including attention), orientation, motor functions, and behavioral planning in response to pain. Surprisingly, there was little or no ACC activation, perhaps because of the relatively mild level of pain evoked.

The effects of analgesia have seldom been imaged with fMRI. A recent PET study reported suppression of nearly all pain-related activations during infusion of an opiate (Casey et al. 2000). Further development of fMRI may permit the study of central mechanisms of analgesic drugs, including the recruitment of descending modulatory pathways.

Two studies (Kiriakopoulos et al. 1997; Rezai et al. 1999) have demonstrated the applicability of fMRI to study the cortical effects of direct CNS stimulation in patients with chronic pain. These studies used novel ways to study the analgesic effects of spinal and deep brain stimulation. Imaging the effects of spinal or thalamic stimulation may also provide insights into normal and altered central connectivity.

SUMMARY

Converging information from fMRI studies, from other imaging methods such as PET, electroencephalography (EEG), and magnetoencephalography (MEG), and from clinical observations and psychophysical testing in patients with cortical lesions indicates that at least four regions are involved in some aspect of the sensory-discriminative and affective-motivational response to pain—the S1 and S2 cortices, the insula, and the ACC (see also Chapter 5). Additional loci in the cerebellum and in the parietal and frontal cortex may also participate in the multidimensional response to pain. The challenge that lies ahead is to probe further into the particular spatiotemporal characteristics of these pain-related activations and to explore the networks responsible for particular aspects of the complex nature of pain.

REFERENCES

Akgören N, Dalgaard P, Lauritzen M. Cerebral blood flow increases evoked by electrical stimulation of rat cerebellar cortex: relation to excitatory synaptic activity and nitric oxide synthesis. *Brain Res* 1996; 710:204–214.

Al-Chaer ED, Quast MJ, Feng Y, et al. Brain imaging of the long term effect of a midline myelotomy on the processing of visceral and somatic pain using fMRI. *Abstracts: 9th World Congress on Pain.* Seattle: IASP Press, 1999, pp 391–392.

Apkarian AV, Darbar A, Krauss BR, et al. Differentiating cortical areas related to pain perception from stimulus identification: temporal analysis of fMRI activity. *J Neurophysiol* 1999; 81:2956–2963.

Baron R, Baron Y, Disbrow E, Roberts TP. Brain processing of capsaicin-induced secondary hyperalgesia: a functional MRI study. *Neurology* 1999; 53:548–557.

Becerra LR, Breiter HC, Stojanovic M, et al. Human brain activation under controlled thermal stimulation and habituation to noxious heat: an fMRI study. *Magn Reson Med* 1999; 41:1044–1057.

Belliveau JW, Kennedy DNJ, McKinstry RC, et al. Functional mapping of the human visual cortex by magnetic resonance imaging. *Science* 1991; 254:716–719.

Berman HH, Kim KHS, Talati A, Hirsch J. Representation of nociceptive stimuli in primary sensory cortex. *Neuroreport* 1998; 9:4179–4187.

Binkofski F, Schnitzler A, Enck P, et al. Somatic and limbic cortex activation in esophageal distention: a functional magnetic resonance imaging study. *Ann Neurol* 1998; 44:811–815.

Bucher SF, Dieterich M, Wiesmann M, et al. Cerebral functional magnetic resonance imaging of vestibular, auditory, and nociceptive areas during galvanic stimulation. *Ann Neurol* 1998; 44:120–125.

Bushnell MC, Duncan GH. Sensory and affective aspects of pain perception: is medial thalamus restricted to emotional issues? *Exp Brain Res* 1989; 78:415–418.

Bushnell MC, Duncan GH, Dubner R, Jones RL, Maixner W. Attentional influences on noxious and innocuous cutaneous heat detection in humans and monkeys. *J Neurosci* 1985; 5:1103–1110.

Bushnell MC, Duncan GH, Hofbauer RK, et al. Pain perception: is there a role for primary somatosensory cortex? *Proc Natl Acad Sci USA* 1999; 96:7705–7709.

Casey KL, Svensson P, Morrow TJ, et al. Selective opiate modulation of nociceptive processing in the human brain. *J Neurophysiol* 2000; 84:525–533.

Cohen MS. Parametric analysis of fMRI data using linear systems method. *Neuroimage* 1997; 6:93–103.

Cohen MS, Bookheimer SY. Localization of brain function using magnetic resonance imaging. *Trends Neurosci* 1994; 17:268–276.

Crease RP. Biomedicine in the age of imaging. *Science* 1993; 261:554–561.

Davis KD, Wood ML, Crawley AP, Mikulis DJ. fMRI of human somatosensory and cingulate cortex during painful electrical nerve stimulation. *Neuroreport* 1995; 7:321–325.

Davis KD, Taylor SJ, Crawley AP, Wood ML, Mikulis DJ. Functional MRI of pain- and attention-related activations in the human cingulate cortex. *J Neurophysiol* 1997; 77:3370–3380.

Davis KD, Kwan CL, Crawley AP, Mikulis DJ. Event-related fMRI of pain: entering a new era in imaging pain. *Neuroreport* 1998a; 9:3019–3023.

Davis KD, Kwan CL, Crawley AP, Mikulis DJ. Functional MRI study of thalamic and cortical activations evoked by cutaneous heat, cold and tactile stimuli. *J Neurophysiol* 1998b; 80:1533–1546.

Davis KD, Kwan CL, Crawley AP, Mikulis DJ. fMRI of cortical and thalamic activations correlated to the magnitude of pain. In: Devor M, Rowbotham MC, Wiesenfeld-Hallin Z (Eds). *Proceedings of the 9th World Congress on Pain,* Progress in Pain Research and Management, Vol. 16. Seattle: IASP Press, 2000, pp 497–505.

DeYoe EA, Bandettini P, Neitz J, Miller D, Winans P. Functional magnetic resonance imaging (fMRI) of the human brain. *J Neurosci Methods* 1994; 54:171–187.

Disbrow E, Buonocore M, Antognini J, Carstens E, Rowley HA. Somatosensory cortex: a comparison of the response to noxious thermal, mechanical, and electrical stimuli using functional magnetic resonance imaging. *Hum Brain Mapp* 1998; 6:150–159.

Duncan GH, Bushnell MC, Bates R, Dubner R. Task-related responses of monkey medullary dorsal horn neurons. *J Neurophysiol* 1987; 57:289–310.

Friston KJ. Modes or models: a critique on independent component analysis for fMRI. *Trends Cogn Sci* 1998; 2:373–376.

Gelnar PA, Krauss BR, Sheehe PR, Szeverenyi NM, Apkarian AV. A comparative fMRI study of cortical representations for thermal painful, vibrotactile, and motor performance tasks. *Neuroimage* 1999; 10:460–482.

Hutchison WD, Davis KD, Lozano AM, Tasker RR, Dostrovsky JO. Pain-related neurons in the human cingulate cortex. *Nat Neurosci* 1999; 2:403–405.

Kim SG, Ugurbil K. Functional magnetic resonance imaging of the human brain. *J Neurosci Methods* 1997; 74:229–243.

Kiriakopoulos ET, Tasker RR, Nicosia S, Wood ML, Mikulis DJ. Functional magnetic resonance imaging: a potential tool for the evaluation of spinal cord stimulation: technical case report. *Neurosurgery* 1997; 41:501–504.

Krauss BR, Grachev I, Szeverenyi NM, Apkarian AV. Imaging the pain of back pain. *Soc Neurosci Abstr* 1999; 25:141.

Kwong KK, Belliveau JW, Chesler DA. Dynamic magnetic resonance imaging of human brain activity during primary sensory stimulation. *Proc Natl Acad Sci USA* 1992; 89:5675–56679.

Lenz FA, Seike M, Lin YC. Neurons in the area of human thalamic nucleus ventralis caudalis respond to painful heat stimuli. *Brain Res* 1993; 623:235–240.

Lenz FA, Gracely RH, Rowland LH, Dougherty PM. A population of cells in the human thalamic principal sensory nucleus respond to painful mechanical stimuli. *Neurosci Lett* 1994; 180:46–50.

Lotze M, Grodd W, Birbaumer N, et al. Does use of a myoelectric prosthesis prevent cortical reorganization and phantom limb pain? *Nat Neurosci* 1999; 2:501–502.

McKeown MJ, Sejnowski TJ. Independent component analysis of fMRI data: examining the assumptions. *Hum Brain Mapp* 1998; 6:368–372.

McKeown MJ, Jung T-P, Makeig S, et al. Spatially independent activity patterns in functional MRI data during the stroop color-naming task. *Proc Natl Acad Sci USA* 1998; 95:803–810.

Miron D, Duncan GH, Bushnell MC. Effects of attention on the intensity and unpleasantness of thermal pain. *Pain* 1989; 39:345–352.

Ogawa S, Lee TM, Kay AR, Tank DW. Brain magnetic resonance imaging with contrast dependent on blood oxygenation. *Proc Natl Acad Sci USA* 1990a; 87:9868–9872.

Ogawa S, Lee T-M, Nayak AS, Glynn P. Oxygenation-sensitive contrast in magnetic resonance image of rodent brain at high magnetic fields. *Magn Reson Med* 1990b; 14:68–78.

Oshiro Y, Fuijita N, Tanaka H. Functional mapping of pain-related activation with echo- planar MRI: significance of the SII-insular region. *Neuroreport* 1998; 9:2285–2289.

Ploghaus A, Tracey I, Gati JS, et al. Dissociating pain from its anticipation in the human brain. *Science* 1999; 284:1979–1981.

Porro CA, Cettolo V, Francescato MP, Baraldi P. Temporal and intensity coding of pain in human cortex. *J Neurophysiol* 1998; 80:3312–3320.

Prichard JW, Brass LM. New anatomical and functional imaging methods. *Ann Neurol* 1992; 32:395–400.

Rees G, Friston K, Koch C. A direct quantitative relationship between the functional properties of human and macaque V5. *Nat Neurosci* 2000; 3:716–723.

Rezai AR, Lozano AM, Crawley AP, et al. Thalamic stimulation and functional magnetic resonance imaging: localization of cortical and subcortical activation with implanted electrodes. *J Neurosurg* 1999; 90:583–590.

Roy CS, Sherrington CS. On the regulation of the blood-supply of the brain. *J Physiol (Lond)* 1890; 11:85–108.

Talairach J, Tournoux P. *Co-planar Stereotaxic Atlas of the Human Brain*. New York: Thieme Medical Publishers, 1988.

Correspondence to: Karen D. Davis, PhD, Toronto Western Hospital, Division of Neurosurgery, MP 14-322, 399 Bathurst Street, Toronto, Ontario M5T 2S8, Canada. Tel: 416-603-5662; Fax: 416-603-5745; email: kdavis@playfair.utoronto.ca.

Pain Imaging, Progress in Pain Research and
Management, Vol. 18, edited by Kenneth L.
Casey and M. Catherine Bushnell, IASP Press,
Seattle, © 2000.

8

Functional Imaging of Animal Models of Pain: High-Resolution Insights into Nociceptive Processing

Robert C. Coghill[a] and Thomas J. Morrow[b,c]

[a]Department of Neurobiology and Anatomy, Wake Forest University School of Medicine, Winston-Salem, North Carolina, USA; [b]Department of Neurology, University of Michigan, Ann Arbor, Michigan, USA; [c]Neurology Research Laboratory, Veterans Affairs Hospital, Ann Arbor, Michigan, USA

RATIONALE FOR ANIMAL IMAGING STUDIES

Functional imaging of pain-related activity of the central nervous system (CNS) provides a powerful method for exploring the complex neural mechanisms that support the pain experience. By allowing the responses of multiple CNS regions to be examined simultaneously in awake, behaving subjects, these techniques have expanded our knowledge of the neurophysiology of pain beyond the limits of traditional single-unit electrophysiological and lesion studies. Most functional imaging studies of pain have used either positron emission tomography (PET) or functional magnetic resonance imaging (fMRI) to examine human subjects, while relatively few imaging studies have focused on animal models of pain. Human studies have an obvious advantage because they allow simultaneous assessment of both experiential/cognitive aspects of pain and brain activation. However, both PET and fMRI studies of humans are subject to several limitations that can be overcome by the use of animal imaging paradigms.

Both PET and fMRI have relatively limited spatial resolutions. Current human PET scanners have a maximal resolution of ~6 mm in all planes, while animal PET scanners can obtain spatial resolutions of ~2 mm (exceeding the theoretical resolution afforded by several PET isotopes). Most fMRI studies of humans typically acquire data with ~4–6 mm spatial resolution, although finer resolutions are possible. However, analysis of fMRI data at fine spatial resolutions (i.e., <4 mm) is complicated both by nonlinear deformation of the brain across the cardiac/respiratory cycle and by submillimetric movement artifacts. Accordingly, neither PET nor fMRI offers the capability to accurately localize the activity of individual nuclei in the brainstem, midbrain, and thalamus. Most animal imaging studies have used film-based autoradiographic techniques to assess the distribution of various radioactive tracers used as indices of neural activity. Depending on the tracer used, autoradiography offers spatial resolution on the order of 20–50 μm. Such resolution is fine enough, for example, to conclusively attribute activation to specific nuclei of the thalamus. This fine spatial resolution, coupled with the availability of tissue sections, allows investigators to correlate activation with histologically defined CNS regions rather than relying on atlas data, which may not be sensitive to individual differences in anatomy.

In addition to limited spatial resolution, human functional imaging studies of chronic pain states are subject to significant variability arising from inter-individual differences in the chronic pain syndrome itself. For example, postherpetic neuralgia, a chronic pain syndrome with a clear etiology, is thought to be composed of different subtypes ranging from those that are sustained by abnormal primary afferent input to those that more closely resemble deafferentation pain (Rowbotham et al. 1998). Furthermore, different patients with a single chronic pain syndrome often have significantly different treatment histories due to individual responses to various drugs. In contrast, inter-individual variation in animal models of chronic pain is considerably reduced by the ability to produce the pain syndrome in a carefully controlled fashion. Other relatively invasive procedures such as single-unit recordings or experimentally induced brain lesions can also be incorporated into the experimental design in animal imaging studies. Taken together, these advantages indicate that animal imaging studies can complement related human studies and provide powerful tools for the investigation of CNS pain mechanisms.

Most functional imaging studies in animals have used tracers of either glucose utilization or cerebral blood flow (CBF) to map pain-induced CNS activation. In general, both methodologies have yielded largely congruent results. The theory and application of each methodology are discussed below.

IMAGING NEURONAL ACTIVITY
VIA THE 2-DEOXYGLUCOSE TECHNIQUE

Since the development of the 2-deoxyglucose (2-DG) method in 1977, several studies have examined neuronal activity during the processing of pain and during analgesic and anesthetic manipulations. Early investigations were hampered by the inadequate image acquisition and analysis technology. Because of these limitations, many investigations were performed in a nonquantitative fashion (i.e., without sampling arterial blood to obtain absolute values of glucose utilization). Nevertheless, quantitative and nonquantitative assessments of activation yielded largely congruent results, confirming electrophysiological findings and providing the tools for studying multifocal neuronal responses simultaneously.

THEORETICAL BASIS OF THE 2-DG METHOD

The 2-DG method for measuring local cerebral metabolic rate of glucose (CMRglc) is the most commonly used functional imaging technique for assessing the effects of pain and of analgesic or anesthetic manipulations on CNS activity in animals. This method rests on the central principle that, after an action potential is produced by a neuron, the sodium-potassium pump is activated to repolarize the cell. This process consumes adenosine triphosphate (ATP). The increased demand for ATP, in turn, increases glucose metabolism (Mata et al. 1980). Thus, glucose uptake serves as a reasonable index of neuronal activity.

Glucose is rapidly metabolized to CO_2 and H_2O, but both are cleared from the CNS too rapidly to allow accurate quantification of tissue radioactivity via conventional autoradiography. This problem was overcome in 1977 by Sokoloff and colleagues with the development of tracer techniques employing a metabolically stable analogue of glucose, 2-deoxyglucose. This compound is taken up and phosphorylated by cells in a manner identical to glucose. However, because it has a hydrogen atom instead of a hydroxyl group on the second carbon, it is not metabolized further and accumulates in cells in proportion to glucose uptake.

The 2-DG method allows the rate of local glucose utilization to be calculated from three variables: (1) the concentration of 2-DG in the plasma, (2) the concentration of glucose in the plasma, and (3) the level of 2-DG in the tissue (Sokoloff et al. 1977). Plasma concentrations of both 2-DG and glucose are obtained from rapid arterial blood sampling, while tissue levels of 2-DG are measured by autoradiography in small animals, or by PET in larger primates and humans. Generally, [14]C- or ^{3}H-labeled 2-DG is used for autoradiography, and ^{18}F-2-DG for PET (Reivich et al. 1979). Autoradiographic analysis of 2-DG accumulation provides a spatial resolution of 100–200 μm, while most PET scanners yield a spatial resolution of ~6 mm (Smith 1983).

The theoretical model underlying the 2-DG method assumes that 2-DG is distributed among three compartments—in the plasma, as free 2-DG in tissue, and as 2-DG-6-phosphate in tissue. However, the rate constants at which 2-DG is transported from the blood to the tissue and then either metabolized to 2-DG-6-phosphate or transported from the tissue back to the blood may not be constant across all physiological or pharmacological conditions. Calculating these constants in every animal is an arduous undertaking. Fortunately, if 2-DG is given in a single bolus rather than as a constant infusion, and if measurement is continued until plasma 2-DG levels fall to near-zero values, terms of the equation containing these rate constants approach zero, eliminating the need to calculate them directly. Accordingly, the experimental duration is determined by the time required for plasma 2-DG levels to reach near-zero values, approximately 30–45 minutes after bolus injection (Sokoloff et al. 1977).

One of the critical assumptions of the theoretical model is that local glucose metabolism, and hence the neuronal activity driving metabolism, remains constant throughout the 30–45-minute experimental period (Sokoloff et al. 1977). This requirement is particularly problematic for studies of acute pain in that stimulation must be carefully tailored to avoid sensitization or habituation. However, in chronic pain models, this relatively long experimental period is ideal for studying ongoing pain that has reached a steady state.

INTERPRETATION OF ALTERATIONS IN GLUCOSE UTILIZATION

The interpretation of localized stimulus-induced alterations in glucose utilization remains controversial. Early in the history of the 2-DG method, cell bodies were assumed to represent the main site of increased glucose utilization within a single neuron (Sokoloff 1999). However, several studies indicate that activation-induced increases in 2-DG uptake are concentrated in regions rich in axonal terminals (Schwartz et al. 1979; Kadekaro et al. 1985). Other lines of evidence indicate that cell bodies are also capable of exhibiting activation-induced increases in glucose metabolism (Yarowsky et al. 1983). Thus, the distribution of 2-DG uptake within a single neuron may include both cell bodies as well as neuron terminals.

Non-neuronal cell types also contribute to stimulus-evoked increases in local glucose utilization. Astrocytes represent one of the primary routes for reuptake of synaptically released glutamate, one of the most widely distributed excitatory neurotransmitters (Magistretti and Pellerin 1999). Glutamate uptake by astrocytes stimulates both glucose uptake and glycolysis, and the lactate produced by this glycolytic reaction helps to sustain the energy demands of neuronal activity (Magistretti and Pellerin 1999). In vivo, there is a one-to-one relationship between glutamate reuptake and glucose use (Sibson et al. 1998). Thus, excitatory neuronal activity is clearly coupled to glucose utilization in a highly regionally-specific fashion (Magistretti and Pellerin 1999). Accordingly, most 2-DG studies of pain have identified increased local glucose utilization in brain and spinal cord regions in which the overall activity is dominated by pain-induced increases in neuronal discharge frequencies.

IMAGING NEURONAL ACTIVITY VIA REGIONAL CEREBRAL BLOOD FLOW

In their classic paper on cerebral blood flow, Roy and Sherrington (1890) described changes in brain volume during electrical stimulation of a peripheral nerve. From this result and experiments showing that metabolites from ischemic brain could duplicate this effect, they concluded that the products of cerebral metabolism can cause variations in the diameter of cerebral vessels and that the brain possesses intrinsic mechanisms for controlling local blood flow during local variations in functional activity. Their hypothesis that changes in localized CBF occur in relation to neuronal activity forms the basis for all the more recent studies of brain function using rCBF imaging in awake humans, including PET and fMRI studies.

Early attempts to identify alterations in global blood flow during different levels of brain activity in humans had disappointing results (Kety and Schmidt 1945; Kety 1950). However, the advent of new radiographic tools for measuring both local CBF and glucose metabolism made it possible to demonstrate that increases in rCBF are tightly and positively coupled to increases in synaptic activity (Sakurada et al. 1978; Sokoloff 1978). More recently, optical imaging studies have revealed highly localized, stimulus-evoked changes in blood flow in the barrel fields of the rodent cerebral cortex (Dowling et al. 1996; Woolsey et al. 1996; Chapter 3). The mechanism coupling rCBF to synaptic activity is still unclear and may involve multiple factors. Although the degree of coupling may vary among different brain regions and under special experimental conditions, it is consistently present under normal conditions (Mraovitch and Seylaz 1987: Mraovitch et al. 1992a,b). Studies comparing local CMRglc and blood flow in the somatosensory system support the view that metabolism and blood flow are augmented to a similar overall degree (Ginsberg et al. 1987). Ginsberg et al. (1987) suggest that the interregional topographic dissimilarities of distribution of flow and metabolism may be explained by the back-diffusion characteristics of the flow tracers employed. It is also possible that changes in regional blood flow occur more rapidly than changes in local metabolic activity, or perhaps we are better able to detect changes in the former than in the latter. Optical imaging studies have shown that localized changes in cortical blood flow occur within a few seconds of a somatosensory stimulus (Woolsey et al. 1996; see Chapter 3). Fox et al. (1988), using unilateral vibrotactile finger stimulation in normal volunteers, found that blood flow increased focally by 30%, with only a slight augmentation of oxidative metabolism.

AUTORADIOGRAPHIC METHODS OF rCBF ASSESSMENT

Most methods for assessing rCBF are derived from the diffusible radiotracer techniques pioneered by Kety (1951, 1960). These techniques are based upon a single-compartment model that describes the flow of tracers between blood and tissue. This model has two critical assumptions: (1) the tracer can freely traverse the blood–brain barrier such that blood and tissue tracer concentrations reach equilibrium after a single capillary transit, and (2) the tissue is homogeneous with respect to flow and other properties. Iodoantipyrine (IAP) and isopropyliodoamphetamine (IMP) are the most widely used tracers of CBF in autoradiographic studies, due in part to their ability to freely move from the blood to the brain (Sakurada et al. 1978; Lear et al. 1982). Although the uptake and distribution of both tracers correspond well with blood flow, IAP and IAMP freely cross the blood–brain barrier in both directions (Sakurada et al. 1978; Lear et al. 1982). The tendency of both tracers to diffuse back out of the tissue after euthanasia and before the tissue has been frozen may result in a significant underestimation of CBF. Significant diffusion of IAP can occur within 30 seconds of euthanasia, leaving investigators minimal time to remove the brain from the skull for freezing (Greenberg et al. 1999). IAMP is somewhat less susceptible to back-diffusion, but is thought to cross the blood–brain barrier via a specific uptake mechanism and thus may not be an accurate index of CBF across all brain regions or all study conditions (Lear et al. 1982).

To circumvent these limitations, a rapid, quantitative autoradiographic technique was recently developed for estimating rCBF during pain perception in rats. This imaging technique employs ^{99m}Tc-exametazime [(RR,SS)-4,8-diaza-3,6,6,9-tetramethylundecate-2, 10-dione bisoxime], a radioligand that is used extensively in human studies to image blood flow with single photon emission computed tomography (SPECT). (Note that this tracer was previously called technetium 99m-d,l-hexamethyl-propyleneamine oxime or [99m]TC-HMPAO). This tracer accumulates in the brain and rapidly compartmentalizes, with no significant redistribution for more than 1 hour (Lear 1988a,b). The high retention and low back-diffusion of ^{99m}Tc stem from its rapid conversion to a nonlipophilic isomer, which makes experimental timing less critical. With timing constraints minimized, it is easy to run multiple subjects through the procedure during a single experiment. In addition, ^{99m}Tc is primarily a gamma-2 emitter (mean energy 140.5 keV) that decays by isomeric transition, with a physical half-life of 6.03 hours. The high energy and short half-life of this radiotracer makes it ideal for use in these animal experiments by minimizing both film exposure time and the storage time required for complete decay of radioactive wastes.

IMPLEMENTATION OF THE [99m]TC-EXAMETAZIME AUTORADIOGRAPHIC METHOD

This radiotracer is produced by adding sodium pertechnetate ^{99m}Tc in isotonic saline to a commercially available radiopharmaceutical kit, Ceretec (Amersham Corp.). This method produces the highly lipophilic complex, ^{99m}Tc-exametazime, which is relatively unstable and rapidly converts to a nonlipophilic isomer, which is not suitable for imaging rCBF. Accordingly, paper chromatography is performed to measure the radiochemical purity of each prepared Ceretec kit and determine the fraction of technetium (^{99m}Tc) label as lipophilic exametazime (Neirinckx et al. 1987; Ballinger et al. 1988). All reconstituted radiotracer kits used should have a lipophilic exametazime content of 90% or higher. After injection into venous circulation, the lipophilic ligand rapidly crosses the blood–brain barrier and diffuses across cell membranes. Because of the unstable nature of the lipophilic form, it rapidly transforms into its nonlipophilic isomer and is trapped intracellularly.

Fig. 1 shows a diagram of the procedure used for rCBF measurement. Briefly, each rat is placed in a soft towel restraint and a flexible intravenous catheter is inserted into its tail vein. The animal then rests quietly in the restraint for approximately 40 minutes to recover from the stress of catheterization. The radiotracer (10–15 mCi) is injected into the tail vein as a bolus over 10–15 seconds. Approximately 2 minutes following tracer injection, the rat is deeply anesthetized, removed from the restraint, and decapitated. The brain is removed from the skull and quick-frozen using powdered dry ice. Standard 20-μm coronal sections are then cut at –18°C. Four consecutive sections are taken at approximately 250-μm intervals and mounted on glass slides to provide sufficient sections through all sampled brain

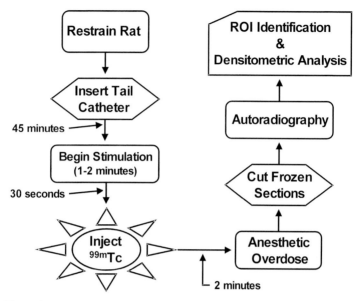

Fig. 1. Flow chart summarizing the steps involved in the measurement of regional cerebral blood flow (rCBF) in rats. ROI = region of interest.

regions for later autoradiographic analysis. Standard autoradiograms are generated by affixing the mounted sections to the emulsion side of Kodak BioMax MR-1 imaging film. When their radioactivity returns to background levels, the slides are stained with cresyl violet. Precise structural identifications are made by comparing the autoradiograms and stained sections to coronal plates from the Paxinos and Watson (1986) stereotactic atlas of the rat brain.

Autoradiograms are analyzed using a microcomputer-assisted video-imaging densitometer (MCID, Imaging Research, Inc.). Each brain section on film is digitized to produce a high-resolution, 256-level grayscale image. Anatomical location of selected regions of interest (ROIs) is determined by overlaying transparent stereotactic atlas templates (adapted from Paxinos and Watson 1986) on digitized brain images displayed on the video monitor and by comparison with the sections stained with cresyl violet. The densitometer system converts sampled film optical densities to apparent tissue radioactivity concentrations (nanocuries per milligram) by comparison with the optical densities of standards also imaged on each film. The average total brain activity is estimated by sampling all pixels in each brain section and averaging the activity across all sections for each animal. Activation index values are calculated for each sampled ROI as percentage difference from the average total activity of the entire brain using the following formula:

AI = [(Sampled ROI Activity – Average Total Brain Activity)/
Average Total Brain Activity] × 100%.

Finally, the within-subject mean AIs for each sampled region are averaged across all subjects in an experimental group to compute within-group means for each ROI (Morrow et al. 1998).

AUTORADIOGRAPHIC IMAGING OF rCBF VERSUS CMRglc

The 2-DG and rCBF imaging methods each have their own merits and limitations. Both techniques allow the simultaneous quantification of activation within multiple CNS regions. However, both use indirect measures (i.e., CBF or CMRglc) to assess neuronal activity. Therefore, anatomical, electrophysiological, and behavioral data should be considered when interpreting the results obtained with either method. The biochemistry and physiology linking glucose utilization and neural activity have been studied more intensively and are better understood than are rCBF responses. Thus, the 2-DG method is more conservative and may be more appropriate for exploratory studies of pain models.

Autoradiographic investigation of rCBF, however, offers several advantages over 2-DG autoradiography. Blood flow autoradiograms have a higher spatial resolution than those produced when imaging metabolism with 2-DG. Due to the diffusion characteristics of 2-DG and the long film exposure times imposed by the low energy of ^{14}C, the spatial resolution of conventional 2-DG is, at best, 100–200 μm (Smith 1983). This resolution is lower than the approximately 20–50-μm resolution of autoradiograms produced using the ^{99m}Tc-exametazime blood flow method.

In the various rCBF methods, the rapid clearance of CBF tracers from the vasculature (a requirement of the single-compartment model of CBF measurement) allows a much finer temporal resolution than is afforded by the 2-DG method. In general, CBF can be fully quantified with a 1-minute uptake period, while the 2-DG method requires a 45-minute uptake period to allow plasma 2-DG to fall to near-zero levels to simplify quantification. To obtain condition-specific images, both methods require constant levels of neural activity during the uptake period. The need for prolonged painful stimuli in 2-DG studies significantly limits the type of stimuli that can be examined. It is clearly unethical to expose unanesthetized animals to severe and inescapable noxious stimuli for 45 minutes. Thus, anesthesia or spinalization (in the case of spinal cord investigations) must be employed when using acute noxious stimuli with the 2-DG method. However, both the 2-DG and

CBF methods are well suited for studies of various chronic pain models in which animals are mildly symptomatic for several hours or even weeks. One disadvantage of the ^{99m}Tc-exametazime rCBF imaging method is that it provides only a semi-quantitative estimate of rCBF, since all data are normalized to the total amount of radiotracer in the brain. Although this approach does not directly measure rCBF, it is sufficiently sensitive to allow detection of regional differences in blood flow, even in unstimulated subjects, as shown in Plate 4. Similar methods have been validated in other laboratories for autoradiographic studies measuring regional glucose metabolism (Porro et al. 1991a,b). Furthermore, normalization to whole brain radioactivity is almost a standard analytic approach for human PET studies of CBF. Normalization avoids the stress of surgery for the placement of the arterial catheter that is required to sample arterial blood for direct blood flow measurement. A disadvantage of the rCBF method is that, because ^{99m}Tc-exametazime is a short half-life tracer and the lipophilic isomer is unstable, the exametazime radioligand kit must be reconstituted just prior to an experiment and used within 30 minutes of preparation. However, the short half-life of the tracer permits minimal storage time before complete decay and subsequent disposal. Finally, each exametazime radioligand kit is mixed with 55 mCi of technetium, a relatively high level of radioactivity that allows for comparatively brief film exposure times. Long-term exposure to this level of radioactivity might be construed as an additional disadvantage of the rCBF method compared to the 2-DG technique.

FUNCTIONAL IMAGING OF PAIN-RELATED CNS ACTIVITY

THE SPINAL CORD

In both the spinal cord and the trigeminal system, multiple types of nociceptive stimuli evoke increases in glucose utilization that follow a laminar/nuclear distribution consistent with the location of regions known to be engaged in various aspects of nociceptive processing (Plates 1 and 2). Prolonged noxious stimulation of the paw of rats and cats produces increased metabolic activity within both superficial (lamina I) and deep (lamina V)

Plate 1. Spatial distribution of nociceptive processing within the rat spinal cord. Studies using 2-DG reveal that progressive increases in noxious heat intensity produce increased activation over progressively larger rostrocaudal expanses of the spinal cord. This progressive recruitment of activity suggests that the number of neurons activated by a painful stimulus serves as one factor utilized by the CNS to encode the intensity of a painful stimulus. The right side of image shows the right side of the spinal cord, ipsilateral to simulation. White outlines indicate regions of interest. From Coghill et al. (1991). ⟶

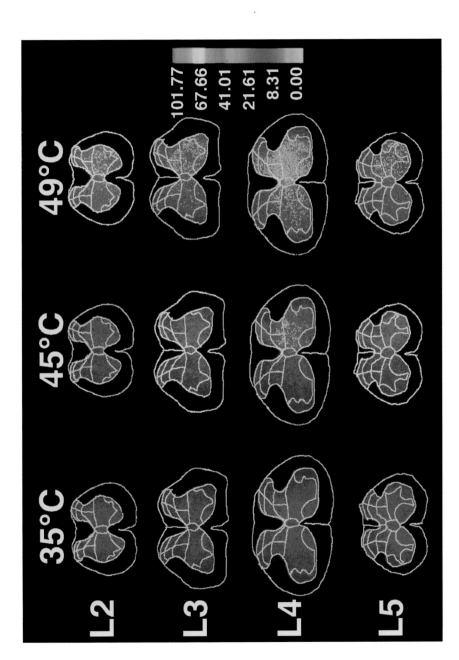

regions of the ipsilateral dorsal horn (Abram and Kostreva 1986; Coghill et al. 1991; Porro et al. 1991b, 1999). Fully quantitative analysis indicates that such noxious stimuli can increase glucose utilization by as much as 56% in the deep dorsal horn, a change far greater than the ~3–8% increases seen in CBF during pain processing in the human brain (Porro et al. 1999). Similarly, electrical stimulation of the tooth pulp, superior sagittal sinus, or the greater occipital nerve increases glucose utilization in the trigeminal nucleus caudalis (medullary dorsal horn) of rats and cats (Shetter and Sweet 1979; Goadsby and Zagami 1991; Goadsby et al. 1997). Many neurons within the nucleus caudalis and laminae I and V of the dorsal horn project to various thalamic nuclei important in somatosensory processes.

Noxious stimulation also increases glucose utilization in several ventral horn regions such as laminae VII and IX (Plates 1 and 2) (Abram and Kostreva 1986; Coghill et al. 1991, 1993a). Lamina VII contains spinothalamic nociceptive neurons with large receptive fields (Giesler et al. 1981). As such, activation within this region probably reflects afferent processing. In contrast, lamina IX contains the cell bodies of motor neurons (Rexed 1954). Accordingly, increased glucose utilization within this region reflects the activation of withdrawal reflexes evoked by noxious stimulation (Coghill et al. 1991, 1993a). Thus, the 2-DG method allows visualization of both afferent and efferent aspects of nociceptive processing.

Temporal aspects of spinal nociceptive processing. During prolonged noxious thermal or chemical stimulation, glucose utilization in the deep dorsal horn increases substantially, while only relatively weak increases are noted within the superficial dorsal horn (Plate 1) (Coghill et al. 1991; Porro et al. 1991b, 1999). The relative paucity of activation in the superficial laminae is surprising, given that a substantial portion of the spinothalamic tract arises from this region and both nociceptive-specific (NS) and wide-dynamic-range (WDR) neurons have been identified in this area (Christensen and Perl 1970; Price et al. 1978; Kenshalo et al. 1979; Craig et al. 1989). However, electrophysiological studies indicate that the responses of NS neurons to prolonged, repetitive thermal stimuli diminish dramatically after ~2 minutes of stimulation, whereas WDR responses are maintained for periods exceeding 20 minutes (Coghill et al. 1993b). Similar differences in temporal profile of activity have been noted in trigeminal neurons in rats during thermal stimulation of the head and in spinal neurons following injection of capsaicin into the rat hindpaw (Simone et al. 1991; McHaffie et al. 1994). Given the preponderance of NS neurons in the superficial laminae and WDR neurons in the deep laminae, the different rates of glucose utilization between these dorsal horn regions may reflect the differential responses of WDR and NS neurons to prolonged noxious stimuli. Furthermore, the different responses of these two spinal regions underscore the close coupling between excitatory neuronal activity and metabolic activity.

Spatial aspects of spinal and trigeminal nociceptive processing. In addition to a gross rostrocaudal organization, sensory processing within the spinal cord dorsal horn is somatotopically organized in a mediolateral dimension. Distal structures are represented medially, and proximal structures laterally. Consistent with this somatotopy, noxious stimulation of the distal portion of the hindlimb of rats increases glucose utilization within medial portions of the lumbar dorsal horn, while formalin injection into the forepaw of rats activates medial portions of the cervical dorsal horn (Plate 1) (Coghill et al. 1991; Porro et al. 1991b).

In contrast to the mediolateral distribution of noxious stimulus-induced activation, the rostrocaudal distribution of increased glucose utilization greatly exceeds the extent of activation that would be predicted from the termination of primary afferents (Molander and Grant 1986; Woolf and Fitzgerald 1986; Coghill et al. 1991; Porro et al. 1991b; Goadsby et al. 1997). For example, noxious thermal or chemical stimulation of a single paw increases glucose utilization throughout almost the entire lumbar or cervical enlargement (Plate 1) (Coghill et al. 1991; Porro et al. 1991b). Additionally, stimulation of a nerve arising solely from the C2 dorsal root ganglion activates both the cervical and trigeminal dorsal horns (Goadsby et al. 1997). Such activation clearly exceeds dermatomal boundaries. The spatially distributed recruitment of neural activity depends on noxious stimulus intensity (Plate 1). Progressive increases in stimulus intensity recruit increasing numbers of spinal cord segments (Coghill et al. 1991).

The extensive spatial recruitment of activity can explain the extensive radiation of some types of pain. In chronic neuropathic pain states, pain has long been known to radiate to body regions far removed from the territory of the injured nerve (Mitchell et al. 1864; Livingston 1943). Functional imaging studies of neuropathic pain models in rats reveal an extensive ipsilateral rostrocaudal recruitment of activity similar to that evoked in studies of acute pain (Plate 3) (Mao et al. 1992). Such results indicate a neural substrate for the unilateral radiation of clinical pain.

Radiation of clinical pain may also involve body regions contralateral to the initial site of injury (Mitchell 1872, 1897; Veldman and Goris 1996). Such bilateral spread of pain has been difficult to explain with conventional evidence. However, bilateral metabolic increases within the spinal cord or trigeminal complex have consistently been found in 2-DG studies of unilateral painful stimuli (Shetter and Sweet 1979; Abram and Kostreva 1986; Coghill et al. 1991; Porro et al. 1991b, 1999; Aloisi et al. 1993; Goadsby et al. 1997). For example, monoarthritis evoked by unilateral injection of complete

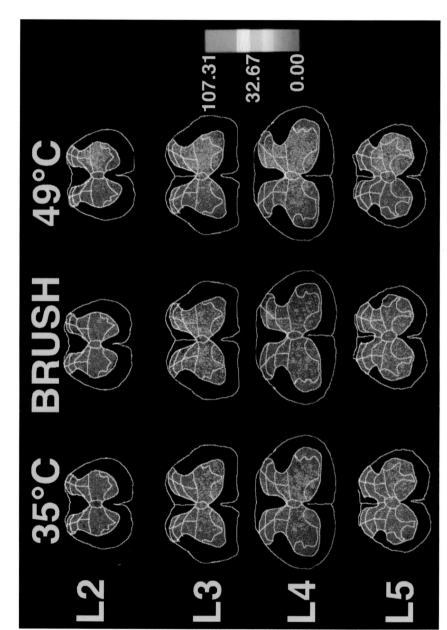

Freund's adjuvant into the tibiotarsal joint of the rat hindpaw produces bilateral increases in glucose utilization (Schadrack et al. 1999). Similarly, in rat models of neuropathic pain, both dorsal horns are activated by a unilateral injury produced by chronic constriction (CCI) of the sciatic nerve (Price et al. 1991; Mao et al. 1992). These bilateral increases in metabolic activity correlate well with bilateral changes in behavioral responses (Aloisi et al. 1993) and are accompanied by bilateral increases in protein kinase C activation, an important component of an intracellular cascade contributing to hyperalgesia (Mao et al. 1993a). The exact mechanism of this bilateral activation is unclear, although polysynaptic, propriospinal interconnections may play a significant role. Nevertheless, this bilateral recruitment of activation can provide an explanation for the bilateral radiation of clinical pain seen in up to 16% of patients with some forms of chronic neuropathic pain (Allen et al. 1999).

Encoding of pain by recruitment of neurons. We usually think of pain as being encoded solely by increases in the discharge frequencies of individual neurons. However, radiation of pain indicates that a second fundamental mechanism, neuron recruitment, contributes significantly to the CNS processing of pain. The importance of neuron recruitment in this process is evident in the encoding of pain by WDR neurons. Multiple, converging lines of evidence indicate that WDR neurons are sufficient to encode pain (Mayer et al. 1975; Price et al. 1978; Maixner et al. 1986; Simone et al. 1991; Coghill et al. 1993b; McHaffie et al. 1994), yet these neurons can respond to both innocuous and noxious stimuli with equal increases in discharge frequencies. Accordingly, an individual WDR neuron cannot provide the CNS with sufficient information to distinguish between innocuous and noxious stimuli. However, if one considers the responses of populations of such neurons, a clearer picture emerges. As noted previously, noxious thermal stimulation of the hindpaw increases glucose utilization over an extensive portion of the lumbar enlargement (i.e., L1–L5). In contrast, innocuous brushing produces more focused and less intense activation within the caudal aspect of L3 (Plate 2) (Coghill et al. 1993a). The differential rostrocaudal spread of metabolic activation indicates that painful and innocuous stimuli recruit substantially different numbers of neurons (Coghill et al. 1993a).

←— **Plate 2.** Differential processing of innocuous and noxious somatosensory information. Noxious stimulation (49°C) produces an extensive rostrocaudal distribution of increased glucose utilization. In contrast, a vigorous brushing stimulus (BRUSH) produces a spatially restricted increase in 2-DG uptake. Together, these results in rats suggest that painful stimuli recruit far more neurons than do innocuous stimuli, and that this recruitment of neurons may contribute to the capacity to distinguish painful from nonpainful stimuli. From Coghill et al. (1993a).

Thus, both the number of neurons activated and their discharge frequency may be used to encode pain intensity.

Studies of human subjects undergoing electrical stimulation of the spinothalamic tract in the anterolateral quadrant of the spinal cord confirm that neuron recruitment contributes directly to the perception of pain (Mayer et al. 1975; Coghill et al. 1993a). Progressive increases in stimulus intensity recruit increasing numbers of neurons, and sensation shifts from an innocuous tingling to pain. Further increases in stimulus intensity and the subsequent recruitment of even more neurons produce more intense pain. Thus, neuron recruitment is a fundamental mechanism used by the CNS to encode pain.

THE BRAIN

Recent advances in functional brain-imaging techniques (PET and fMRI) now provide powerful tools with which to assess simultaneously the activation of multiple brain regions during pain and other sensory experiences in humans. Studies in humans using PET have revealed unique patterns of rCBF associated with the perception of pain (Talbot et al. 1991; Casey et al. 1994, 1996; Coghill et al. 1994, 1999; Coghill 1999). The identification of these pain-related cerebral activation patterns suggests exciting new ideas regarding the role of specific cortical and subcortical structures in the perception of acute and chronic pain. Such studies help clarify the function of the pain network as a whole, providing information that was previously unattainable from clinical data or from stimulation, lesion, or electrophysiological experiments. Animal imaging studies not only have confirmed human findings, but have permitted investigations that are not possible with present human imaging techniques.

Ascending transmission of nociceptive information. Both lateral and medial thalamic regions receive direct input from spinal regions demonstrated to be activated by nociceptive stimuli in animal imaging studies. Lateral thalamic nuclei such as the ventroposterior lateral nucleus (VPL), ventroposterior inferior nucleus (VPI), and medial part of the posterior complex (POm) receive input from both superficial and deep dorsal horn regions, while several medial nuclei receive input from ventral horn regions (Willis and Westlund 1997). Pathways from lamina I to both the nucleus submedius (Sm) and the posterior portion of the ventromedial nucleus (VMpo) also have been identified (Craig and Burton 1981; Craig 1999). Human imaging studies generally identify pain-induced activation within the thalamus. However, these studies lack the spatial resolution to conclusively localize pain-induced activation to a single nucleus within the thalamus. In contrast, animal imaging studies of both acute and chronic nociceptive states have identified activation within multiple individual thalamic nuclei.

Studies of acute pain using 2-DG have shown statistically significant activation within the VPL and ventrolateral nucleus (VL) following formalin injection into the rat paw (Porro et al. 1999). In rCBF studies of both the early and late phases of formalin-induced pain, the response of somatosensory relay nuclei is less reliably detected, but there are trends toward activation (Fig. 2; Morrow et al. 1998). The use of relatively large regions of interest in Morrow et al.'s CBF investigation may have decreased sensitivity by increasing partial volume effects (i.e., averaging spatially distinct activated zones with adjacent inactive zones). In studies of chronic pain, however, both rCBF and 2-DG techniques have revealed activation of various thalamic relay nuclei. Both rCBF and glucose utilization are increased in the VPL and PO thalamic nuclei in CCI rat models of chronic neuropathic pain (Fig. 2; Mao et al. 1993b; Paulson et al. 2000). Similarly, glucose utilization within the PO and SM is increased during adjuvant-induced arthritis (Neto et al. 1999).

Several medial thalamic nuclei that receive direct spinal input (Willis and Westlund 1997; Craig 1999) are also activated in animal models of pain. The VM is the most consistently responsive structure and is activated in the formalin, CCI, and adjuvant arthritis models (Fig. 2; Mao et al. 1993b; Porro et al. 1999; Neto et al. 1999; Paulson et al. 2000). The central lateral nucleus also exhibits increased glucose utilization during CCI (Mao et al. 1993b).

Both CCI and adjuvant arthritis models of chronic pain are characterized by bilateral increases in thalamic activation, consistent with findings in the spinal cord (Mao et al. 1993b; Neto et al. 1999; Paulson et al. 2000). Bilateral thalamic processing thus provides a route for information from a unilateral injury to reach bilateral cerebral cortical regions. Bilateral thalamic activation has also been recorded in human studies of rCBF changes evoked by acute pain (Casey et al. 1994, 1996; Coghill 1999). However, human PET studies of chronic pain generally have detected contralateral decreases in thalamic CBF, a paradoxical finding in need of further investigation (Di Piero et al. 1991; Hsieh et al. 1995; Iadarola et al. 1995).

A number of pathways other than the spinothalamic tract are capable of transmitting nociceptive information from the spinal cord to the forebrain. The spinoreticulothalamic pathway and the spinoparabrachial-amygdaloid pathway are two examples (Peschanski and Besson 1984; Bernard et al. 1989; Villanueva et al. 1996). The dorsal medullary reticular formation and its main thalamic targets, the parafascicular and VM nuclei, are activated via the spinoreticulothalamic pathway in 2-DG studies of formalin pain and adjuvant arthritis (Neto et al. 1999; Porro et al. 1999). The spinoparabrachial-amygdaloid pathway mediates the increased glucose utilization in the lateral

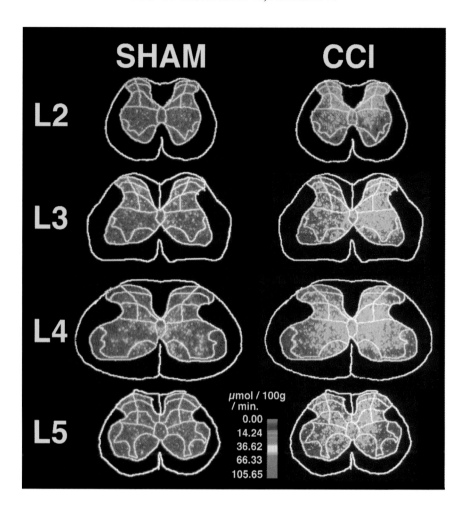

Plate 3. Distribution of spinal cord activation produced during a rat model of neuropathic pain. Chronic constriction injury (CCI, right column) of the right sciatic nerve produces extensive, bilateral increases in glucose utilization as compared with sham-operated rats (left column). Images are oriented as in Plate 1. From Mao et al. (1992).

parabrachial nucleus during formalin pain and CCI (Porro et al. 1991a, 1999; Mao et al. 1993b) and in the amygdala during CCI and adjuvant arthritis (Mao et al. 1993b; Neto et al. 1999). Activation of the spinoparabrachial-amygdaloid pathway may be involved in coordinating nociceptive, emotional, and autonomic responses to noxious stimulation (Mao et al. 1993b).

Processing of nociceptive information by the cerebral cortex. The rat somatosensory cortex shows statistically reliable changes in both CMRglc and rCBF following formalin injection and CCI and during adjuvant-induced arthritis (Mao et al. 1993b; Morrow et al. 1998; Neto et al. 1999;

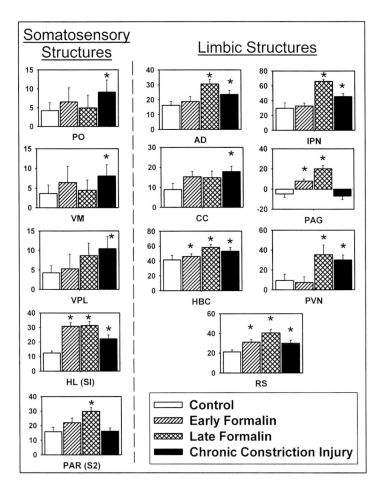

Fig. 2. Regional cerebral blood flow (rCBF) within select regions of interest (ROIs) expressed as the bilateral mean activation index (AI). The graphs display mean AI values from rats at early and late phases of the formalin test, from rats 2 weeks after a unilateral chronic constriction injury (CCI), and from unstimulated controls. Bars are presented only for ROIs showing a significant difference in relative blood flow in at least one of the experimental groups as compared to controls (* $P < 0.05$, ANOVA). For formalin-stimulated rats, an apparent time-dependent increase in AI occurred for several ROIs between the early phase (2 minutes after formalin) as compared to the late phase (15 minutes after formalin). Only HL (in the early-phase formalin) and VPL (in the CCI group) showed any significant side-to-side difference in activation (contralateral greater than ipsilateral), with this lateralized AI difference always superimposed on a significant bilateral increase. Data shown are from Morrow et al. (1998) and Paulson et al. (2000). AD = anterior dorsal nucleus (thalamus); CC = cingulate cortex; HBC = habenular complex; HL (S1) = hindlimb area of somatosensory cortex; IPN = interpeduncular nucleus; PAG = periaqueductal gray (midbrain); PAR (S2) = secondary somatosensory region of parietal cortex; PO = posterior group (thalamus); PVN = paraventricular nucleus (hypothalamus); RS = retrosplenial cortex; VM = ventromedial nucleus (thalamus); VPL = ventroposterior lateral nucleus (thalamus).

Porro et al. 1999; Paulson et al. 2000). This activation is somatotopically organized. The forepaw region is most intensely activated after formalin injections into the forepaw, and the hindlimb region is most responsive after hindlimb injections in rats (Fig. 2; Mao et al. 1993b; Morrow et al. 1998; Neto et al. 1999; Porro et al. 1999; Paulson et al. 2000).

In contrast with human studies, bilateral activation of the somatosensory cortex is consistently observed in both acute and chronic rodent pain models (Mao et al. 1993b; Morrow et al. 1998; Neto et al. 1999; Porro et al. 1999; Paulson et al. 2000). This activation of cerebral cortical regions is consistent with the bilateral changes observed in the spinal cord and thalamus. A significant change occurs in the spatial distribution of activation within the somatosensory cortex during the shift from acute to prolonged pain. In the early phase of formalin pain, rCBF within the somatosensory cortex is significantly greater in the hemisphere contralateral to stimulation. In the late phase of formalin pain, activation within the somatosensory cortex of both hemispheres is nearly equally elevated, such that no significant differences are evident between sites (Morrow et al. 1998). Furthermore, activation of the somatosensory cortex in chronic pain models is considerably more diffuse than in the acute pain model; both hindpaw and forepaw regions are activated following injury limited to the hindpaw (Mao et al. 1993b; Neto et al. 1999). This dispersion of activation away from the somatotopic focus is consistent with the wide rostrocaudal distribution of spinal activation and may represent a substrate for the perceptual radiation of pain.

Both acute and chronic pain evoke increases in glucose utilization and/ or rCBF in the cingulate cortex (Fig. 2; Mao et al. 1993b; Neto et al. 1999; Porro et al. 1999; Paulson et al. 2000). In humans, activation within this complex region is significantly related to perceived pain intensity and most likely contributes to many differing processes associated with pain such as attention, affect, and motor control (Devinsky et al. 1995; Coghill 1999). The increase in rCBF in cingulate cortex is also consistent with activation of one of its major inputs, the thalamic anterior dorsal nuclei (Fig. 2, Plate 4). The retrosplenial cortex is robustly activated in animal models of acute and chronic pain (Mao et al. 1993b; Morrow et al. 1998; Neto et al. 1999; Paulson et al. 2000) (Plate 4). The role of this brain area in nociception is unclear, but it may be important in emotion and memory (Maddock 1999). Both the cingulate and retrosplenial cortices are consistently activated bilaterally.

Other cerebral cortical areas, such as the insula and ventrolateral orbitofrontal cortex (VLO), are involved in nociceptive processes. Both show increased glucose utilization during the late phase of formalin-induced pain (Porro et al. 1999). Nociceptive neurons have been identified in the VLO of the rat (Backonja and Miletic 1991).

Sensory-motor integration. The motor processes that mediate escape from potentially injurious stimuli represent a critical component of nociception. For escape responses to be generated, sensory information must be integrated with ongoing motor activity. Several brain regions may mediate this integration. For example, the caudate putamen is consistently activated during 2-DG studies of formalin-evoked pain, CCI, and adjuvant arthritis (Mao et al. 1993b; Neto et al. 1999; Porro et al. 1999). Nociceptive neurons constitute approximately 97% of the somatosensory neurons identified in this region (Chudler et al. 1993). These neurons include both WDR and NS types, and frequently have large receptive fields, sometimes encompassing the entire body (Chudler et al. 1993). These areas may work in conjunction with the superior colliculus to coordinate escape responses (McHaffie et al. 1989; Chudler et al. 1993). Both WDR and NS neurons have been identified in the superior colliculus in single-unit electrophysiological studies (McHaffie et al. 1989). Given the importance of the superior colliculus in sensory-motor integration and orientation, pain-induced increases in this region may reflect processes related to nocifensive behavior (McHaffie et al. 1989). However, increased activation within deep layers of the superior colliculus has been detected only in 2-DG studies of CCI (Mao et al. 1993b).

Descending modulation of nociception. Several brain regions modulate the flow of nociceptive information via descending pathways (Reynolds 1968; Mayer et al. 1971; Watkins and Mayer 1982). Most of these regions are composed of relatively small nuclei that cannot be investigated reliably with human imaging techniques. However, animal imaging studies have demonstrated activation of medullary, midbrain, and diencephalic sites involved in the descending modulation of pain.

The medullary reticular formation is involved in both nociception and descending pain modulation (Watkins and Mayer 1982). Several reticular nuclei show increased glucose utilization both during acute pain evoked by formalin injection and in models of chronic pain evoked either by CCI of the sciatic nerve or by adjuvant arthritis. These regions include the parvocellular reticular nucleus, ventral gigantocellular reticular nucleus, paragigantocellular nucleus, and nucleus raphe magnus (Porro et al. 1991a, 1999; Mao et al. 1993b; Neto et al. 1999). Both the lateral paragigantocellular and gigantocellular reticular nuclei are involved in autonomic regulation of cardiovascular function, so their activation may be related to changes in sympathetic activity during pain (Chan et al. 1980; Chan and Kuo 1980; Chen and Chan 1980; Blair 1987). Pontine reticular nuclei also show higher glucose utilization following formalin injection, CCI, or induction of adjuvant monoarthritis (Porro et al. 1991a; Mao et al. 1993b; Neto et al. 1999).

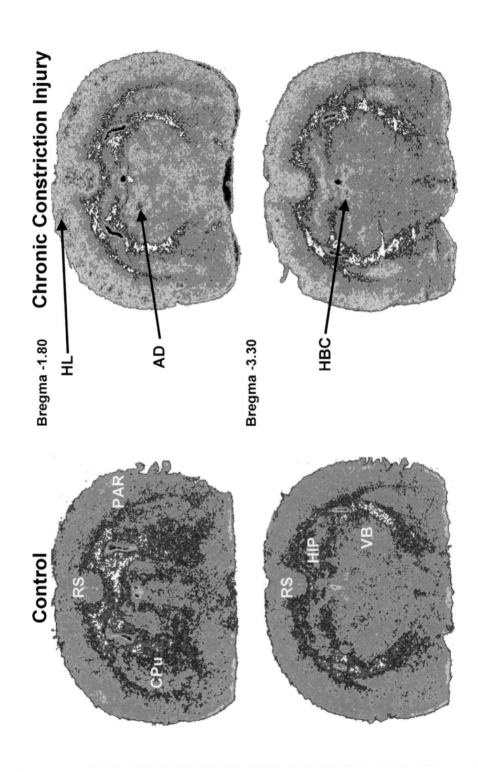

Control

Chronic Constriction Injury

Bregma -1.80

Bregma -3.30

HL

AD

HBC

RS

PAR

CPu

RS

HIP

VB

Several midbrain regions play a significant role in pain modulation. For example, the periaqueductal gray matter (PAG) responds during both formalin pain and CCI (Fig. 2; Porro et al. 1991a; Mao et al. 1993b; Morrow et al. 1998). The PAG was one of the first supraspinal regions to be implicated in descending modulation of pain, so its activation is consistent with the activation of medullary structures involved in pain inhibition (Watkins and Mayer 1982). The interpeduncular nucleus also shows increased CBF during both formalin pain and CCI (Morrow et al. 1998; Paulson et al. 2000). In contrast to the PAG, stimulation of the interpeduncular nucleus is known to modulate antinociceptive circuitry in the nucleus raphe magnus, and may produce hyperalgesia (Hentall and Budhrani 1990).

Additional sites within the diencephalon have been implicated in the modulation of pain. Of these, both the paraventricular nucleus of the hypothalamus (PVN) and the habenular complex show increased activation during CCI and during the late phase of formalin pain (Fig. 2, Plate 4) (Morrow et al. 1998; Porro et al. 1999; Paulson et al. 2000). Electrical simulation of the habenular complex markedly attenuates nociception in the formalin test, and effects of PVN lesions suggest that this structure is involved in the production of stress-induced analgesia (Cohen and Melzack 1986, 1993).

FUTURE DIRECTIONS IN FUNCTIONAL IMAGING STUDIES OF ANIMAL MODELS OF PAIN

A fundamental issue in the neurobiology of pain concerns the plastic changes of the activity of central networks following tissue and nerve injury. These changes may be studied at several levels, from subcellular to behavioral, and by different methods. The 2-DG and rCBF imaging techniques are well suited for investigating the time profiles and circuitry of CNS activation during pain states. However, although animal imaging provides a powerful tool for investigating mechanisms of pain in animals, its use has been limited to relatively few studies, primarily investigating spontaneous tonic pain

---

← **Plate 4.** Color-enhanced digitized brain images showing the pattern of rCBF in a control rat and a rat with chronic constriction injury (CCI). Sections are taken at select anteroposterior levels according to the stereotactic atlas of Paxinos and Watson (1996). Although each image represents only a single histological section from the brain of one animal, white and gray matter are clearly delineated and multiple brain regions are easily identified due to differences in regional blood flow. Note that CCI produces increases in forebrain rCBF as compared to control, even in the absence of stimulation. AD = anterior dorsal nucleus (thalamus); CPu = caudate putamen; HBC = habenular complex; HIP = hippocampus; HL = hindlimb area of S1 somatosensory cortex; PAR = secondary somatosensory (S2) region of parietal cortex; RS = retrosplenial cortex; VB = thalamic ventrobasal nuclei.

induced by inflammation or damage to the peripheral or central nervous system. Both behavioral studies in animals and clinical experience in humans show that the most clinically important consequences of chronic inflammation or CNS damage are the development of an increased responsiveness to noxious stimuli (hyperalgesia) and the perception as painful of previously innocuous mechanical or thermal stimuli (allodynia). Future animal imaging studies should investigate the mechanisms of hyperalgesia and allodynia in many models of neuropathic pain. A systematic comparison of the spatial and temporal profiles of brain activity should clarify the functional role of individual brain regions or circuits in various pain states. By determining which CNS structures are critical in each animal model of pain, we may be able to find out whether a unique CNS network is critical for the production and maintenance of neuropathic pain.

Coghill et al. (1999), using PET in humans, showed that the processing of pain intensity is highly distributed among several cerebral structures. However, no animal imaging studies have attempted to identify which brain structures process information related to stimulus intensity. Without such studies, it will be impossible to fully evaluate the plastic changes in the CNS that occur as consequence of pathological pain states. Studies similar to that of Coghill et al. (1999) should be conducted with animal models. The rCBF method is the best approach because, compared to 2-DG, it requires only a brief period of sensory stimulation.

Improvements are needed in the methods used to image brain activity in animals. Unlike human PET or fMRI, which use a scanner and computer automation to analyze the enormous quantity of image data, 2-DG and rCBF imaging methods in animals rely on manual ROI identification and densitometric analysis of autoradiograms. Animal imaging techniques are therefore tedious, requiring extensive investigator input and a significant investment of time. Statistical parametric mapping techniques, as used in the analysis of PET images, would greatly enhance the productivity and precision of film-based animal imaging studies. Ideally, investigators would use images digitized from film autoradiograms of animal brain sections, perform two-dimensional warping of each image to a comparable section from standard brain atlas, average the warped images across multiple samples and across multiple animals, and finally apply parametric mapping and associated Z-score analysis to the averaged images. Of course, the most significant advance in animal imaging would be the development of an automated small-animal scanner like that used in PET or fMRI, but with the high resolution of film autoradiograms.

The major shortcoming of all neuroimaging methods, including PET and fMRI, is their inability to distinguish excitation from inhibition. Although the word *activation* is used extensively to describe imaging data, this term is misleading. *Activation* does not mean *excitation,* as might initially be inferred. The term *activation* relates only to changes in overall levels of underlying neuronal activity and cannot provide information about the *valence* of this activity. Recent advances in the identification and mapping of changes in receptor expression may provide the key to solving the problem of the activation valence, at least for film-based animal imaging models. Future imaging studies not only may include rCBF or 2-DG images, but may additionally map out changes in the expression of specific receptor types, some of which have known excitatory or inhibitory function. Such an approach could help to relate the activation identified by 2-DG or rCBF to underlying excitatory and inhibitory processes.

In summary, animal imaging studies complement comparable research in humans using PET and fMRI. By presenting a "snapshot view" of activation in multiple brain structures simultaneously, these studies can provide critical insights into the network of structures responsible for pain and analgesia mechanisms. By identifying new brain regions activated during pain or by analgesic interventions, such studies can offer new directions to electrophysiological, anatomical, and pharmacological investigations into CNS mechanisms of nociception. Animal imaging studies offer a global view of the CNS network(s) involved in pain processing and provide a method for examining how nervous system lesions, brain stimulation, pharmacological interventions, or the presence of pain itself can alter the function of these networks. Animal imaging thus can provide a view into the plasticity within the CNS network for pain.

ACKNOWLEDGMENTS

T.J. Morrow is supported by NIH PO1 HDO33986 and the U.S. Department of Veterans Affairs.

REFERENCES

Abram SE, Kostreva DR. Spinal cord metabolic response to noxious radiant heat stimulation of the cat hind footpad. *Brain Res* 1986; 385:143–147.

Allen G, Galer BS, Schwartz L. Epidemiology of complex regional pain syndrome: a retrospective chart review of 134 patients. *Pain* 1999; 80:539–544.

Aloisi AM, Porro CA, Cavazzuti M, Baraldi P, Carli G. 'Mirror pain' in the formalin test: behavioral and 2-deoxyglucose studies. *Pain* 1993; 55:267–273.

Backonja M, Miletic V. Responses of neurons in the rat ventrolateral orbital cortex to phasic and tonic nociceptive stimulation. *Brain Res* 1991; 557:353–355.

Ballinger JR, Reid RH, Gulenchyn KY. Radiochemical purity of [^{99m}Tc]HM-PAO. *J Nucl Med* 1988; 29:572–573.

Bernard JF, Peschanski M, Besson JM. A possible spino (trigemino)-ponto-amygdaloid pathway for pain. *Neurosci Lett* 1989;100:83–88.

Blair RW. Responses of feline medial medullary reticulospinal neurons to cardiac input. *J Neurophysiol* 1987; 58:1149–1167.

Casey KL, Minoshima S, Berger KL, et al. Positron emission tomographic analysis of cerebral structures activated specifically by repetitive noxious heat stimuli. *J Neurophysiol* 1994; 71:802–807.

Casey KL, Minoshima S, Morrow TJ, Koeppe RA. Comparison of human cerebral activation pattern during cutaneous warmth, heat pain, and deep cold pain. *J Neurophysiol* 1996; 76:571–581.

Chan SH, Kuo JS. Interaction of gigantocellular reticular nucleus with reflex bradycardia and tachycardia in the cat. *Brain Res* 1980; 182:457–460.

Chan SH, Kuo JS, Chen YH, Hwa JY. Modulatory actions of the gigantocellular reticular nucleus on baroreceptor reflexes in the cat. *Brain Res* 1980; 196:1–9.

Chen YH, Chan SH. The involvement of gigantocellular reticular nucleus in clonidine-promoted hypotension and bradycardia in experimentally-induced hypertensive cats. *Neuropharmacology* 1980; 19:939–945.

Christensen BN, Perl ER. Spinal neurons specifically excited by noxious or thermal stimuli: marginal zone of the dorsal horn. *J Neurophysiol* 1970; 33:292–307.

Chudler EH, Sugiyama K, Dong WK. Nociceptive responses in the neostriatum and globus pallidus of the anesthetized rat. *J Neurophysiol* 1993; 69:1890–1903.

Coghill RC. Brain mechanisms supporting the pain experience: a distributed processing system. In: Max M (Ed). *Pain 1999— An Updated Review.* Seattle: IASP Press, 1999, pp 67–76.

Coghill RC, Price DD, Hayes RL, Mayer DJ. Spatial distribution of nociceptive processing in the rat spinal cord. *J Neurophysiol* 1991; 65:133–140.

Coghill RC, Mayer DJ, Price DD. The roles of spatial recruitment and discharge frequency in spinal cord coding of pain: a combined electrophysiological and imaging investigation. *Pain* 1993a; 53:295–309.

Coghill RC, Mayer DJ, Price DD. Wide dynamic range but not nociceptive specific neurons encode multidimensional features of prolonged repetitive heat pain. *J Neurophysiol* 1993b; 69:703–716.

Coghill RC, Talbot JD, Meyer E, et al. Distributed processing of pain and vibration in the human brain. *J Neurosci* 1994; 14:4095–4108.

Coghill RC, Sang CN, Maisog J Ma, Iadarola MJ. Pain intensity processing within the human brain: a bilateral, distributed mechanism. *J Neurophysiol* 1999; 82:1934–1943.

Cohen SR, Melzack R. Habenular stimulation produces analgesia in the formalin test. *Neurosci Lett* 1986; 70:165–169.

Cohen SR, Melzack R. The habenula and pain: repeated electrical stimulation produces prolonged analgesia but lesions have no effect on formalin pain or morphine analgesia. *Behav Brain Res* 1993; 54:171–178.

Craig AD. Functional anatomy of supraspinal pain processing with reference to the central pain syndrome. In: Max M (Ed). *Pain 1999— An Updated Review.* Seattle: IASP Press, 1999, pp 87–96.

Craig AD, Burton H. Spinal and medullary lamina I projection to nucleus submedius in medial thalamus: a possible pain center. *J Neurophysiol* 1981; 45:443–466.

Craig AD Jr, Linington AJ, Kniffki KD. Cells of origin of spinothalamic tract projections to the medial and lateral thalamus in the cat. *J Comp Neurol* 1989; 289:568–585.

Devinsky O, Morrell MJ, Vogt BA. Contributions of anterior cingulate cortex to behaviour. *Brain* 1995; 118:279–306.

Di Piero V, Jones AK, Iannotti F, et al. Chronic pain: a PET study of the central effects of percutaneous high cervical cordotomy. *Pain* 1991; 46:9–12.

Dowling JL, Henegar MM, Liu D, Rovainen CM, Woolsey TA. Rapid optical imaging of whisker responses in the rat barrel cortex. *J Neurosci Methods* 1996; 66:113–122.

Fox P, Raichle ME, Mintun MA, Dence C. Nonoxidative glucose consumption during focal physiologic neural activity. *Science* 1988; 241:462–464.

Giesler GJ, Yezierski RP, Gerhart KD. Spinothalamic tract neurons that project to medial and/or lateral thalamic nuclei: evidence for a physiologically novel population of spinal cord neurons. *J Neurophysiol* 1981; 46:1285–1286.

Ginsberg MD, Dietrich WD, Busto R. Coupled forebrain increases of local cerebral glucose utilization and blood flow during physiologic stimulation of a somatosensory pathway in the rat: demonstration by double-label autoradiography. *Neurology* 1987; 37:11–19.

Goadsby PJ, Zagami AS. Stimulation of the superior sagittal sinus increases metabolic activity and blood flow in certain regions of the brainstem and upper cervical spinal cord of the cat. *Brain* 1991; 114:1001–1011.

Goadsby PJ, Knight YE, Hoskin KL. Stimulation of the greater occipital nerve increases metabolic activity in the trigeminal nucleus caudalis and cervical dorsal horn of the cat. *Pain* 1997; 73:23–28.

Greenberg JH, LoBrutto C, Lombard KM, Chen J. Postmortem diffusion of autoradiographic blood flow tracers. *Brain Res* 1999; 842:184–191.

Hentall ID, Budhrani VM. The interpeduncular nucleus excites the on-cells and inhibits the off-cells of the nucleus raphe magnus. *Brain Res* 1990; 522:322–324.

Hsieh JC, Belfrage M, Stone-Elander S, Hansson P, Ingvar M. Central representation of chronic ongoing neuropathic pain studied by positron emission tomography. *Pain* 1995; 63:225–236.

Iadarola MJ, Max MB, Berman KF, et al. Unilateral decrease in thalamic activity observed with positron emission tomography in patients with chronic neuropathic pain. *Pain* 1995; 63:55–64.

Kadekaro M, Crane AM, Sokoloff L. Differential effects of electrical stimulation of the sciatic nerve on metabolic activity in spinal cord and dorsal root ganglion in the rat. *Proc Natl Acad Sci USA* 1985; 82:6010–6013.

Kenshalo DR, Leonard RB, Chung JM, Willis WD. Responses of primate spinothalamic neurons to graded and to repeated noxious heat stimuli. *J Neurophysiol* 1979; 42:1370–1389.

Kety SS. Circulation and metabolism of the human brain in health and disease. *Am J Occup Ther* 1950; 8:205–217.

Kety SS. The theory and application of the exchange of inert gas at the lungs and tissues. *Pharmacol Rev* 1951; 3:1–41.

Kety SS. Measurement of local blood flow by the exchange of an inert diffusible substance. *Methods Med Res* 1960; 8:228–236.

Kety SS, Schmidt CF. The determination of cerebral blood flow in man by use of nitrous oxide in low concentrations. *Am J Physiol* 1945; 143:53–66.

Lear JL. Initial cerebral HM-PAO distribution compared to LCBF: use of a model which considers cerebral HM-PAO trapping kinetics. *J Cereb Blood Flow Metab* 1988a; 8:S31–S37.

Lear JL. Quantitative local cerebral blood flow measurements with technetium-99m HM-PAO: evaluation using multiple radionuclide digital quantitative autoradiography. *J Nucl Med* 1988b; 29:1387–1392.

Lear JL, Ackermann RF, Kameyama M, Kuhl DE. Evaluation of [123I]isopropyliodoamphetamine as a tracer for local cerebral blood flow using direct autoradiographic comparison. *J Cereb Blood Flow Metab* 1982; 2:179–185.

Livingston WK. *Pain Mechanisms*. New York: MacMillan Co, 1943.

Maddock RJ. The retrosplenial cortex and emotion: new insights from functional neuroimaging of the human brain. *Trends Neurosci* 1999; 22:310–316.

Magistretti PJ, Pellerin L. Cellular mechanisms of brain energy metabolism and their relevance to functional brain imaging. *Philos Trans R Soc Lond B Biol Sci* 1999; 354:1155–1163.

Maixner W, Dubner R, Bushnell MC, Kenshalo DR, Oliveras J-L. Wide-dynamic-range dorsal horn neurons participate in the encoding process by which monkeys perceive the intensity of noxious heat stimuli. *Brain Res* 1986; 374:385–388.

Mao J, Price DD, Coghill RC, Mayer DJ, Hayes RL. Spatial patterns of spinal cord [14C]-2-deoxyglucose metabolic activity in a rat model of painful peripheral mononeuropathy. *Pain* 1992; 50:89–100.

Mao J, Mayer DJ, Hayes RL, Price DD. Spatial patterns of increased spinal cord membrane-bound protein kinase C and their relation to increases in ^{14}C-2-deoxyglucose metabolic activity in rats with painful peripheral mononeuropathy. *J Neurophysiol* 1993a; 70:470–481.

Mao J, Mayer DJ, Price DD. Patterns of increased brain activity indicative of pain in a rat model of peripheral mononeuropathy. *J Neurosci* 1993b; 13:2689–2702.

Mata M, Fink DJ, Gainer H, et al. Activity-dependent energy metabolism in rat posterior pituitary primarily reflects sodium pump activity. *J Neurochem* 1980; 34:213–215.

Mayer DJ, Wolfle TJ, Akil H, Carder B, Liebeskind JC. Analgesia from electrical stimulation in the brainstem of the rat. *Science* 1971; 174:1351–1354.

Mayer DJ, Price DD, Becker DP. Neurophysiological characterization of the anterolateral spinal cord neurons contributing to pain perception in man. *Pain* 1975; 1:51–58.

McHaffie JG, Kao C-Q, Stein BE. Nociceptive neurons in the rat superior colliculus: response properties, topography, and functional implications. *J Neurophysiol* 1989; 62:510–525.

McHaffie JG, Larson MA, Stein BE. Response properties of nociceptive and low-threshold neurons in rat trigeminal pars caudalis. *J Comp Neurol* 1994; 347:409–425.

Mitchell SW. *Injuries of Nerves and Their Consequences*. Philadelphia: J.B. Lippincott, 1872, p 38.

Mitchell SW. *Clinical Lessons on Nervous Diseases*. Philadelphia: Lea Brothers, 1897.

Mitchell SW, Morehouse GR, Keen WW. *Gunshot Wounds and Other Injuries of Nerves*. Philadelphia: Lippincott, 1864.

Molander C, Grant G. Laminar distribution and somatotopic organization of primary afferent fibers from hindlimb nerves in the dorsal horn. A study by transganglionic transport of horseradish peroxidase in the rat. *Neuroscience* 1986; 19:297–312.

Morrow TJ, Paulson PE, Danneman PJ, Casey KL. Regional changes in forebrain activation during the early and late phase of formalin nociception: analysis using cerebral blood flow in the rat. *Pain* 1998; 75:355–365.

Mraovitch S, Seylaz J. Metabolism-independent cerebral vasodilation elicited by electrical stimulation of the centromedian-parafascicular complex in rat. *Neurosci Lett* 1987; 83:269–274.

Mraovitch S, Calando Y, Goadsby PJ, Seylaz J. Subcortical cerebral blood flow and metabolic changes elicited by cortical spreading depression in rat. *Cephalalgia* 1992a; 12:137–141.

Mraovitch S, Calando Y, Pinard E, Pearce WJ, Seylaz J. Differential cerebrovascular and metabolic responses in specific neural systems elicited from the centromedian-parafascicular complex. *Neuroscience* 1992b; 49:451–466.

Neirinckx RD, Canning LR, Piper IM, et al. Technetium-99m d,l-HM-PAO: a new radiopharmaceutical for SPECT imaging of regional cerebral blood perfusion. *J Nucl Med* 1987; 28:191–202.

Neto FL, Schadrack J, Ableitner A, et al. Supraspinal metabolic activity changes in the rat during adjuvant monoarthritis. *Neuroscience* 1999; 94:607–621.

Paulson PE, Morrow TJ, Casey KL. Bilateral behavioral and regional cerebral blood flow changes during painful peripheral mononeuropathy in the rat. *Pain* 2000; 84:233–245.

Paxinos G, Watson C. *The Rat Brain in Stereotaxic Coordinates*. New York: Academic Press, 1986.

Peschanski M, Besson JM. A spino-reticulo-thalamic pathway in the rat: an anatomical study with reference to pain transmission. *Neuroscience* 1984; 12:165–178.

Porro CA, Cavazzuti M, Galetti A, Sassatelli L. Functional activity mapping of the rat brainstem during formalin- induced noxious stimulation. *Neuroscience* 1991a; 41:667–680.

Porro CA, Cavazzuti M, Galetti A, Sassatelli L, Barbieri GC. Functional activity mapping of the rat spinal cord during formalin- induced noxious stimulation. *Neuroscience* 1991b; 41:655–665.

Porro CA, Cavazzuti M, Baraldi P, et al. CNS pattern of metabolic activity during tonic pain: evidence for modulation by beta-endorphin. *Eur J Neurosci* 1999; 11:874–888.

Price DD, Hayes RL, Ruda M, Dubner R. Spatial and temporal transformations of input to spinothalamic tract neurons and their relation to somatic sensations. *J Neurophysiol* 1978; 41:933–947.

Price DD, Mao JR, Coghill RC, et al. Regional changes in spinal cord glucose metabolism in a rat model of painful neuropathy. *Brain Res* 1991; 564:314–318.

Reivich M, Kuhl D, Wolf A, et al. The [18F]fluorodeoxyglucose method for the measurement of local cerebral glucose utilization in man. *Circ Res* 1979; 44:127–137.

Rexed B. A cytoarchitectonic atlas of the spinal cord in the cat. *J Comp Neurol* 1954; 100:297–379.

Reynolds DV. Surgery in the rat during electrical analgesia induced by focal brain stimulation. *Science* 1968; 164:444–445.

Rowbotham MC, Petersen KL, Fields HL. Is postherpetic neuralgia more than one disorder? *Pain Forum* 1998; 7:231–237.

Roy CS, Sherrington CS. On the regulation of the blood-supply of the brain. *J Physiol* 1890; 11:85–108.

Sakurada O, Kennedy C, Jehle J, et al. Measurement of local cerebral blood flow with iodo [^{14}C] antipyrine. *Am J Physiol* 1978; 234:H59–H66.

Schadrack J, Neto FL, Ableitner A, et al. Metabolic activity changes in the rat spinal cord during adjuvant monoarthritis. *Neuroscience* 1999; 94:595–605.

Schwartz WJ, Smith CB, Davidsen L, Savaki H, Sokoloff L. Metabolic mapping of functional activity in the hypothalamo-neurohypophysial system of the rat. *Science* 1979; 205:723–725.

Shetter AG, Sweet WH. Relative cerebral glucose metabolism evoked by dental-pulp stimulation in the rat. *J Neurosurg* 1979; 51:12–17.

Sibson NR, Dhankhar A, Mason GF, et al. Stoichiometric coupling of brain glucose metabolism and glutamatergic neuronal activity. *Proc Natl Acad Sci USA* 1998; 95:316–321.

Simone DA, Sorkin LS, Oh U, et al. Neurogenic hyperalgesia: central neural correlates in the responses of spinothalamic tract neurons. *J Neurophysiol* 1991; 66:228–246.

Smith CB. Localization of activity-associated changes in metabolism of the central nervous system with the deoxyglucose method: prospects for cellular resolution. In: Barker JL, McKelvy JF (Eds). *Current Methods in Cellular Neurobiology.* New York: John Wiley, 1983, pp 269–317.

Sokoloff L. Local cerebral energy metabolism: its relationships to local functional activity and blood flow. *Ciba Found Symp* 1978; 171–197.

Sokoloff L. Energetics of functional activation in neural tissues. *Neurochem Res* 1999; 24:321–329.

Sokoloff L, Reivich M, Kennedy C, et al. The [^{14}C] deoxyglucose method for the measurement of local cerebral glucose utilization: theory, procedures, and normal values in the conscious and anesthetized albino rat. *J Neurochem* 1977; 28:897–916.

Talbot JD, Marrett S, Evans AC. Multiple representations of pain in human cerebral cortex. *Science* 1991; 251:1355–1358.

Veldman PHJM, Goris RJ. Multiple reflex sympathetic dystrophy. Which patients are at risk for developing a recurrence of reflex sympathetic dystrophy in the same or another limb? *Pain* 1996; 64:463–466.

Villanueva L, Bouhassira D, Le Bars D. The medullary subnucleus reticularis dorsalis (SRD) as a key link in both the transmission and modulation of pain signals. *Pain* 1996; 67:231–240.

Watkins LR, Mayer DJ. Organization of endogenous opiate and nonopiate pain control systems. *Science* 1982; 216:1185–1192.

Willis WD, Westlund KN. Neuroanatomy of the pain system and of the pathways that modulate pain. *J Clin Neurophysiol* 1997; 14:2–31.

Woolf CJ, Fitzgerald M. Somatotopic organization of cutaneous afferent terminals and dorsal horn neuronal receptive fields in the superficial and deep laminae of the rat lumbar spinal cord. *J Comp Neurol* 1986; 251:517–531.

Woolsey TA, Rovainen CM, Cox SB, et al. Neuronal units linked to microvascular modules in cerebral cortex: response elements for imaging the brain. *Cereb Cortex* 1996; 6:647–660.

Yarowsky P, Kadekaro M, Sokoloff L. Frequency-dependent activation of glucose utilization in the superior cervical ganglion by electrical stimulation of cervical sympathetic trunk. *Proc Natl Acad Sci USA* 1983; 80:4179–4183.

Correspondence to: Robert C. Coghill, PhD, Department of Neurobiology and Anatomy, Wake Forest University School of Medicine, Winston-Salem, NC 27157-1010, USA.

Index

Page numbers for figures are in *italic*.
Page numbers for color plates are
followed by *pl*.
Page numbers for tables are followed by t.

A

Action potentials, 3
Activation, defined, 196, 235
Acute pain
  as clinical problem, 12
  fMRI in, 201–203, 202t, 203t, 205
Adenosine, in metabolic coupling, 36–37
Adenosine triphosphate (ATP), 32, 37,
  166
Affective dimensions of pain
  anterior cingulate cortex in, 135–138
  components, 131–132
  dissociation from sensation, 135–138
  emotions in, 138–139
  insula in, 138
Afferents, nociceptive
  ascending pathways, 4, 5
  central processes, 3–4
  physiology, 3
Allodynia
  anterior cingulate cortex in, 142
  in central nervous system injuries, 14
  in complex regional pain syndromes,
    12–14
  dynamic tactile, 142
Analgesia
  endogenous, 9–10
  fMRI in, 206–207
  forebrain mechanisms, 143
  hypnotic suggestion, 8, 147
  motor cortex stimulation, 143, 145
  neurophysiology, 8–9
  PET imaging, 143–147
  psychological interventions, 147
  thalamic stimulation, 143, 145
  vibration in
    frequency discrimination, 80–81, *83*
    vs. same-site flutter, 71–72, 74, *75*
    wind-up and, 78, 80–81
Animal models
  functional imaging, 211–239
  future directions, 233–235
  limitations, 234
  utilization, 235

somatosensory cortex activation, 228,
  229, 230
Anterior cingulate cortex (ACC)
  in allodynia, 142
  hypnosis and, 136
  neuroanatomy, 129–130
  in nociceptive processing, 230
  noxious stimulation and, 49
  in pain perception, 135–138
  regional cerebral blood flow in pain,
    127
  in visceral pain, 141
Arachidonic acid, 39–40
Arterial spin labeling (ASL), 168–169,
  170pl
Asymbolia, pain, 7
Attention, 147, 206
Autoradiographic imaging, 216–220

B

Bicommissural line, in brain, 108
Block fMRI, 176, *178,* 178–179
Blood oxygenation, 31, 33–35
Blood-oxygenation-level-dependent
    (BOLD) signal
  arterial blood, 172
  in brain activation, 167
  in fMRI, 17, 161, 171–172, *174pl*
  magnetic field strength, 164
  sensitivity, 35
Brain
  bicommissural line, 108
  functional imaging
    clinical pain, 139–142
    image analysis techniques, 97
    methods, 226
  functional specialization, 124, *137pl*
  nociceptive processing
    ascending, 226–228
    in cerebral cortex, 228, 230
    descending, 231, 233
    sensory-motor integration, 231
  pain center, 126
  pain signature, 127–131
  stereotaxy, 108
Brain activation studies, 95–121
  anatomic standardization, *107pl,* 109
  in animal models, 211–239
  clinical pain, 139–142

241